Oncologic Emergencies

Oncologic Emergencies

Edited by

Patrick G. Johnston, MD PhD FRCP FRCPI
Professor of Oncology,
The Queen's University of Belfast and
Belfast City Hospital

Roy A.J. Spence, OBE JP MA MD FRCS
Consultant Surgeon, Belfast City Hospital;
Honorary Professor, The Queen's University
of Belfast and Honorary Professor,
University of Ulster

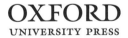
OXFORD
UNIVERSITY PRESS

OXFORD
UNIVERSITY PRESS

Great Clarendon Street, Oxford OX2 6DP

Oxford University Press is a department of the University of Oxford.
It furthers the University's objective of excellence in research, scholarship,
and education by publishing worldwide in

Oxford New York

Auckland Bangkok Buenos Aires Cape Town
Chennai Dar es Salaam Delhi Hong Kong Istanbul Karachi
Kolkata Kuala Lumpur Madrid Melbourne Mexico City Mumbai Nairobi
São Paulo Shanghai Taipei Tokyo Toronto
and an associated company in Berlin

Oxford is a registered trade mark of Oxford University Press
in the UK and in certain other countries

Published in the United States
by Oxford University Press Inc., New York

A catalogue record for this title is available from the British Library

Library of Congress Cataloging in Publication Data
Oncological emergencies/edited by Patrick G. Johnston, Roy A.J. Spence.
(Oxford medical publications)
1. Cancer—Complications.   2. Medical emergencies.   I. Johnston, Patrick G., MD PhD
FRCP FRCPI.   II. Spence, Roy A.J. (Roy Archibald Joseph)   III. Series.
[DNLM: 1. Emergencies.   2. Neoplasms—complications. QZ 200 O5808 2002]
RC262 .O522 2002   616.99′4025–dc21   2001050051

ISBN 0 19 850867 0 (PBk. : alk. paper)

10 9 8 7 6 5 4 3 2 1

Typeset by Newgen Imaging Systems (P) Ltd., Chennai, India
Printed in Great Britain
on acid-free paper by
T.J. International Ltd., Padstow, Cornwall

Preface

One in three of our population will develop cancer in their lifetime and one in five will die from this disease. Virtually every doctor and nurse, either in family or hospital practice, will come into contact with patients with cancer at some point in their career. With the increasing use of radiotherapy and the exponential increase in chemotherapy in cancer patients, many patients now present with complications of their treatment. Furthermore, some cancers present acutely as an emergency with complications such as raised intracranial pressure and spinal cord compression. These patients present to their family doctor/internist, Accident and Emergency Departments, or as an acute hospital admission, either as an emergency due to the disease itself, or as a complication of the treatment of the disease.

We were prompted to write this textbook by our colleagues both in family practice/internal medicine and in specialist hospital practice who are seeing an increasing number of patients presenting either with a complication of the cancer or as a sequel to their treatment. In these emergency situations it is essential that treatment is appropriate and prompt in order to be life-saving. We have therefore edited this textbook "Oncologic Emergencies" with this in mind.

We are most grateful to our colleagues in Europe and in the USA, who are busy clinicians and clinical academics and who frequently encounter patients presenting as emergencies. We have endeavored to cover the broad spectrum of oncologic emergencies in the major systems ranging from cardiovascular emergencies to neurologic emergencies, bone problems through to acute pain and psychiatric problems. We have given particular emphasis to the acute infectious and hematologic emergencies which are extremely common and life-threatening. We have also included a chapter on drug-related emergencies which are not uncommon.

Each chaper gives a background to the complications whether cancer- or treatment-related and clearly outlines the modern approach to treatment.

For ease of reference the book contains many algorithims as guidelines for the management of various emergency situations which we hope will be of use to the practising clinician. Each chapter is referenced with 10–15 up-to-date papers for further reading.

We hope that this text will be of interest to doctors who have contact with cancer patients who are treating such patients with either cancer-related or treatment-related complications. The book should be of interest to doctors in family practice, Emergency Room doctors and those dealing with acute hospital admissions. It should also be of interest to doctors in training in medicine, particularly those in the area of oncology.

The book should be of interest to postgraduate nurses in both hospital and family practice, and senior medical students.

We trust the reader will find this text to be an important and up-to-date educational resource and one that will ultimately benefit the cancer patient who presents as an emergency.

P.G.J. & R.A.J.S.

Acknowledgements

The authors are pleased to acknowledge the enormous help received from Oxford University Press in the development and writing of this text. We particularly wish to acknowledge the advice, help, and encouragement given to us by Ms Catherine Barnes from Oxford University Press. We would also like to acknowledge the help of Miss Anne Wilkie who did much work in helping collate the text.

We are grateful to our contributors, each of whom is an expert in their own area, from Europe and USA. Our colleagues are extremely busy both clinically and academically and have given of their time to produce what we believe are excellent chapters in their respective specialized areas.

We would also particularly acknowledge the help of Mr Alister Hamilton, Consultant Orthopaedic Surgeon, Belfast, who gave advice in the preparation of the text and illustrations in the Bone Emergencies chapter (Chapter 8).

We would wish to particularly acknowledge the help of our two colleagues, Drs Richard Kennedy and Ultan McDermott, Specialist Registrars in the Department of Oncology, Queen's University, Belfast. Drs Kennedy and McDermott did much work in helping collate the various contributions; they gave us considerable help in proof reading and gave advice on the content and presentation of the text. Their help has been greatly appreciated and is gratefully acknowledged.

Above all, we acknowledge the support and patience of our respective families and we dedicate this book to our wives and children and to the cancer patient.

R.A.J.S. & P.G.J.

Contents

Contributors

Dr Manish Agrawal, Clinical Associate, Medicine Branch, National Cancer Institute, Bethesda, MD 20889

Dr Stephen J. Chanock, National Cancer Institute, Bldg 10, Rm 13N240, Bethesda, MD 20892

Dr Kenneth J. Cohen, Assistant Professor of Oncology, Assistant Professor Pediatrics, The John Hopkins University School of Medicine, The John Hopkins Hospital, Baltimore, Maryland, USA

Dr Bernadette Corcoran, Consultant Palliative Medicine, Belfast City Hospital, Belfast BT9 7AB

Dr Kevin Cullen, Professor of Oncology, Georgetown University, 2nd Floor, Corridor B, 3800 Reservoir Road, NW, Washington DC, 20007, USA

Dr Ruth Eakin, Consultant Oncologist, Belvoir Park Hospital, Hospital Road, Belfast BT8 5JR

Dr Martin M. Eatock, Consultant Medical Oncologist, Belfast City Hospital, Belfast

Dr Tracey Evans, Oncology Fellow, Partners/Dana-Farber Cancer Care, Massachusetts General Hospital, Boston, MA

Dr Juan Gea-Banacloche, National Cancer Institute, Bldg 10, Rm 13N240, Bethesda, MD 20892

Mr Chris Hagan, Specialist Registrar in Urology, Belfast City Hospital

Dr Lee J. Helman, Chief, Pediatric Oncology Branch, National Cancer Institute, National Institutes of Health, Bethesda, Maryland, USA

Dr Mohamed Hussein, Georgetown University, 2nd Floor, Corridor B, 3800 Reservoir Road, NW, Washington DC, 20007, USA

Professor Patrick G. Johnston, Professor of Oncology, Queen's University Belfast/Belfast City Hospital

Dr Markus Jörger, Fellow in Medical Oncology, University Hospital, Zurich, Switzerland

Mr Patrick F. Keane, Consultant Urologist, Belfast City Hospital

Dr Chris B. Kelly, Consultant Psychiatrist, Queen's University Belfast/Belfast City Hospital, Department of Mental Health, Whitla Medical Building, 97 Lisburn Road, Belfast BT9 7BL

Dr Sheila Kelly, Consultant in Palliative Medicine, Marie Curie Centre, Kensington Road, Belfast BT5 6NF

Dr M. John Kennedy, Consultant Medical Oncologist, St James's Hospital, Dublin

Dr Richard Kennedy, Macmillan Specialist Registrar, Department of Oncology, University Floor, Belfast City Hospital BT9 7AB

Dr Samir N. Khleif, Senior Investigator, Medicine Branch, National Cancer Institute, Consultant, Medical Oncology, Naval Hospital Bethesda, Bethesda, MD 20889

Dr Timothy Kinsella, Vincent K. Smith Chair, Professor and Chairman, Department of Radiation Oncology, Director of Radiation Oncology, University Hospitals of Cleveland, School of Medicine, 11100 Euclid Avenue, Cleveland, Ohio 44106-6068, USA

Dr Thomas Lynch, Associate Professor of Medicine, Harvard Medical School, Medical Director, MGH Thoracic Oncology Center, Massachusetts General Hospital, Boston, MA

Professor Shaun R. McCann, Consultant Hematologist, St James's Hospital, Dublin and Professor of Haematology, University of Dublin, Trinity College

Professor Roy J. McClelland, Professor of Mental Health, Queen's University Belfast/ Belfast City Hospital, Department of Mental Health, Whitla Medical Building, 97 Lisburn Road, Belfast BT9 7BL

Dr Ultan McDermott, Specialist Registrar, Department of Oncology, Belfast City Hospital, Belfast BT9 7AB

Dr Niamh O'Connell, Lecturer in Haematology, St James's Hospital and University of Dublin, Trinity College, Dublin

Dr Bernard Pestalozzi, Associate Professor of Oncology, University of Zurich, Ramistrasse 100, CH 8091, Zurich, Switzerland

Dr Aamrah R. Shah, Registrar in Oncology, St James's Hospital, Dublin

Professor Roy Spence, Consultant Surgeon, Belfast City Hospital/Honorary Professor, Queen's University Belfast/Honorary Professor, University of Ulster

Dr Thomas J. Walsh, Senior Investigator, Immunocompromised Host Section, National Cancer Institute, Bldg 10, Rm 13N240, Bethesda, USA

Dr Richard H. Wilson, Fellow, Medicine Branch, National Cancer Institute, Bethesda, USA

Chapter 1

Cardiovascular Emergencies

Aamrah R. Shah and M. John Kennedy

1.1 Introduction

Cardiovascular emergencies occur commonly in cancer patients. Complications of cancer and its therapy, including pericardial effusion and tamponade, cardiac masses, extrinsic compression of the heart and great vessels by tumor masses, and cardiomyopathy leading to heart failure are frequently encountered clinical problems.

Cardiac complications of cancer or its therapy are protean. Tumors may cause arrhythmias due to mediators they secrete or direct mechanical irritation of the heart or pericardium. Pericardial effusion and tamponade may also follow surgery, radiation, or chemotherapy. Chemotherapy can lead to angina, myocardial infarction, arrhythmia, and/or sudden death. Radiation can cause acute pericardial disease, acute valvular insufficiency, effusive constrictive pericarditis, and myocardial infarction. Thus, the cardiovascular complications of cancer, and its therapy, can pose considerable difficulties in the management of patients with cancer.

1.2 Cardiomyopathy and heart failure

1.2.1 Cancer-related cardiomyopathy

Although cancer-related cardiomyopathy leading to heart failure is rare, metabolically active mediators are commonly associated with certain neoplastic diseases. Such mediators may have a direct effect on the cardiovascular system. Carcinoid heart disease is the result of long-term release of biologically active compounds that stimulate the production of a distinctive fibromuscular plaque which can destroy the integrity of the cardiac valves and may lead to right-sided heart failure.

Patients with pheochromocytoma may develop catacholamine-induced cardiomyopathy, which can be reversible if the tumor is resected or catacholamine levels are controlled. Cardiac amyloidosis may develop in patients with multiple myeloma and rarely in Hodgkin's disease, and may cause restrictive cardiomyopathy.

1.2.2 Treatment-related cardiotoxicity

Cytotoxic antibiotics of the anthracycline class are the best known potentially cardiotoxic chemotherapeutic agents. Alkylating agents, antimetabolites and antimicrotubular agents have also been associated with cardiotoxicity (Table 1.1). A number of risk factors may predispose a patient to cardiotoxicity (Table 1.2) and may help the clinician sense the potential for cardiotoxicity before therapy is initiated. Patients should be screened for risk factors, and an attempt to modify them should be made. Monitoring for cardiac events and their treatment will usually depend on the signs and symptoms anticipated and exhibited. Patients may be asymptomatic with the only manifestations being electrocardiographic changes. Treatment of chemotherapy-induced cardiac events is symptomatic. Agents that can be used prophylactically are few, although dexrazonane, a cardio-protective agent specific for anthracycline chemotherapy, has shown promising results. Prompt measures such as discontinuation or modification of chemotherapy or use of appropriate drug therapy should be initiated when indicated.

Anthracycline-induced cardiomyopathy

Anthracyclines and the anthracenedione mitoxantrone cause a progressive cardiomyopathy due to myocardial cell loss and fibrosis. The pathogenesis of anthracycline-induced cardiomyopathy is probably multi-factorial with a significant role being played by free radical mediated myocyte damage. The incidence of cardiomyopathy due to anthracycline therapy increases in a dose-related fashion. A safe cumulative dose for patients without

Table 1.1 Chemotherapy agents associated with congestive cardiac failure (CCF)

Anthracyclines
Doxorubicin
Daunorubicin
Epirubicin
Idarubicin
Mitoxantrone

Alkylating agents
Cyclophosphamide
Ifosfamide
Cisplatin
Mitomycin

Antimetabolites
Fluorouracil
Cytarabine

Antimicrotubular agents
Paclitaxel
Vinca alkaloids

Miscellaneous
Cladrabine
Asparginase
Tretinoin
Pentostatin

Table 1.2 Risk factors for anthracycline-induced cardiomyopathy

- Age >70
- Female gender
- Cumulative dose, rate and schedule of drug administration
- Combination therapy
- Mediastinal radiotherapy
  (Previous or concomitant)
- Previous cardiac disease
  (Coronary, valvular or myocardial)
- Hypertension
- Liver disease
- Whole body hyperthermia

Table 1.3 Anthracycline-induced cardiotoxicity

Drug	Onset	Incidence	Clinical course
Doxorubicin	Within a week	EKG changes 20–30%	Acute or subacute
Daunorubicin	After a single dose or a course	Arrhythmias 0.5–3%	Sinus tachycardia Arrhythmias Pericarditis Myocarditis
	Early 0–231 days (within a year)	At < 400 mg/m^2: 0.14% 500 mg/m^2: 7%	CHF
	Late 4–15 years after completion		CHF
Epirubicin	Unknown	Unknown	CHF
Idarubicin		At cumulative dose 150–290 mg/m^2: 5%	CHF Arrhythmias Angina, MI
Mitoxantrone	Weeks	6% at 60 mg/m^2 15% at 120 mg/m^2	Arrhythmias CHF MI EKG change

previous anthracycline exposure is 150 mg/m^2. Daunorubicin, idarubicin, and epirubicin are somewhat less toxic than doxorubicin (Table 1.3). Long after anthracycline therapy, radiation to the heart can cause a recall phenomenon which may result in cardiac failure.

Clinical syndromes of anthracycline-induced cardiotoxicity   Acute or subacute injury can occur immediately after treatment. This is uncommon and may manifest as a transient arrhythmia, a pericarditis–myocarditis syndrome, or acute left ventricular failure. Anthracyclines can induce chronic cardiotoxicity resulting in cardiomyopathy and heart failure. Presentation may be with tachycardia, decreased exercise tolerance, clinical fluid overload, heart failure or arrhythmias.

Late-onset cardiotoxicity presents with ventricular dysfunction, arrhythmias, including non-sustained ventricular tachycardia and sudden death. This syndrome may manifest years to decades (>15 years) after anthracycline treatment has been completed.

Trastuzumab-induced cardiotoxicity

Trastuzumab is a monoclonal antibody which binds to and inhibits the Her-2/neu receptor, a proto-oncogene product which is overexpressed in about 30 percent of human breast cancers. Randomized trials have indicated that it can cause acute heart failure when used concomitantly with anthracyclines. It is unclear whether it can induce heart failure in patients who have never received an anthracycline. The incidence of heart failure when it is administered with doxorubicin at conventional doses approached 25 percent. Trastuzumab also appears to cause heart failure when administered subsequent to anthracycline therapy although the incidence is less (5–7 percent). The exact mechanism of trastuzumab-induced cardiac failure is unclear and it appears to be partially reversible with therapy. Patients should be carefully monitored during therapy and should have a baseline ejection fraction determined to detect underlying asymptomatic left ventricular dysfunction. If underlying left ventricular dysfunction is significant, alternative therapy should be considered. In view of the significance of this toxicity, and the evolving role of trastuzumab, it is imperative to perform long-term cardiac follow-up of women receiving this therapy.

Diagnostic approach   The potential life long cardiotoxic effect of conventional anthracycline therapy highlights the need for ongoing monitoring of treated patients.

1. Electrophysiological abnormalities may result in non-specific ST- and T-wave changes, decreased QRS voltage and prolongation of the QT interval on the electrocardiogram.

2. Sinus tachycardia is the most common rhythm disturbance, but arrhythmias including ventricular, supraventricular and junctional tachycardia have been reported. None of these changes is specific for anthracycline-induced cardiotoxicity.

3. Radionuclide angiocardiography is extensively used in monitoring early anthracycline-induced cardiotoxicity and has proven value in reducing the incidence of cardiac failure from anthracycline-induced cardiotoxicity.

4. Two-dimensional echocardiography is the other primary non-invasive technique used to monitor toxicity, and is particularly useful in children. Resting left ventricular ejection fraction and fractional shortening are the most commonly evaluated

end-points. However, as with radionuclide measurements, cardiac compensation in the face of substantial anthracycline-induced cardiac injury often maintains normal left ventricular ejection fraction until the cardiomyopathic changes are relatively well established.

5. Echocardiography may also demonstrate some degree of mitral insufficiency due to papillary muscle dysfunction caused by the cardiomyopathy.

The diagnostic test with the greatest specificity and sensitivity for anthracycline-induced cardiomyopathy is endomyocardial biopsy. Typical histopathological changes include loss of myofibrils, distension of the sarcoplasmic reticulum, and vacuolization of the cytoplasm. These histologic markers are used to grade injury on a scale of one to three. A biopsy score of 2.5 or higher mandates discontinuation of therapy.

Management As anthracycline-induced cardiomyopathy is irreversible the best treatment is prevention. This can be accomplished by careful monitoring of the ventricular ejection fraction. Strategies used in an attempt to prevent cardiomyopathy are given in Table 1.4.

Therapeutic options An algorithm for the management of anthracycline-induced cardiomyopathy is shown in Fig. 1.1. The mainstay of treatment for established anthracycline-induced ventricular dysfunction, as for the other types of cardiomyopathy, is limited to conventional therapy for heart failure with agents such as diuretics, inotropes, digitalis, and angiotensin converting enzyme inhibitors. Long-term therapy with such agents, along with cardioselective β-blockers, seems to be of benefit.

Arrhythmias should be treated if symptomatic. As with other forms of clinical heart failure, the overall prognosis for patients with anthracycline-induced ventricular failure (both early and late onset) is poor. Heart transplantation may be a viable alternative in rare selected patients. Prevention continues to be the primary strategy to decrease mortality due to anthracycline-induced cardiotoxicity. The decision to continue anthracycline therapy should be based on the potential benefit of response versus the risk of developing a fatal cardiac failure.

Table 1.4 Monitoring parameters and prevention of anthracycline-induced cardiotoxicity

- The use of anthracycline analogues
- Limits on the amount of drug used
- Alternative drug delivery methods
- Administration in combination with cardio-protective agents
- Infusion rather than bolus therapy
- Avoid drug interactions that increase cardiotoxicity (e.g. paclitaxel)
- Cardioprotectants e.g. dexrazonane (ICF-187)

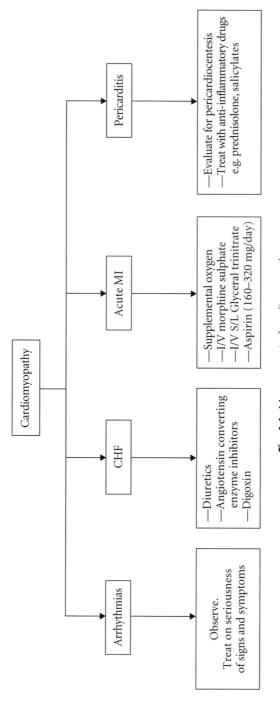

Fig. 1.1 Management of cardiomyopathy.

1.3 **Arrhythmias**

Arrhythmias in cancer patients may be due to direct mechanical irritation or invasion, or may be a consequence of myocardial damage from cancer or its therapy. Rhythm disturbances that occur as a result of pathological processes within the heart behave in a manner similar to dysrhythmias that occur as a complication of the acute phase of a myocardial infarction. Dysrhythmias due to cardiomyopathy may follow anthracycline chemotherapy, or radiation injury, and occasionally infiltrative processes, such as amyloidosis and metastasis may be causal. Rhythm disturbances observed include atrial flutter, atrial fibrillation, supraventricular tachycardia (SVT), ventricular tachyarrhythmia, left bundle branch block, bigeminy, trigeminy, premature ventricular contractions, ventricular tachycardia (VT) and ventricular fibrillation. The most common of these is SVT. Atrial fibrillation may complicate thoracic and upper abdominal surgery, or may be secondary to underlying neoplastic lung disease.

Treatment-related arrhythmia   Most chemotherapy-related disturbances of rhythm are of short duration and of little clinical importance (Table 1.5). However, when dysrhythmia results in significant hemodynamic embarrassment, or when it is anticipated that a rhythm disturbance may become life-threatening, active intervention is required.

Management   An algorithm to manage arrhythmias is shown in Fig. 1.2. Recognizing the potential malignant dysrhythmia and withdrawing the offending drug is often the

Table 1.5 Chemotherapy agents associated with arrhythmias

Anthracyclines
Daunorubicin
Idarubicin
Mitoxantrone

Alkylating agents
Ifosfamide
Cisplatin
Carmustine
Busulphan

Antimetabolites
Fluorouracil

Antimicrotubules
Paclitaxel
Teniposide
Vinca alkaloids

Miscellaneous
Amsacrine
Asparginase
Tretinoin
Pentostatin

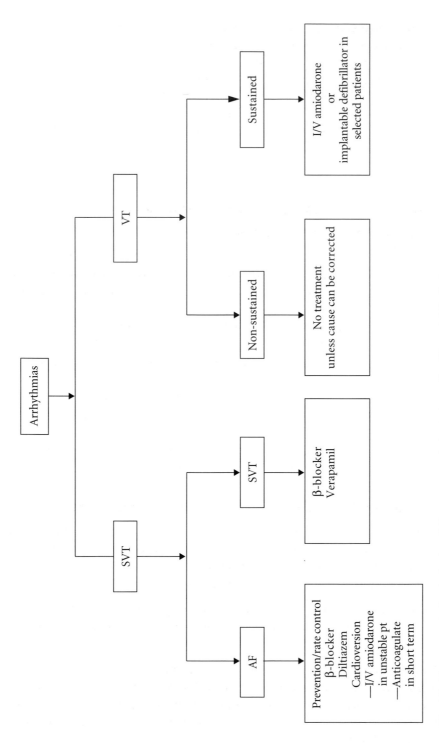

Fig. 1.2 Management of arrhythmias. SVT = supraventricular tachycardia; AF = atrial fibrillation; VT = ventricular tachycardia.

most appropriate therapy. β-blockers and maintenance of potassium and magnesium homeostasis may be helpful in preventing recurrences. Overdrive pacing, intravenous magnesium or isoproterenol administered as an infusion may sometimes be necessary to convert rare dysrhythmias such as torsades des pointes.

Atrial fibrillation may be treated with verapamil, diltiazem or a β-blocker. Cardioversion may be necessary. Patients should be anticoagulated in the short term. Treatment for SVT is controversial but options include β-blockers, verapamil or diltiazem. Non-sustained VT is not an indication for treatment unless the cause can be corrected. Amiodarone is remarkably effective for this dysrhythmia.

1.4 Pericardial effusion and cardiac tamponade

1.4.1 Cancer-related tamponade

Exudative effusion is the most common manifestation of metastatic disease to the pericardium. Five to ten percent of patients dying with disseminated malignancies have cardiac or pericardial metastases, though far fewer have symptomatic pericardial disease. Although malignant pericardial effusions are not particularly common, they are of great importance because of the potential for acute cardiac tamponade and death. The rate of accumulation and the distensibility of the pericardial sac determine the hemodynamic effect and the symptoms of these effusions. Effusions due to tumors most often progress to tamponade due to bleeding.

Common causative malignancies include breast, lung, lymphoma involving the mediastinum, leukemia, and melanoma. As fluid builds up in the pericardial sac, it inhibits passive diastolic filling of the normally low-pressure right heart. This produces the classical physical signs of cervical and abdominal venous hypertension and accounts for the diagnostic echocardiographic findings of right atrial and right ventricular diastolic collapse.

1.4.2 Treatment-related pericardial effusion/tamponade

Chemotherapy-related effusions are rare. Table 1.6 outlines some of the chemotherapeutic agents responsible for pericardial effusion/tamponade. Endocardial fibrosis and cardiac tamponade associated with busulphan, cytarabine, and tretinoin are extremely rare, with only a few published case reports in the literature.

Clinical presentation   The clinical presentation may be dramatic and can include syncope, chest pain, or palpitations. More subtle symptoms include dyspnea, chest heaviness, or simple fatigue.

Clinical assessment   Full physical examination may reveal components of the often-described clinical triad of hypotension, tachycardia, and muffled heart sounds. These physical findings, along with distended neck veins and a pulsus paradoxus, lead to a clinical diagnosis of tamponade. In the absence of therapy, patients may progress to a low-output shock state.

Table 1.6 Chemotherapeutic agents causing pericardial effusion/tamponade

Alkylating agents
Busulphan

Antimetabolites
Cytarabine

Miscellaneous
Tretinoin

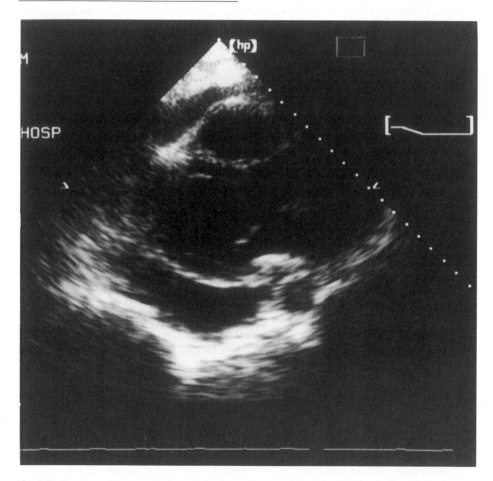

Fig. 1.3 Parasternal long-axis view of the heart by two-dimensional echocardiography shows a large pericardial effusion (P).

Diagnostic evaluation   Widening of the cardiac silhouette may be observed on chest X-ray. A pleural effusion is seen in a third of cases. Electrocardiography may reveal sinus tachycardia, low voltage QRS, electrical alternance or a wandering baseline. Transthoracic echocardiography is diagnostic and can be used to evaluate right and left ventricular

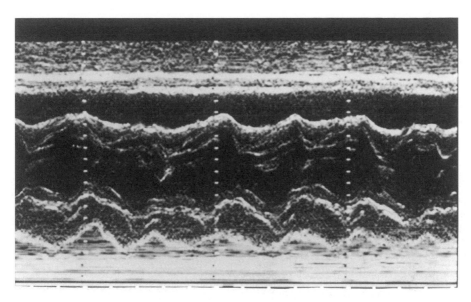

Fig. 1.4 M-mode echocardiography showing a pericardial effusion.

function and the presence or absence of right ventricular and atrial diastolic collapse (Figs 1.3 and 1.4). Equalization of diastolic pressures in all cardiac chambers, determined by right heart catheterization, is pathognomonic.

Treatment   Volume expansion and vasopressor support is applied (if necessary) to maintain blood pressure. Adequate oxygenation must be maintained. Diuretics are usually contraindicated. Suspected or proven tamponade is best treated by pericardiocentesis which is accomplished easily under local anesthesia. General anesthesia for an urgent drainage procedure or window in this setting is dangerous and should be avoided. A single tap, however, is unlikely to prevent reaccumulation unless the underlying cause can be addressed. Operative treatment of a malignant pericardial effusion may be required for recurrence of a symptomatic malignant effusion. The most aggressive approach to management of symptomatic pericardial effusion has been a limited anterior thoracotomy with anterior pericardiectomy. This may now be achieved with less invasive video-assisted surgery. The role of pericardial sclerosis is controversial. Doxycycline, bleomycin, or thiotepa has been used as pericardial sclerosants with success. Thiotepa is not associated with severe pain and is reasonably effective, particularly in breast cancer, and infrequently causes pericardial constriction. Despite sclerosis or a pericardial window, pericardial effusion and tamponade can recur.

1.5 **Cardiac masses**

Primary and secondary tumors of the heart are rare. Most primaries develop in the left atrium and mitral valve. Tumors may spread to the heart via the vascular system. They

Table 1.7 Cardiac tumors

Benign
Myxomas
Rhabdomyomas
Lipomas
Fibroelastomas
Primary malignant cardiac tumors
Sarcomas
Osteosarcomas, Chondrosarcomas (rare)
Mesotheliomas
Pheochromocytomas
Metastatic
Ewing's sarcoma may metastasize to endocardial surface of heart

may grow in from the inferior vena cava (hepatic, renal, and adrenal tumors; and tumors metastatic to the liver or kidney) or extend into the superior vena cava (thyroid, lung, breast, thymoma, and lymphoma).

Metastatic tumors can involve the heart by direct extension, as well as by hematogenous spread (Table 1.7). Cardiac function can also be compromised by masses within the pericardial space.

Clinical features   Any of the above can present as acute cardiac compromise due to obstruction of the right ventricular outflow tract, thromboembolic events, and arrhythmias. Lymphoma in the mediastinum may compress the right ventricular outflow tract.

Management   Non-invasive techniques such as echocardiography and gated magnetic resonance imaging may be diagnostic. The potential for thromboembolic events is high and should be treated by anticoagulation. Dysrhythmias should be treated symptomatically. Lymphomas and testicular tumors should be treated with chemotherapy. Benign remnants may subsequently require surgical resection as they can serve as a nidus for thrombus formation.

1.6 **Radiation-induced heart disease**

With the widespread use of mediastinal irradiation to control or cure many neoplasms, the population of patients surviving for a substantial period is steadily increasing. There is strong evidence of radiation-induced damage to the heart and great vessels in many such patients. The spectrum of involvement includes the three layers of the heart as well as the coronary vessels, the valvular and sub-valvular apparatus, and the conduction system.

Clinical features   The spectrum of cardiac disease observed is outlined in Table 1.8.

Table 1.8 Spectrum of radiation-induced heart disease

Pericardium
Acute pericarditis
Pericardial effusion
Constrictive pericarditis
Myocarditis

Fibrosis with cardiomyopathy
Endocardium
Endocardial fibrosis

Valvular dysfunction
Predominantly left-sided valvular lesions
Regurgitation more common than stenosis

Coronary artery disease
Angina and myocardial infarction
Sudden death syndrome
Coronary spasm
Conduction system
Atrioventricular block

Pericardial disease   Pericardial disease is the most common manifestation of radiation-induced cardiotoxicity. Clinical presentations include acute pericarditis, pericardial effusion with or without tamponade, and constrictive pericarditis. Most cases of acute pericarditis occur within the first year after radiation therapy. Clinical features include fever, pleuritic chest pain, pericardial friction rub, and some enlargement of the cardiac silhouette on the chest radiograph. All patients respond to bed rest, non-steroidal anti-inflammatories and mild diuretics. Symptomatic pericardial effusion presents relatively early, within 15 months after irradiation, whereas the mean time of presentation for constrictive pericarditis is 48 months. Patients with pericardial effusion may develop constriction in later years.

Myocardium and endocardium   Patients receiving mediastinal irradiation can develop myocardial fibrosis either as a result of direct injury or due to radiation-induced coronary artery disease. The most conspicuous change is diffuse interstitial fibrosis observed chiefly in the right ventricle, presumably because of the commonly used anterior radiation field.

Coronary artery disease   Coronary artery disease in patients with prior mediastinal irradiation can mimic atherosclerotic disease. The proximal epicardial vessels and the coronary ostia are the most commonly involved sites. Affected patients commonly present with angina or myocardial infarction. Sudden death and coronary spasm may also occur.

Valvular dysfunction   Radiation-associated valvular disease has been well described but the exact clinical incidence is not known. Affected valves have diffuse cusp or leaflet fibrosis and left-sided valves appear to be more frequently involved. Both regurgitation and stenosis are common in the aortic area, but regurgitant lesions are the only ones described in the mitral area.

Conduction system   The conduction system is the least commonly involved of all the cardiac structures in patients with radiation-induced cardiac toxicity. The most common manifestation is complete atrioventricular block.

Management   Investigations and management of radiation induced heart disease are outlined in Fig. 1.5. As radiation-induced heart disease occurs in a substantial number of patients with prior mediastinal irradiation, screening of asymptomatic patients should be considered, though the extent to which these patients benefit from systematic screening is controversial.

Recommendations are that electrocardiography and stress testing be done at 5-year intervals as a relatively cost-effective screening mechanism for patients with previous mediastinal irradiation.

Radiation-induced heart disease must be considered in any patient who has had mediastinal irradiation of more than 3500 cGy and is found to have cardiac symptomatology. Newer radiation techniques with cardiac shielding may decrease the incidence. Pericardial disease is the most common manifestation, and anterior pericardiectomy is advisable when a patient develops symptomatic pericardial effusion. Concomitant pericardiectomy should be considered in a patient undergoing operation for radiation-induced coronary or valvular disease to avoid later complications. Percutaneous transluminal coronary angioplasty has a high restenosis rate, and stent implantation may improve the long-term patency.

1.7 **Thromboembolic complications**

Thrombosis is a common complication of malignancy. Factors that may affect the risk of thromboembolism vary widely from patient to patient and include type of tumor, nutritional status, type of chemotherapy, response to chemotherapy (e.g. tumor lysis syndrome), liver and renal function, and performance status. Circulating tumor cells may adhere to the vascular endothelium and form a nidus for clot formation. Tumors may also penetrate vessels promoting clot formation. A systemic hypercoagulable state and external compression of vessels by tumor masses impeding blood flow are some of the factors that can initiate thrombus formation. Tumors most commonly involved with venous thromboembolism are the mucin secreting adenocarcinomas and intracranial malignancies (Table 1.9).

A variety of clinical syndromes are associated with the hypercoagulable state of malignancy and of its treatment and include disseminated intravascular coagulation, venous and arterial thromboembolism, cerebrovascular events, pulmonary embolism, intestinal infarction and other ischemic vascular crises.

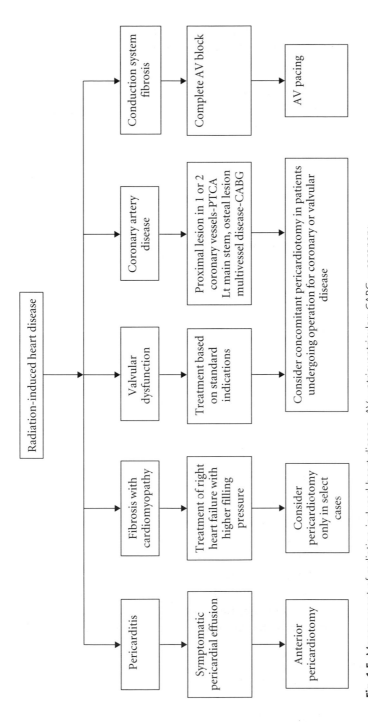

Fig. 1.5 Management of radiation-induced heart disease. AV = atrioventricular; CABG = coronary artery bypass graft; PTCA = percutaneous transluminal coronary angioplasty.

Table 1.9 Tumors associated with thromboembolism

Cancers with procoagulant activity
Hepatoma
Lung
Renal cell
Colorectal
Chondrosarcoma
Liposarcoma
Neuroblastoma
Melanoma
Non-lymphoid leukemia
Lymphoblastic leukemia

Cancers with vascular invasion and mechanical causes
Renal cell carcinoma
Germ cell tumor
Hepatocellular
Gastric
Lung
Adrenocortical

Cancers with increased risk post-operation
Lung
Pancreas
Ovary
Stomach

1.7.1 Treatment-related thromboembolism

Chemotherapeutic agents associated with venous thromboembolism are listed in Table 1.10. Chemotherapy agents also increase endothelial cell reactivity to platelets, a phenomenon which may underlie thrombotic thrombocytopenic purpura and hemolytic uremic syndrome. Many chemotherapy agents can cause phlebitis, notably the anthracyclines, nitrosoureas, mitomycin, epipodophyllin, dacarbazine, and fluorouracil.

Pulmonary embolism

Neoplastic cells generate thrombin and procoagulants, and vessel wall injury and stasis may increase the risk for pulmonary embolism, a common complication of cancer. In addition the presence of an upper extremity central venous catheter is a risk factor for the development of upper extremity deep venous thrombosis and subsequent pulmonary embolism.

Clinical assessment　The clinical manifestations of pulmonary embolism are outlined in Table 1.11. Clinical examination may reveal:

1. Tachypnea and tachycardia.
2. Crepitations heard over the involved area, a pleural friction rub and evidence of pleural effusion.

Table 1.10 Chemotherapeutic agents associated with thromboembolism

- Mitomycin
- Bleomycin
- Cisplatin
- Methyl-CCNU
- Cytosine arabinoside
- Cyclosporine A

Table 1.11 Clinical manifestations of pulmonary embolism

Acute minor pulmonary embolism
Usually no hemodynamic disturbance in acute minor pulmonary embolism
Dyspnea
Pleuritic chest pain
Apprehension
Cough and hemoptysis

Acute major pulmonary embolism
Severe dyspnea
Dull central chest pain
Cyanosis
Gallop rhythm
Raised venous pressure
Tachypnea
Syncope or death

3. Splinting of the involved side may manifest in elevation of the diaphragm and generalized decreased breath sounds. Cardiac examination may reveal signs of right ventricular failure, including a right-sided third heart sound, the murmur of pulmonary
regurgitation, or increased intensity of the pulmonary component of the second
heart sound.

Diagnostic evaluation   Baseline full blood count, coagulation studies and arterial
blood gas analysis may demonstrate an increased alveolar–arterial oxygen gradient.
Most patients have a normal chest X-ray or non-specific findings. However, the chest
X-ray may show evidence of splinting (a raised diaphragm and basilar atelectasis).
Pleural effusion or pulmonary infiltrates may be seen after infarction of the lung.
A lobar consolidation similar to bacterial pneumonia may be present. Vascular changes
occur frequently in acute pulmonary embolism, but are difficult to interpret. Peripheral
pruning is sometimes evident. With large central pulmonary emboli, a sausage-shaped
dilatation of the involved pulmonary artery may be observed.

Characteristic EKG abnormalities are seen in only about 25 percent of patients with
massive pulmonary embolism. These include $S_1 Q_3 T_3$ pattern, right bundle branch

block, p-pulmonale and right axis deviation. Other non-specific changes include sinus tachycardia, atrial fibrillation, and T-wave inversion in the anteroseptal leads (V_1–V_3).

Ventilation–perfusion (V/Q) scintigraphy is useful in evaluating suspected pulmonary embolism. Unfortunately most patients do not have a high-probability scan and a definite diagnosis is made in only a minority of patients.

Pulmonary angiogram remains the standard test. Where the index of clinical suspicion is moderate or high and the isotope scan is equivocal, pulmonary angiogram should be considered.

Spiral computed tomography (CT) is increasingly helpful in detecting pulmonary embolism. A sensible approach will be to order V/Q first, followed by Doppler U/S for patients with low- or intermediate-probability (non-diagnostic) scans.

Increased levels of D-dimers have been found in 90 percent of patients with pulmonary embolism documented on V/Q lung scanning. Levels, however, are also elevated for up to a week post-operatively or in myocardial infarction, sepsis, and other systemic illnesses. A negative D-dimer assay in conjunction with a negative imaging study may help rule out pulmonary embolism. Once standardized, these assays may become useful screening tests.

Therapeutic options   An algorithm for the management of pulmonary embolism may be found in Fig. 1.6. Apart from supportive therapy (analgesia and oxygen), three immediate treatment options for pulmonary embolism are anticoagulation with heparin, thrombolytic therapy, and pulmonary embolectomy.

Unfractionated heparin is the first line treatment for hemodynamically stable pulmonary embolus. Limited studies on treatment with low molecular weight heparin have shown it to be as safe and effective as unfractionated intravenous heparin. Loading with an oral anticoagulant is usually undertaken simultaneously. When warfarin is started during active thrombosis the levels of protein C and protein S fall, creating a thrombogenic potential. Oral loading with warfarin should therefore be covered by simultaneous heparin for 4–5 days. Oral anticoagulation is given to achieve an international normalization ratio (INR) of 2–3. The ideal duration of therapy is unknown. Occlusion of two or more lobar vessels on pulmonary angiogram or greater than 50 percent loss of perfusion on lung scan may result in significant hemodynamic instability. Mortality is 85 percent in the first 6 hours after such an event. These patients are treated with anticoagulation and supportive care. Hemodynamic instability secondary to massive pulmonary embolism is an indication for thrombolytic therapy. Currently three thrombolytic agents, urokinase, streptokinase, and tissue plasminogen activator (TPA) are approved for use in pulmonary embolism. Tissue plasminogen activator has the benefit of being infused over a short time period and causing more rapid thrombolysis. In patients with massive pulmonary embolism so severely compromised hemodynamically that they may not survive the hour or two required to derive benefit from thrombolysis, or in patients with some contraindication to thrombolysis, pulmonary embolectomy may be life-saving.

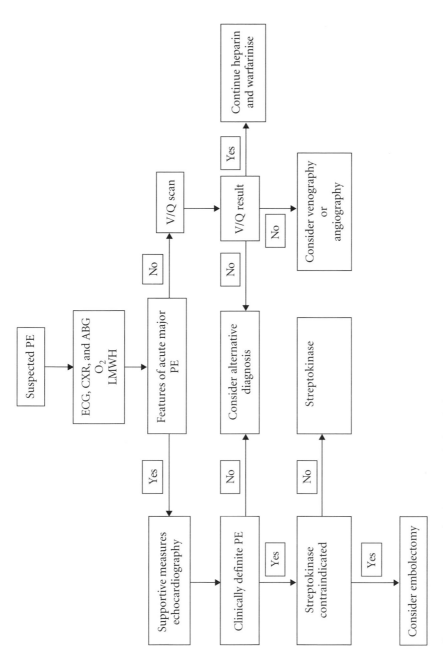

Fig. 1.6 Management of pulmonary embolism (PE). ABG = arterial blood gas; LMWH = low molecular weight heparin; V/Q = ventilation/perfusion scan.

Superior vena cava syndrome

The superior vena cava (SVC) is formed by the union of right and left brachiocephalic veins and empties into the superior-posterior right atrium. The vessel is relatively thin-walled and lies within a non-distensible space in the mediastinum. This makes it susceptible to extrinsic compression by primary tumors or lymph nodes. Malignant causes represent 85–97 percent of all cases of SVC syndrome. Bronchogenic carcinoma is the most common cause of SVC syndrome. Breast cancer may account for as many as 10 percent of cases. Other causes are given in Table 1.12. Superior vena cava obstruction may be due to iatrogenic causes such as thrombus formation in the presence of pacemaker wires or indwelling central lines. This possibility must be considered in the initial work up of oncology patients, who frequently have hypercoagulable states in the presence of such devices.

Clinical features   These are summarized in Table 1.13. The clinical presentation of SVC syndrome may be acute or subacute. While a slowly progressive occlusion of the SVC may allow substantial collateral blood flow to develop, an acute obstruction of blood flow from the head and upper extremities will cause increased venous pressure with resulting symptoms. Dyspnea is the most common presenting symptom and a high percentage of patients complain of swelling of the trunk or extremities.

   Cough, chest pain, dysphagia, and headache are common. Physical examination will reveal facial or upper extremity edema, tearing (chemosis) and dyspnea in many patients. The extent of jugular venous distension is variable. Cyanosis, paralysis of the true vocal cords, Horner's syndrome, and blurred vision are uncommon (Table 1.13). Occult SVC syndrome (compression of the SVC noted on CT without clinical manifestations) is uncommon.

Diagnostic approach   Diagnostic tests are summarized in Table 1.14. As the therapeutic approach will be determined by the underlying histologic diagnosis, tissue must

---

Table 1.12 Primary diagnosis in SVC syndrome

Bronchogenic carcinoma
Small cell
Non-small cell

Lymphoma

Metastatic carcinoma
Breast

Primary mediastinal tumors
Thymoma
Thymic carcinoid
Germ cell tumors

SVC thrombosis

Table 1.13 Clinical features of SVC syndrome

Symptoms	Signs
Facial edema	Jugular venous distention
Dyspnea	Facial and upper body plethora
Cough	Upper extremity swelling
Distorted vision	Chemosis
Orthopnea	Mental changes
Hoarseness	Stupor and coma
Headache	Papilledema
Nasal stuffiness	Syncope
Tongue swelling	Cyanosis
Nausea	
Light headedness	
Stridor	

Table 1.14 Diagnostic procedures used in SVC syndrome

Non-invasive
Plain radiograph
Venogram with contrast
Radionucleotide venogram
Computerized axial tomogram (contrast enhanced)

Invasive
Induced sputum cytology
Bronchoscopy
Mediastinoscopy
Thoracotomy
Median sternotomy

be obtained for examination in previously undiagnosed patients. This may prove hazardous in a symptomatic patient. Very rarely is immediate treatment administered on an empirical basis and only when tracheal obstruction is present. Lymphoma is most likely to cause tracheal obstruction and is more commonly observed in children.

In a patient with clinical evidence of SVC obstruction, routine studies include chest X-ray, CT and magnetic resonance imaging (MRI) scans, venography, and nuclear flow studies. The chest radiograph is abnormal in 80 percent of cases and shows widening of the upper mediastinal shadow. Right-sided pleural effusion is present in approximately 25 percent of patients. Computed tomography imaging provides more accurate information on the location of the obstruction and may guide attempts at biopsy by mediastinoscopy, bronchoscopy, or fine needle aspiration.

Venography may prove helpful in establishing the pattern of collateral flow but requires a more invasive procedure and use of iodinated contrast material. It may be associated with an increased risk of thrombus formation and has therefore largely been replaced by radionuclide studies. Contrast venography may however be useful when surgical reconstruction is contemplated. Radionuclide studies have several advantages over contrast venography. The tracer (typically Technetium-99-m labeled microspheres) is not thrombogenic. The study may also aid in the determination of collateral flow and guide in the determination of radiotherapy portals. Gallium single photoemission CT (SPECT) may be of value in selected cases.

Management A management algorithm is suggested in Fig. 1.7. Patients with clinical SVC syndrome often gain significant symptomatic improvement from conservative treatment measures including elevation of the head of the bed and supplemental oxygen. Corticosteroids and diuretics will often reduce edema. These manoeuvres usually allow time to evaluate the pathology specimen prior to initiating therapy before proceeding to definite treatment.

Small cell lung cancer (SCLC) may be managed initially with multi-agent chemotherapy and significant improvement occurs in most cases within 24–48 hours. Radiotherapy is an effective treatment modality for most malignant causes of SVC syndrome notably non-small cell lung cancer. High dose fractions (defined as doses >3 Gy/day) compared to conventional-dose treatment of 2 Gy/day produce an improved response. Chemotherapy as a single modality for particularly sensitive tumor types, such as SCLC, lymphomas, and germ cell tumors is the treatment of choice.

Recurrent non-responsive superior vena cava obstruction (SVCO) may recur following either radiotherapy or chemotherapy. In patients where there is no scope for more radiotherapy and when the tumor has become resistant to chemotherapy, the prognosis is extremely poor. Occasionally a patient may maintain a good performance status despite recurrent SVCO. In such cases it may be appropriate to consider the insertion of a superior vena caval stent. It has a response rate of 68–100 percent and a recurrence rate of 4–45 percent. Pulmonary edema may complicate stent placement and anticoagulation is required. Thrombosis occurs in 30–50 percent of patients so treated.

Thrombolytic therapy with either urokinase or streptokinase may be required for patients who show evidence of clot formation within the SVC. Thrombolysis can be initiated within five to seven days of onset of symptoms. Thrombolytics may also be given through the catheter. Surgical reconstruction of the SVC may be a useful way to palliate symptoms in carefully selected patients.

Hepatic veno-occlusive disease

Hepatic veno-occlusive disease (HVOD) is a non-thrombotic obliteration of the small intrahepatic branches of the hepatic veins by collagenous and reticular intimal thickening. It is a major early complication of bone marrow transplantation (BMT) and essentially all preparative chemoradiotherapy regimens have been implicated in

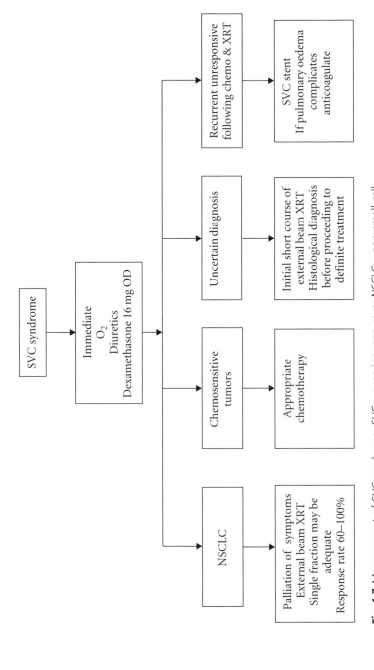

Fig. 1.7 Management of SVC syndrome. SVC = superior vena cava; NSCLC = non-small cell lung cancer; XRT = radiation therapy; OD = once daily.

HVOD. It may vary from mild and reversible to life-threatening and lethal. Clinical features of HVOD include

- Painful hepatomegaly
- Weight gain
- Ascities
- Hyperbilirubinemia

Bearman *et al.* developed a mathematical model for predicting fatal outcome after BMT based on serum bilirubin and weight gain from day 7 before through day 16 after transplantation. Severe HVOD is lethal in the majority of patients and methods to prevent this complication have been actively pursued. Attel *et al.* conducted a prospective, randomized trial of continuous low-dose heparin for the prevention of HVOD after BMT. Heparin was found to be effective in preventing HVOD, which occurred in 13.7 percent of the control group versus 2.5 percent of the heparin group. Unfortunately, there is no proven standard therapy for established HVOD. Treatment of severe HVOD with recombinant human TPA has produced conflicting results.

Thrombotic microangiopathic syndrome

A thrombotic microangiopathic syndrome characterized by renal insufficiency, microangiopathic hemolytic anemia, and thrombocytopenia has been described after treatment with antineoplastic agents. Mitomycin is the most common agent responsible. Table 1.10 lists other types of chemotherapeutic agents associated with this syndrome. Clinically, essentially all patients with this syndrome have a triad of anemia, thrombocytopenia, and renal dysfunction. Most die of renal failure within a few months after the diagnosis of thrombotic microangiopathy is established.

Management Several modalities, including steroids, antiplatelet agents, plasma exchange and plasmapheresis have not been effective in treating this disorder. Snyder *et al.* reported a multicenter study of the treatment with protein A immunoadsorption of plasma. Response to therapy was observed in 25 of 55 patients, with an estimated 1-year survival of 61 percent in responders. This new modality may be the preferred treatment in patients with chemotherapy-induced thrombotic microangiopathic syndrome.

Suggested reading

Abner, A. (1993) Approach to the patient who presents with superior vena cava obstruction. *Chest*, 103, 394–7S.

Arkel, Y.S. (2000) Thrombosis and cancer. *Semin Oncol*, 27, 362–74.

Attel, M., Huguet, F., Rubie, H., Haynh, A., Charlet, J.P., Payen, J.L., *et al.* (1992) Prevention of hepatic veno-occlusive disease after bone marrow transplantation by continuous infusion of low dose heparin: A prospective, randomised trial. *Blood*, 79, 2834–40.

Baker, G.L. and Barnes, H.J. (1992) Superior vena cava syndrome. *Am J Crit Care*, 1, 54–64.

Becker, K., Erckenbrecht, J.F., Haussinger, D., and Frieling, T. (1999) Cardiotoxicity of the antiproliferative compound fluorouracil. *Drugs*, 57(4), 475–84.

DeCamp, M.M., Mentzer, S.J., Swanson, S.J., and Sugerbaker, D.J. (1997) Malignant effusive disease of the pleura and pericardium. *Chest*, 112, 291–5S.

Doll, D.C. and Yarbro, J.W. (1994) Vascular toxicity associated with chemotherapy and hormone therapy, 6, 345–50.

Feldman, A.M., Lorell, B.H., and Reis S.E. (2000) Trastuzumab in the treatment of metastatic breast cancer, Anticancer therapy versus cardiotoxicity. (Editorial). *Circulation*, 102, 272–4.

Forni, M. and Armand, J.P. (1994) Cardiotoxicity of chemotherapy. *Curr Opin Oncol*, 6, 340–4.

Hochster, H., Wasserheit, C.W., and Speyer, J. (1995) Cardiotoxicity and cardioprotection during chemotherapy. *Curr Opin Oncol*, 7, 304–9.

Keefe, D.L. (2000) Cardiovascular emergencies in the cancer patient. *Semin Oncol*, 27, 244–55.

Ko, J.C., Yang, P.C., Yuan, A., Chang, D.B., Yu, C.J., Wu, H.D., *et al.* (1994) Superior vena cava syndrome: Rapid histologic diagnosis by ultrasound-guided transthoracic needle aspiration biopsy. *Am J Respir Crit Care Med*, 149, 783–7.

Markman, M., Kennedy, A., Webster, K., Kulp, B., Peterson, G., and Belinson, J. (1998) Paclitaxel administration to gynaecologic cancer patients with major cardiac risk factors. *J Clin Oncol*, 16, 3483–5.

Pai, V.B. and Nahata, M.C. (2000) Cardiotoxicity of chemotherapeutic agents, incidence, treatment and prevention. *Drug Saf*, 4, 263–302.

Perez, E.A. (1998) Paclitaxel and cardiotoxicity. (Editorial) *J Clin Oncol*, 16, 3481–2.

Physician's Desk Reference (2000) Herceptin. *Micromedex® Healthcare Series*, vol. 106.

Salmon, D.J., Leyland-Jones, B., Shak, S., Fuchs, H., *et al.* (2001) Use of chemotherapy plus a monoclonal antibody against HER2 for metastatic breast cancer that over expresses HER2. *N Eng J Med*, 344, 783–92.

Shah, K., Lincoff, A.M., and Young, J.B. (1996) Anthracycline induced cardiomyopathy. *Ann Intern Med*, 125, 47–58.

Singla, P.K. and Iliskovic, N. (1998) Doxorubicin-induced cardiomyopathy. *N Engl J Med*, 339, 900–5.

Snyder, Jr H.W., Mittletman, A., Oral, A., Messenschmidt, G.L., Henry, D.H., Korec, S., *et al.* (1993) Treatment of cancer chemotherapy associated thrombocytopenia purpura/haemolytic uremic syndrome by protein A immunoadsorbance of plasma. *Cancer*, 71, 1882–92.

Sonnenblick, M. and Rosin, A. (1991) Cardiotoxicity of interferon. A review of 44 cases. *Chest*, 99, 557–61.

Veeragundham, R.S. and Goldin, M.D. (1998) Surgical management of radiation-induced heart disease. *Ann Thorac Surg*, 65, 1014–19.

Chapter 2

Neurologic Emergencies

Manish Agrawal and Samir N. Khleif

2.1 Introduction

Approximately 15–20 percent of patients with cancer develop neurologic complications during the course of their illness. The incidence of neurologic complications of cancer is increasing in frequency as the disease is being controlled for longer periods of time producing an increased opportunity for metastases to the nervous system to develop. Neurologic complications in patients with cancer are either direct effects of tumor as in compression of/spread to brain, spinal cord, leptomeninges, or peripheral nerves or result from treatments such as chemotherapy, biologic, or radiation therapy. These complications are diverse, varying from acute and life-threatening to more insidious with long-term effects. Virtually any tumor can directly involve the nervous system, however, due to their high prevalence, lung, breast, and prostate tumors are the most frequent culprits.

The presentation and management of neurologic emergencies with cancer will be discussed in this chapter. This will cover both emergencies due to direct tumor involvement as well as those related to therapy. At the end of the chapter we will discuss the ophthalmologic complications of cancer.

2.2 Tumor-related neurologic complications

2.2.1 Epidural cord compression

In most patients back pain is benign and self-limited. However, in patients with cancer, back pain can be the first sign of epidural cord compression (ECC). Epidural spinal cord compression is compression of the thecal sac by tumor in the epidural space. This compression occurs either at the levels of the spinal cord or cauda equina. Epidural cord compression occurs in 5–14 percent of patients with cancer. Cord compression most commonly occurs at the thoracic spine (59–78 percent), followed by the lumbosacral (21–43 percent) and the cervical spine (4–15 percent). Although any type of cancer can cause cord compression, breast, prostate, and lung are the most common (Table 2.1).

Tumor causes cord compression in one of three ways: the most common mechanism (85 percent) is when a hematogenously disseminated metastasis to a vertebra erodes into the epidural space; the next most common mechanism (10–12 percent) is when

Table 2.1 Primary sites of tumors causing cord compression (adapted from Fuller *et al.*)

Tumor type	Frequency (%)
Breast	29
Lung	17.2
Prostate	14.2
Lymphoma	5.0
Renal	4.2
Myeloma	4.0
Other	24

paravertebral tumors gain access to the epidural space via the intervertebral foramina; and finally (1–3 percent) are caused by a direct metastasis to the epidural space.

Early diagnosis of this condition is crucial to minimize lasting neurologic dysfunction. Failure to diagnose cord compression when pain is the only symptom may result in progressive and irreversible paraplegia and incontinence. The most important prognostic factor for the preservation of neurologic function is the degree of function at the start of therapy. In patients who are ambulatory at the start of therapy 80 percent will remain so after therapy, whereas only 5 percent of paraplegic patients are ambulatory after treatment. Thus any patient with a known malignancy and new back pain should have at least a plain X-ray of the affected area.

Clinical presentation   Over 90 percent of patients with ECC present with pain (Tables 2.2 and 2.3). Initial growth of the cancer in the vertebral body causes local pain as a result of the stretching of the periosteum. Further growth compresses adjacent neural and vascular structures causing neurologic signs and radicular pain. Pain may begin from hours to months before other neurologic symptoms or signs develop. The pain is localized in the back at the midline. The pain due to ECC is unlike the pain pattern from degenerative spine disease in that it usually worsens at night (Table 2.4). It is also unlike the pain of a herniated disc in that it is exacerbated by recumbence and improved by the upright position. In addition, this pain is frequently accompanied by radicular pain due to invasion of radicular structures. The radicular pain from a cervical lesion usually radiates down the upper extremities while that from a lumbar lesion usually radiates down the lower extremities. Radicular pain from a thoracic lesion usually radiates in a band around the chest or abdomen.

Limb weakness is the second most common symptom after pain and precedes sensory loss and sphincter disturbance (Tables 2.2 and 2.3). The weakness usually begins in the legs, regardless of the spinal compression site. There is more weakness proximally than distally early in the course. As the cord compression progresses, an upper motor neuron

Table 2.2 First symptom of spinal cord compression (adapted from DeAngelis and Posner)

Signs and symptoms	Percentage of patients (%)
Pain	94
Weakness	3
Ataxia	2
Sensory loss	0.5
Autonomic dysfunction	0

Table 2.3 Neurologic signs and symptoms of spinal cord compression at diagnosis (adapted from Fuller *et al.*)

Signs and symptoms	Percentage of patients (%)
Pain	91
Weakness	79
Sensory dysfunction	67
Autonomic dysfunction	49

Table 2.4 Causes of spinal cord dysfunction in patients with cancer (from Quinn and DeAngelis *et al.*)

Epidural cord compression (ECC)
Tumor
Abscess
Hematoma
Disc herniation
Vertebral hemangioma

Intramedullary process
Metastases
Abscess
Hematoma
Syrinx

Myelopathy
Radiation
Intrathecal chemotherapy
Paraneoplastic

Leptomeningeal metastases

Spinal arachnoiditis

pattern with weakness develops and it is accompanied by spasticity, positive Babinski's sign, and exaggerated reflexes. Untreated cord compression progresses to a more profound weakness, proximally and distally, leading to eventual paraplegia.

Sensory abnormalities usually develop shortly after weakness. Paresthesias in ECC begin in the toes and ascend in a stocking-like fashion. Autonomic dysfunction occurs late and is never the sole presenting symptom of cord compression. Autonomic abnormalities include impotence, urinary incontinence or retention, and fecal incontinence or retention. Occasionally ataxia with back pain may be the initial presentation of cord compression.

Cauda equina compression causes a dermatomal sensory loss that is usually bilateral, involves the perianal area, the posterior thigh, or the lateral aspect of the leg. Early deficits in cauda equina involvement include mild decrease in distal vibratory and proprioceptive sensation and more advanced deficits include loss of light touch and pinprick sensation. Cauda equina compression alone produces a lower motor neuron pattern characterized by hypotonia, areflexia, muscle atrophy, and fasciculations.

Diagnosis   Over 85 percent of cord compressions due to solid tumors will have an abnormal spine radiograph (Fig. 2.1). The most common findings are vertebral body erosion and collapse, subluxation, and pedicle erosion. If the cord compression is via the intervertebral foramina there may not be an abnormal spine radiograph or bone scan.

Magnetic resonance imaging (MRI) is the best diagnostic tool for cord compression. It is non-invasive and provides anatomic resolution of the vertebrae and surrounding structures. The entire spine should be imaged because of the high incidence of asymptomatic multilevel disease (20–49 percent). A definitive diagnosis requires a T2-weighted MRI that shows a mass impinging on the thecal sac (Fig. 2.2).

A CT-Myelogram will be necessary as an alternative to MRI when patients are unable to undergo MRI (because of aneurysm clips, cardiac pacemakers, ferromagnetic implants, severe scoliosis, or severe claustrophobia).

Treatment   The goal of treatment is palliative and directed at maintaining ambulation, decreasing tumor bulk, and relieving pain. The initial pain may be severe and patients may require parenteral narcotic analgesics for adequate control.

Corticosteroids should be administered promptly to patients in whom there is a high clinical suspicion of ECC. Corticosteroids have substantial pain-relieving qualities in addition to their oncolytic, anti-inflammatory, and anti-edema effects. The dosage of dexamethasone is controversial. Dexamethasone 10 mg bolus with 16 mg/day is appropriate if the patient is neurologically stable; doses as high as 100 mg bolus with 96 mg/day are used if there is progressive loss of function. An intermediate dose may be as equally effective with fewer side effects, but no well-randomized clinical trials exist to support this.

Within 24 hours of the initiation of steroid treatment radiation therapy should be initiated. Only symptomatic regions or asymptomatic sites with significant epidural disease are treated. The standard treatment is 3000 cGy over 10 fractions with a margin of two vertebral bodies above and below the site.

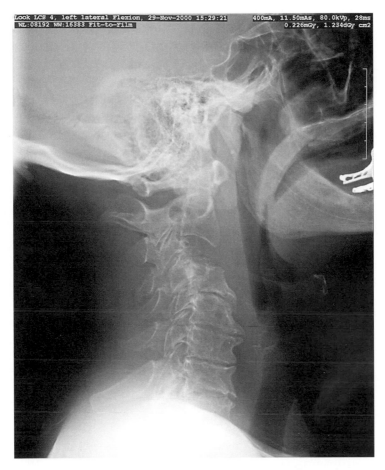

Fig. 2.1 A sixty-five-year-old man with non-small cell lung cancer. Plain radiograph of C-spine reveals complete obliteration of C3 vertebrae from metastasis.

Vertebral body resection followed by stabilization or decompressive laminectomy are surgical options for cord compression. Surgery is limited to patients with no prior history of cancer, patients with progressive neurologic decline during or after radiation therapy, or with spinal instability or bone fragments contributing to pain or neurologic findings. Aggressive resection carries significant morbidity and mortality. The mortality ranges from 6 to 10 percent.

2.2.2 Increased intracranial pressure

Increased intracranial pressure and its disastrous effect of cerebral herniation can be a result of one or a combination of several intracranial oncologic-related complications. They include brain metastases, intracranial hemorrhage, cerebral infarction, and a variety of other less common intracranial processes (venous sinus thrombosis, meningitis, head trauma, and abscess).

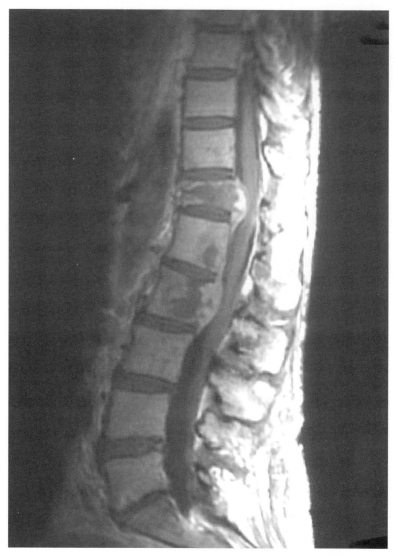

(A)

Fig. 2.2 Metastatic colon carcinoma to the lumbar and thoracic spine. Sagittal T1-weighted before (A) and after (B) intravenous administration of contrast. On the pre-contrast scan abnormal low signal intensity lesions are identified in the body of T12, L1, and L2 vertebrae. A pathological fracture is noted at T12. On the post-contrast scan heterogeneous enhancement is noted in the involved vertebrae. In addition, abnormal enhancement is noted in soft tissue masses at T12 and L2 that compromise the spinal canal at these two levels. These masses represent extension of the tumor into the epidural space. On the T2-weighted scan (C) the abnormal lesions demonstrate abnormal increase signal intensity. There is good delineation of the epidural tumors which at T12 displace the conus of the cord posteriorly.

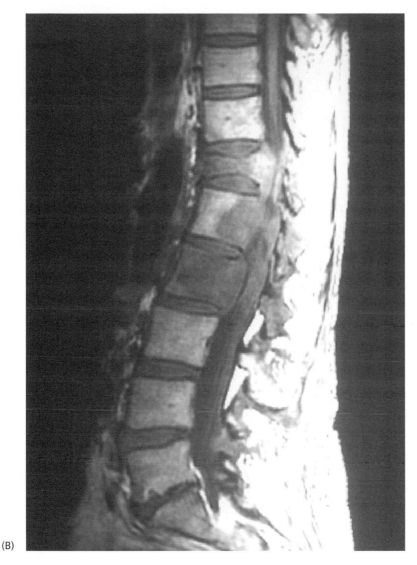

(B)

Fig 2.2 (continued)

Metastases to the brain are the most common intracranial tumors in adults and are ten times more common than primary brain tumors. Brain metastases occur in 20–40 percent of adult cancer patients. These lesions can appear at any time in the course of a cancer, however, they usually present in the setting of a known cancer within 6 months to 2 years after the diagnosis. The cancers most likely to metastasize to the brain are lung, breast, and melanoma (Table 2.5). Secondary brain lesions mainly result from hematogenous spread and are most commonly seen at the junction of the gray and white matter where the caliber of the blood vessels change. They can affect any

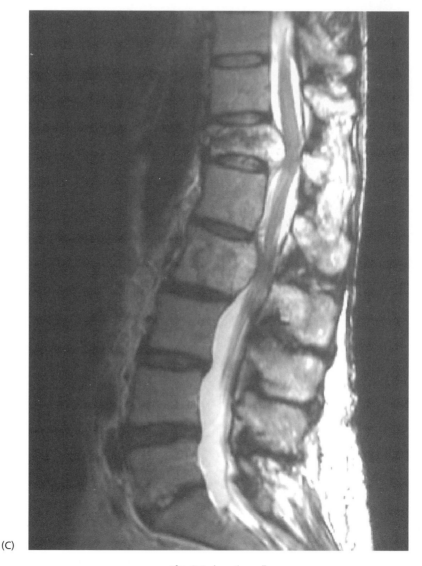

(C)

Fig. 2.2 (continued)

part of the brain. The cerebrum is the most frequently affected (80 percent), the cerebellum is affected in 15 percent, and the brainstem is affected in 5 percent. Brain metastases disrupt the function of adjacent neural tissue by direct displacement of brain structures, edema, irritation of the overlying gray matter, and compression of the vasculature.

Cancer patients may suffer from either hemorrhagic cerebrovascular or ischemic events. Intracerebral hemorrhage in patients with cancer is most commonly due to hemorrhage into a metastatic tumor, followed by thrombocytopenia and leukostasis. Lung cancer is the most common cause of a hemorrhagic brain metastasis. Other tumors have a greater propensity to bleed than lung cancer but occur less commonly such as melanoma,

Table 2.5 Primary sites of metastatic brain tumors (from Newton 1999)

Tumor type	Frequency (%)
Lung	50–60
Breast	15–20
Melanoma	5–10
Gastrointestinal	4–6
Genitourinary	3–5
Other	3–5
Unknown	4–8

Table 2.6 Signs and symptoms of brain metastases at presentation (from DeAngelis and Posner)

Signs and symptoms	Percentage of patients (%)
Headache	24
Hemiparesis	20
Cognitive disturbances	14
Seizures	12
Ataxia	7
Other	16
No symptoms	7

germ cell tumor, choriocarcinoma, and renal cell carcinoma (Table 2.5). Cerebral hemorrhage from coagulopathies occurs more commonly in patients with hematologic malignancies than in patients with solid tumors. Platelet transfusion is recommended when platelet counts fall below 10 000 per μl because the risk for spontaneous intracerebral hemorrhage is high. Disseminated intravascular coagulation, liver dysfunction, and cancer therapy (which will be discussed later) are other processes that increase the risk for intracerebral hemorrhage.

Patients with cancer are at increased risk for cerebral infarction for several reasons including (a) accelerated atherosclerosis takes place decades following head and neck radiation therapy which included cervical or cerebral vessels in the field; (b) higher tendency for disseminated intravascular coagulation, septic cerebral infarction, compression of vascular structures by a metastasis, and non-bacterial thrombotic endocarditis.

Clinical presentation Patients with increased intracranial pressure present with headache, altered mental status, and focal weakness (Table 2.6). The headaches due to brain metastases are usually generalized, occur during sleep and progressively become more severe over weeks. If hemorrhage occurs in a brain metastasis, symptom onset is sudden with severe headache or seizures. Focal neurologic signs, such as aphasia, hemiplegia, hemisensory loss, and visual abnormalities can follow within minutes.

An exam should focus on signs of brain herniation. They include impairment of consciousness, papilledema, pupillary abnormalities, eye movement abnormalities, posturing, nausea, vomiting, and stiff neck. Late signs include hypertension, bradycardia, and the Cushing reflex.

Diagnosis A computed tomography scan without contrast can quickly visualize acute hemorrhage, edema due to a mass, mass effect, or hydrocephalus (Fig. 2.3). An MRI is superior to CT at imaging anatomic detail of the intracranial process. The differential diagnosis of a brain lesion besides metastatic tumor includes primary brain tumor, abscess, infarct, and hemorrhage (Fig. 2.4). Metastatic tumors are usually rounded, well-circumscribed, non-infiltrative masses surrounded by a large amount of edema.

Treatment Therapy to lower intracranial pressure (ICP) must begin immediately to prevent herniation if there is clinical evidence of raised ICP. The basic treatment for increased intracranial pressure is the same regardless of the underlying etiology. Once the emergent elevated ICP is lowered, more definitive treatment directed towards the underlying cause can be given.

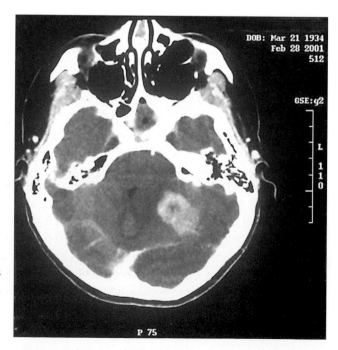

Fig. 2.3 Sixty-seven-year-old woman with breast cancer with new headaches and unsteady gait. CT of head reveals contrast enhancing mass lesion with edema and mass effect.

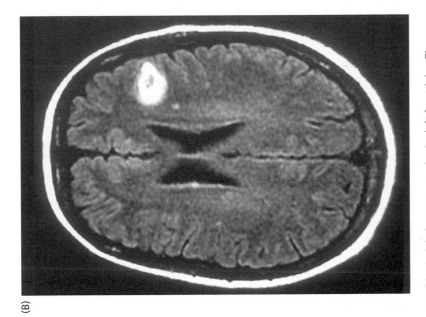

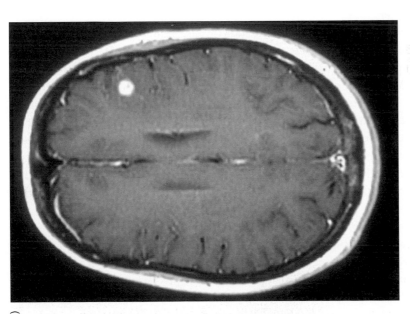

Fig.2.4 Metastatic melanoma to brain. Axial post-contrast T1-weighted MRI scan of brain (A) shows a mass in the left front lobe. The mass, with disrupted blood–brain barrier, demonstrated abnormal enhancement and its borders are well outlined. On (B) an MRI scan with FLAIR technique shows the same mass with a zone of edema in the surrounding brain parenchyma. The edema is hyperintense with respect to normal brain. The tumor margins are obscured by the edema.

Hyperventilation is the most rapid method to decrease ICP. The patient must be intubated and ventilated to a pCO_2 between 25 and 30 mm Hg. A decrease in pCO_2 will cause vasoconstriction, decreasing cerebral blood volume and thus ICP. The effects of hyperventilation will only last a few hours before the kidney's compensation brings the body back to equilibrium.

Mannitol is a hyperosmotic used to lower the ICP. Mannitol works by creating an osmotic gradient between the blood and brain causing water from the brain to follow the gradient into the blood. The effect is seen within minutes and lasts for several hours. 20–25 percent solution of mannitol is given at a dose of 0.5–2.0 g/kg intravenously over 20–30 minutes. Repeated doses may be required.

Dexamethasone is helpful in lowering ICP by decreasing the amount of intracranial vascular edema. Its onset of action is within hours and persists for several days. The doses of dexamethasone are institution-dependent—no definitive data on what dose to be used in a situation. The most common recommended doses are an initial bolus of 10 mg with a maintenance dose of 4 mg every 6 hours. Higher doses are recommended by some authors. This includes loading doses of up to a 100 mg followed by a maintenance dose of 40–100 mg/day dose. These larger doses are typically used in patients with rapidly progressive neurologic symptoms; in this case dexamethasone would need to be tapered over the course of radiation therapy. Steroids are most useful when raised ICP is due to brain metastases or abscess. If the elevated ICP is unrelated to the metastatic brain disease, steroids are not effective and should not be used in intracerebral hemorrhage except in patients with increased ICP from an hemorrhagic metastatic tumor.

Anticonvulsant drugs such as phenytoin or carbamazepine are required in patients with seizures. There are no data to support their prophylactic benefit.

If there is continued neurologic deterioration despite maximal medical treatment, neurosurgical intervention may be necessary. The interventions include evacuation of a hematoma or abscess, resection of a metastasis, or ventriculostomy.

All the medical interventions are temporary until definitive treatment can begin. Two randomized prospective studies have shown that surgery plus whole-brain irradiation is the treatment of choice for patients with surgically accessible single brain metastases. Both the studies showed a dramatic difference in long-term survival in those patients treated with surgery plus radiation versus those that received radiation alone.

Patients with multiple brain metastases or patients that are not candidates for surgery should receive whole-brain irradiation. The most common regimen is 3000 cGy of radiation delivered in ten treatments over a period of 2 weeks. Stereotactic radiosurgery is another form of radiation therapy that allows for more precise focusing of the radiation beam which limits damage to adjacent brain tissue. Cranial radiation can acutely cause an increase in edema and should be started in conjunction with other treatments of uncontrolled elevation of ICP.

A concern in those patients with acute intra-cerebral hemorrhage is management of severe hypertension. It is recommended that mean arterial pressure greater than 125–135 mm Hg be treated. The ideal antihypertensive agent should be short-acting, easily titrated, and likely to avoid cerebral vasodilation with its associated increase in ICP (e.g. labetalol or nitroprusside). Correction of coagulation abnormalities is an essential treatment of ICH. Platelet transfusions should be given until counts are greater than 50,000 per μl, elevation of prothrombin time (PT) should be normalized with vitamin K and fresh-frozen plasma.

2.2.3 Leptomeningeal metastases

Leptomeningeal metastases are the spread of cancer cell into the cerebrospinal fluid (CSF) of the subarachnoid space bathing the brain, spinal cord, and spinal nerve roots. They occur in about 5 percent of cancer patients. Leptomeningeal metastases occur most commonly in cancers of the breast, lung, melanoma, acute lymphocytic leukemia, and lymphoma (Table 2.7).

Clinical presentation   Leptomeningeal metastases should always be suspected in a cancer patient with neurologic signs and symptoms indicating dysfunction in more than one anatomic site within the nervous system. Patients with leptomeningeal metastases usually present with signs and symptoms due to several mechanisms. One mechanism is local injury to the brain, spinal cord, spinal roots, and cranial nerves travelling through the spinal fluid causing cranial nerve palsies, weakness, paresthesia, pain, and encephalopathy. Another is interruption of blood supply to neural tissue causing infarction and focal signs findings or seizures. A third mechanism is obstruction of normal CSF flow pathways leading to hydrocephalus and increased intracranial pressure. Finally, leptomeningeal metastases can interfere with normal neural metabolism causing encephalopathy.

Table 2.7 Frequency of leptomeningeal metastases in different tumor types (adapted from DeAngelis and Posner)

Cancer	Percent developing leptomeningeal metastases (%)
SCLC	9–25
Melanoma	23
ALL	11
NHL	4–10
Breast	5
AML	<5

"Numb Chin Syndrome" is a classical symptom that should raise high suspicion of leptomeningeal metastases in patients with cancer. It is more common with leukemias and lymphomas; however it may be a presenting symptom in breast cancer.

The signs and symptoms of leptomeningeal spread can indicate spinal, cranial nerve and brain involvement (Table 2.8). The spine is affected in 75 percent of patients with leptomeningeal metastases. Signs and symptoms due to spine involvement include neck or back pain, asymmetric reflexes, and extremity weakness. The pain is prominent and can present as neck stiffness. Weakness is also common and is usually bilateral with a lower motor neuron pattern. Cranial nerve palsies occur in more than 50 percent of the patients. Common symptoms of cranial nerve palsies include diplopia, visual loss, dysphagia, hearing loss and facial numbness. Finally, the brain is involved in half of the patients with leptomeningeal metastases. Common symptoms include headache, cognitive changes, gait abnormalities, seizures, and nausea and vomiting.

Diagnosis

The diagnosis is made by lumbar puncture. An MRI of the brain should be obtained prior to the lumbar puncture to rule out increased intracranial pressure. At least 4 cc of CSF should be collected and taken to the laboratory immediately to minimize the time for autolysis of malignant cells. CSF cytologic studies are positive in 45–50 percent of patients after one lumbar puncture and in more than 90 percent after three lumbar punctures. Therefore, three samples should be taken because 10 percent of patients with leptomeningeal involvement have persistently negative cytologic examinations of their CSF. The CSF protein is usually elevated, there is a pleocytosis, and the glucose concentration is low.

Table 2.8 Signs and symptoms of leptomeningeal metastases (from Newton, 1999)

Signs and symptoms	Percentage of patients (%)
Reflex asymmetry	60–70
Weakness	45–70
Mental status changes	40–60
Cranial nerve palsy	40–50
Headache	30–45
Spinal/radicular pain	20–40
Sensory deficits	20–35
Gait difficulties	15–30
Nausea/vomiting	10–30
Cerebellar signs	15–25
Bowel/bladder dysfunction	15–20
Seizures	16

Contrast-enhanced MRI of the brain and spine reveals the presence of meningeal tumor in only 30–50 percent of patients where one exists. Communicating hydrocephalus can also be a sign of leptomeningeal metastases, because meningeal tumor often impairs CSF pathways. Radiologic studies may reveal hydrocephalus without a mass lesion, or diffuse contrast enhancement of the meninges.

Treatment   Treatment must include the entire neuroaxis and is a combination of radiation therapy and intrathecal chemotherapy. Radiation therapy can be directed to bulky and symptomatic sites or to the entire neuraxis. Intrathecal therapy via an Omaya reservoir or repeated lumbar punctures with methotrexate (10–15 mg twice weekly or 2 mg daily for 5 days every other week), cytarabine (25–100 mg two or three times weekly), or thiotepa (10 mg two or three times weekly) increases the median survival to 3–6 months. Without treatment, the median survival is 4–6 weeks with death due to progressive neurologic dysfunction.

2.3 Therapy-related neurologic complications

2.3.1 Radiotherapy

Cranial radiation

Acute complications   Acute encephalopathy although rare, can occur within two weeks of the onset of irradiation. The elderly patients with large or multifocal tumors, or those who receive large doses per fraction are at higher risk of developing this complication.

The patient typically presents with headache, nausea, drowsiness, fever, and worsening of neurologic signs. The mechanism is thought to be a radiation-induced breakdown of the blood–brain barrier resulting in cerebral edema, which causes increased intracranial pressure. If new symptoms or worsening of pre-existing symptoms occur during cranial radiation, corticosteroids should be started promptly. Corticosteroids (dexamethasone 10–16 mg bolus with 16 mg maintenance per day) are the mainstay for the treatment of acute complications of radiotherapy. Rarely, high-risk patients such as those with severe mass effect and increased intracranial pressure can develop brain herniation during radiotherapy. Therefore, these patients should be pretreated with high dose steroids before beginning irradiation to reduce the risk of brain herniation.

Early complications   Early-delayed complications occur between 2 weeks and 3–4 months after the completion of radiotherapy. The mechanism of these complications is thought to be temporary demyelination from radiation injury to oligodendroglia. The complications include the somnolence syndrome, symptoms simulating local recurrence, and brain stem encephalopathy.

Patients can present with somnolence syndrome, particularly those that have received whole-brain irradiation. Patients usually complain of hypersomnia, drowsiness, irritability, and sometimes headache and fever. There can also be attention deficits and alteration of recent memory function. Improvement occurs over weeks to months and steroids can reduce the duration of somnolence syndrome.

Sometimes an early-delayed complication is confused with recurrence of the lesion being radiated. About 15 percent of patients present with focal symptoms and have imaging with CT or MRI which suggest tumor recurrence with an increase in the size of the low-density lesion. Clinical suspicion and resolution of symptoms may be the only clues. Improvement occurs spontaneously and steroids may accelerate its resolution.

A very rare complication, which may also result from cranial irradiation is brain stem encephalopathy of the posterior fossa. Most of these patients recover spontaneously, but some may develop stupor, coma, and death.

Delayed complications   The two main delayed complications of brain irradiation are radiation necrosis and cognitive dysfunction. They can occur from 4 months to 15 years after radiotherapy. The likelihood of delayed damage to the brain depends on the dose per fraction, the total dose delivered, the total volume of the brain irradiated, the presence of other systemic diseases that enhance the side effects of irradiation (e.g. diabetes, hypertension), concomitant chemotherapy, and the patient's age.

Radiation necrosis usually begins one to two years after the completion of radiotherapy. Although focal necrosis following radiosurgery can occur earlier than one year post-treatment, patients typically present with focal neurologic signs mimicking a new tumor. Brain imaging with CT or MRI can show increased hypodensity affecting predominantly the white matter. Hence, it may be difficult to differentiate necrosis from recurrent tumor. PET can help but the only way to confirm the diagnosis is with biopsy. Resection of the area of necrosis yields the best results. Most patients transiently respond to steroids but durable responses are rare.

Cognitive dysfunction and leukoencephalopathy without necrosis is the most frequent complication of long-term survivors. It is also known as 'diffuse radiation injury.' Patients present with subtle neuropsychological impairment to severe dementia. The symptoms generally occur within 4 years of irradiation and are mainly characterized by attention deficits, memory dysfunction, and immediate problem solving ability. At late stages patients can develop severe intellectual loss, emotional lability and apathy, and gait disturbances. Characteristic MRI changes are seen as bilateral increases in T2 signal throughout the white matter. Radiation-induced dementia is a diagnosis of exclusion. The clinical course is progressive deterioration (80 percent of cases), occasional cases of stabilization and rarely improvement. There is no effective therapy for this condition.

The three important factors which affect the risk of developing cognitive dysfunction/dementia are (a) the extent and dose of radiation; at safe doses and focal therapy, the risk is low; (b) concurrent chemotherapy; and (c) age—older patients and children are more sensitive to the diffuse neurotoxicity of radiotherapy.

Other rare long-term complications of radiation therapy include (a) secondary tumors, such as meningiomas, sarcomas, gliomas, and malignant schwannomas which can appear years after treatment; (b) cerebrovascular events—stenosis and occlusion of large vessels in the brain may appear years after treatment with radiation and present as transient ischemic attacks or strokes; and (c) endocrinopathies. These are usually due to hypothalamic dysfunction and occasionally from direct damage to the glands themselves.

Spinal cord radiation

Complications involving the spinal cord after radiation therapy are uncommon and usually subacute. Lhermitte's sign, transient electric shock-like sensations with neck flexion, can occur 2–4 months after radiation treatment to the cervical cord and usually resolves over 3–6 months.

The more severe form of spinal cord complication is delayed progressive myelopathy. It can occur months to years after radiation therapy and its incidence is affected by the total radiation dose and dose per fraction. This is an irreversible condition, which begins as a Brown–Séquard syndrome and progresses over weeks to months to paraparesis or quadriparesis. MRI may show spinal cord swelling, hypersignal within the cord, and contrast enhancement. There is no effective treatment for this condition.

A less common form of myelopathy is motor-neuronal syndrome, which is due to injury to the anterior horn cells after pelvic irradiation. Months to years after irradiation, patients can develop a subacute flaccid, asymmetrical paraparesis that affects both distal and proximal muscles, with accompanying atrophy, fasciculations, and areflexia. There are no sensory deficits or sphincter dysfunction. The myelogram and MRI are normal. The deficit usually stabilizes after a few months.

Peripheral nerve irradiation

An early-delayed injury of brachial plexus can result from irradiation for the treatment of breast carcinoma. Patients present with paresthesias in the hand and forearm, sometimes associated with pain and accompanied by weakness and atrophy in C6-T1 distribution. Most patients recover within a few weeks.

A late-delayed radiation plexopathy can occur after irradiation of either the brachial or lumbosacral plexus. This disorder usually occurs a year or more after radiation therapy with doses of 60 Gy or more. Brachial plexopathy is characterized by paresthesias, loss of sensation and weakness of muscles in the upper or lower plexus. There is usually accompanying lymphedema and palpable induration in the supraclavicular fossa. The important differential diagnosis is between radiation damage versus recurrent tumor. Severe pain usually indicates tumor rather than radiation fibrosis. The clinical course can vary from stabilization after months to years of slow deterioration to some cases progressing rapidly to rendering the arm useless. Lumbosacral plexopathy causes a slowly progressive weakness of one or both legs without pain.

2.3.2 **Chemotherapy**

Many chemotherapeutic agents cause neurotoxicity (Table 2.9). The particular agent, the route administered (intravenous or intrathecal), and the dose level (low dose or high) are all important factors in predicting the risk of neurotoxicity.

Table 2.9 Neurotoxicity of chemotherapy

Chemotherapeutic agent	Clinical complication
Asparaginase	Sagittal sinus thrombosis
Cisplatin	Peripheral neuropathy-painful numbness and tingling in the extremities, loss of DTRs, loss of propioception Ototoxicity Cranial nerve neuropathies Lhermitte's sign Encephalopathy
Cytosine arabinoside	Aseptic meningitis—after IT injection Pancereballar dysfunction at high doses Guillain–Barré-like syndrome at high doses Encephalopathy High doses (40mg/m^2/day)—severe encephalopathy, cortical blindness, dementia, and coma
5-Fluorouracil	Pancerebellar syndrome at high doses Encephalopathy Optic neuropathy
Ifosfamide	Encephalopathy with somnolence
Methotrexate	Aseptic meningitis—2–4 hours after IT injection Transverse myelopathy 30 min–48 hours after IT injection Stroke-like syndrome
Nitrosoureas	Necrotizing encephalopathy at high doses of BCNU or infusion into carotid artery
Paclitaxel and Docetaxel	Peripheral neuropathy
Procarbazine	Encepatholopathy
Thiotepa	Encephalopathy at high doses—somnolence, seizures, coma
Vincristine	Peripheral neuropathy—paresthesias in the fingertips and feet, motor weakness including foot drop Cranial nerves Autonomic dysfunction

Intrathecal therapy (IT)

Methotrexate   Acute aseptic meningitis occurs in 10 percent of patients receiving intrathecal methotrexate. Patients usually present with meningismus, confusion, fever, lethargy, headache, nausea, vomiting and pleocytosis. This entity usually occurs within 4–6 hours after intrathecal injection and resolves over several days. Dexamethasone can relieve some of the symptoms.

A rare complication of intrathecal methotrexate is transverse myelopathy. With this condition, patients present with rapidly developing sensory changes, paraplegia, and bladder dysfunction. The symptoms usually begin 30 min to 48 hours after intrathecal therapy (IT) treatment. The mechanism is thought to be an idiosyncratic reaction to the drug.

Patients who have received high cumulative dose of IT can also develop a chronic encephalopathy. These patients usually present with cognitive impairment, dementia, spasticity, and seizures.

Cytarabine (Ara-C)   Acute aseptic meningitis can occur after intrathecal treatment with Ara-C presenting similarly to those patients treated with methotrexate. In rare cases intrathecal methotrexate can also cause a myelopathy.

Thiotepa   Intrathecal thiotepa can induce a severe radiculomyelopathy.

High dose chemotherapy

High dose Ara-C (3 g/m^2 every 12 hours for six doses) causes neurotoxicity in 10–25 percent of patients. Most commonly patients present with pancerebellar dysfunction. The syndrome usually begins several days after the initiation of therapy and lasts for several days. Patients usually begin to recover after about 14 days and recovery may be incomplete in about 20 percent of patients. This syndrome is thought to be due to the loss of cerebellar Purkinje's cells and neurons in the deep cerebellar layers. High dose cytosine arabinoside has also been reported to produce a peripheral neuropathy mimicking the Guillain–Barré syndrome. Discontinuation of the drug usually allows for recovery.

Methotrexate   High dose methotrexate can cause an early-delayed neurologic reaction in about 4 percent of patients. The disorder usually occurs 7–10 days after the third or fourth treatment and is characterized by stupor or coma, and often associated with multifocal neurologic signs that change hour to hour. Most patients recover completely and do not usually have a recurrence even if methotrexate is re-instituted.

5-fluorouracil   High dose 5-fluorouracil has also been associated with pancerebellar dysfunction that begins during or following therapy and gradually resolves over several weeks.

Fludarabine   Doses greater than 40 mg/m^2 per day can cause a severe encephalopathy causing cortical blindness, dementia and sometimes coma. Magnetic resonance imaging and pathologic examination show a necrotizing leukoencephalopathy, most severe in the occipital lobes.

Nitrosoureas   High doses in patients with primary central nervous system tumors can cause ocular toxicity and encephalopathy. After intracarotid treatment, patients present with seizures and slowly progressive neurologic dysfunction.

Etoposide   High dose etoposide has also rarely been associated with acute encephalopathy.

Standard dose chemotherapy

Acute encephalopathy   Cisplatin, vincristine, asparaginase, procarbazine, 5-FU, cytosine arabinoside, ifosfamide/mesna, tamoxifen have all been associated with acute encephalopathy. Patients typically present with insomnia, rapidly followed by confusion with either stupor or agitation. Generalized seizures and myoclonus can also occur.

Stroke-like episodes   These usually occur after treatment with high dose methotrexate and rarely with cisplatin. The clinical presentation is one of acute encephalopathy with fluctuating motor deficit that resolves spontaneously.

Chronic encephalopathy   Methotrexate, BCNU, Ara-C, fludarabine, agents that can cause chronic encephalopathy. A subcortical dementia characterized by apathy, intellectual and memory loss, frontal syndrome, sleep disorders, incontinence and gait disorders. It usually develops months to years after treatment. Progressive deterioration is typical.

Neuropathy   An acute or subacute Guillain–Barré-like syndrome can be seen after suramin (similar to that of high dose Ara-C). This neuropathy is slowly reversible after drug discontinuation. A sensorimotor axonal neuropathy is characterized by distal paresthesias, loss of deep tendon reflexes, followed by distal extremity weakness. Vincristine is the classic culprit. Discontinuation of the drug usually allows for recovery. A purely sensory neuropathy following cisplatin or taxanes is a classic complication. After cisplatin associated neuropathy, patients are characterized by loss of position sense and ataxia, whereas taxane neuropathy affects pinprick and tactile sensation. Recovery is delayed and slow. Finally autonomic dysfunction characterized by constipation, orthostatic hypotension, and urinary retention can be seen after treatment with vincristine.

2.4 Ophthalmic complications and cancer

Patients with cancer may experience loss of vision by the direct effects of tumor infiltration of the anterior visual pathways. It can also occur by indirect effects of cancer such as opportunistic infections, cerebrovascular thromboembolic disorders, nutritional and metabolic complications, side effects of treatment and finally as a paraneoplastic syndrome.

2.4.1 Optic nerve involvement

This condition is seen more in hematologic malignancies than in solid tumors. Non-Hodgkin's lymphoma presents with infiltration of the optic nerve in 0.5 percent of patients sometime during the course of their disease. In most of these cases the infiltration occurs from spread of a CNS tumor. Children with acute leukemia will have evidence of optic nerve infiltration in 4 percent of the cases. The condition is less common in solid tumors; the most common solid tumors to spread to the optic nerve are adeno-carcinomas, breast and lung in women and lung and bowel in men. Other tumors that can metastasize to the optic nerve include cancer of the stomach, pancreas, uterus, ovary, prostate, kidney, and tonsillar fossa. Tumors can metastasize to the optic nerve by hematogenous dissemination, invasion from the orbit, from the choroid, and from the CNS. The nerve is affected more than the sheath alone. Contiguous spread of primary tumors from the paranasal sinuses, brain, and adjacent intraocular structures are much less common. Because the optic nerve is anatomically close to the paranasal sinuses, it can be infiltrated by cancer that arises in the sinuses or the nasopharynx.

Patients with carcinomatosis meningitis will have optic nerve involvement in 15–40 percent. Visual loss may occur at the same time as other signs of meningitis or as the first sign of the disease. Usually both eyes are affected. The optic neuropathy that occurs in the setting of meningeal carcinomatosis is usually a diagnostic quartet of (a) headaches, (b) blindness, (c) sluggish papillary reflexes and (d) normal optic discs.

Clinical presentation   Patients typically present with evidence of optic neuropathy. The visual loss is severe and any type of field defect may be present. A relative afferent papillary defect is usually present unless the patient has bilateral optic nerve metastases or the opposite nerve has been damaged by some other condition.

Diagnosis   Any person with known cancer with or without other evidence of metas-tases, who develops optic neuropathy should be suspected of having cancer involve-ment of the optic nerve until proven otherwise. CT scanning will show an enhancing nerve and on MRI, the nerve is usually enlarged. In patients with leukemia, optic disc swelling can also be due to increased ICP by CNS involvement of the tumor.

Treatment   Most metastatic tumors to the optic nerve will have at least a temporary response to radiation therapy. It is particularly rapid and dramatic in patients with leukemic infiltration of the optic nerve. In most of these patients visual function returns to normal.

2.4.2 **Other rare conditions**

Secondary carcinomas   Metastasis of cancer to the eye and orbit usually occurs by hematogenous dissemination because there are no intraocular lymphatic channels. Tumor is carried there via the internal carotid artery to the ophthalmic artery to the ocu-lar region. The uvea is the most common location of ocular metastases presumably because of its extensive vascularity and slow blood flow. The posterior choroid is the most common location of intraocular metastasis. In women breast cancer is the most com-mon primary malignancy metastatic to the eye accounting for 62–77 percent of patients. In men, lung cancer is the most common primary that metastatizes to the eye accounting for 26–49 percent of cases. Most patients present with blurring of vision to frank blind-ness. The treatment is palliative and usually consists of external beam irradiation.

Cancer-associated retinopathy This condition is characterized by progressive photoreceptor degeneration with subsequent visual deterioration. This is thought to be a non-metastatic effect of the primary tumor as a result of a tumor cell product that is directly toxic to the retina or a tumor antigen that stimulates an autoimmune response within certain retinal cells.

Acknowledgement

The authors would like to thank Drs. Brian Fuller and Mazen Al-Hakim for a critical review of this chapter and Dr. Nicolas Patronas for providing some of the radiographs.

Suggested reading

Byrne, T.N. (1992) Spinal cord compression from epidural metastases. *N Engl J Med*, **327**, 614–19.

Chamberlain, M.C. (1998) Leptomeningeal metastases: a review of evaluation and treatment. *J Neurooncol*, **37**, 271–84.

DeAngelis, L.M. and Posner, J.B. (2000) Neurologic complications. In *Cancer medicine*, 5th edn (ed. J.F. Holland, E. Frei, R.C. Bast, *et al.*) B.C. Decker, Hamilton, Ontario.

Eliassi-Rad, B., Daniel, M.A., and Green, W.R. (1996) Frequency of ocular metastases in patients dying of cancer in eye bank populations. *Br J Ophthalmol*, **80**, 125–8.

Fuller, B.G., Heiss, J.D., and Oldfield, E.H. (2001) Spinal cord compression. In *Cancer: principles and practice of oncology*, 6th edn (ed. Devita, Hellman, and Rosenberg) Lippincott Williams & Wilkins.

Glantz, M.J., Cole, B.F., Friedberg, M.H., *et al.* (1996) A randomized, blinded, placebo-controlled trial of divalpex sodium prophylxis in adults with newly diagnosed brain tumors. *Neurology*, **46**, 985–91.

Jacobson, D.M. (1996) Paraneoplastic disorders of neuro-ophthalmologic interest. *Curr Opin Ophthalmol*, **7**, 30–8.

Keime-Guibert, F., Napoliano, M., and Delattre, J. (1998) Neurological complications of radiotherapy and chemotherapy. *J Neurol*, **245**, 695–708.

Loblaw, D.A. and Laperriere, N.J. (1998) Emergency treatment of malignant extradural spinal cord compression: an evidence based guideline. *J Clin Oncol*, **16**, 1613–24.

Miller, N.R. and Newman, N.J. (1999) Compressive and infiltrative optic neuropathies. In *The essentials: Walsh & Hoyt's Clinical-Neuro-Ophthalmology*, 5th edn (ed. N.R. Miller, N.J. Newman) Williams & Wilkins, Baltimore, MD.

Mintz, A.H., Kestle, J., Rathbone, M.P., *et al.* (1996) A randomized trial to assess the efficacy of surgery in addition to radiotherapy in patients with a single cerebral metastasis. *Cancer*, **78**, 1470–6.

Newton, H.B. (1999) Neurologic complications of systemic cancer. *Am Fam Physician*, **59**(4), 878–86.

Patchell, R.A. (1996) The treatment of brain metastases. *Cancer Invest*, **14**, 169–77.

Patchell, R.A., Tibbs, P.A., and Walsh, J.W. (1990) A randomized trial of surgery in the treatment of single metastases to the brain. *N Engl J Med*, **322**, 494–500.

Posner, J.B. (1995) *Neurologic complications of cancer*, (1st edn) F. A. Davis, Philadelphia.

Quinn, J.A. and DeAngelis, L.M. (2000) Neurologic emergencies in cancer patient. *Semin Oncol*, 27(3), 3111–21.

Rees, J. (2000) Neurologic manifestations of malignant disease. *Hosp Med*, 61(5), 319–25.

Schiff, D., Batchelor, T., and Wen, P.Y. (1998) Neurologic emergencies in cancer patients. *Neurol Clin*, 16, 449–83.

Shust, M.A. (1994) Oncologic disease. In *Ocular manifestations of systemic disease*, 1st edn (ed. B.H. Blaustein) Churchill Livingstone, New York, NY.

Vecht, C.J., Haaxma-Reiche, H., Noordijk, E.M., *et al.* (1993) Treatment of single brain metastasis: radiotherapy alone or combined with neurosurgery? *Ann Neurol*, 33, 583–90.

Chapter 3

Metabolic Emergencies

Mohamed Hussein and Kevin Cullen

3.1 Hypercalcemia

Hypercalcemia associated with malignancy is the most common cause of hypercalcemia seen in hospitalized patients and one of the most common metabolic complications of malignancies. Twenty to forty percent of all patients with cancer will develop hypercalcemia in the course of disease. The likelihood of hypercalcemia in patients with malignant disease is influenced by the duration of the disease, site of malignancy and the presence or absence of metastases. It varies among different types of tumors. Among solid tumors, breast cancer, lung and head and neck are the most often complicated by hypercalcemia. Among hematologic disorders multiple myeloma and lymphoma are the most often associated with hypercalcemia. Tumor-induced hypercalcemia is associated with a poor prognosis irrespective of the response of serum calcium to treatment.

Hypercalcemia generally develops as a late complication of malignancy; its appearance has grave prognostic significance. Currently available hypocalcemic agents have little effect in decreasing the mortality rate among patients with hypercalcemia of malignancy. The patients with hypercalcemia who responded to specific antineoplastic treatment are found to have a slightly greater survival advantage over non-responders.

3.1.1 Pathophysiology

Normal calcium homeostasis is a balance of intestinal absorption of calcium, bone resorption and formation, and renal excretion of calcium. In the normal individual, bone resorption and formation are closely balanced, so that renal excretion of calcium is almost equal to intestinally absorbed calcium. Bone resorption is stimulated by parathyroid hormone (PTH) and inhibited by calcitonin. Intestinal calcium absorption occurs both actively and passively. Active absorption of calcium is saturable and regulated primarily by 1,25-dihydroxy-vitamin D_3 [1,25-$(OH)_2D_3$]. Other hormones, such as PTH and steroids, participate indirectly in regulation of the active intestinal absorption of calcium by modulating renal production of 1,25-$(OH)_2D_3$. Renal calcium reabsorption is increased by PTH.

The pathogenesis of hypercalcemia of malignancy comprises increased net bone resorption and enhanced renal tubular reabsorption of calcium. There are three major mechanisms involved in its pathogenesis:

First, humoral hypercalcemia of malignancy is the main etiology in patients without bone metastases and is mediated by PTH-related protein (PTH-RP) secreted by cancer cells. Parathyroid hormone-related protein hypercalcemic effects are due to its strong sequence homology with native PTH in the bioactive amino terminal region and its ability to interact with G-protein-linked 7-transmembrane PTH/PTH-RP receptor. High levels of PTH-RP are commonly found in patients with solid tumors, especially squamous carcinomas. Several studies have shown that patients with high levels of PTH-RP are resistant to treatment with bisphosphonates.

The second mechanism is the induction of local osteolysis by a variety of different mediators secreted by tumor cells and other cells at the site of metastasis. These mediators include PTH-RP, prostaglandins (especially E series), cytokines including transforming growth factors (TGF) and interleukins. Disregulated TGF secretion may be responsible for the mixed lytic and blastic appearance of skeletal metastases in osteotrophic cancers such as breast and prostate cancers while interleukin release is the main mechanism of hypercalcemia in multiple myeloma.

The third mechanism is increased production of serum $1,25\text{-}(OH)_2D_3$ level by alpha-vitamin D_3 hydroxylase. This mechanism may be most important in patients with Hodgkin's disease, non-Hodgkin's lymphoma, multiple myeloma and occasionally in other solid tumors. Hypercalcemia induced by this mechanism usually responds to corticosteroid therapy.

Although very rare, parathyroid carcinoma with markedly elevated PTH should be considered in patients presenting with very severe refractory hypercalcemia which could be life-threatening if the disease is not controlled.

Many factors may precipitate hypercalcemia in patients with malignancy. Immobility is associated with an increase in resorption of calcium from bone. In addition, anorexia, nausea, and vomiting exacerbate dehydration and reduce renal calcium excretion. Hormonal therapy (estrogens, anti-estrogens such as tamoxifen and androgens) and thiazide diuretics which increase renal calcium reabsorption may precipitate and exacerbate hypercalcemia.

3.1.2 **Clinical manifestations**

Hypercalcemia of malignancy presents with non-specific symptoms such as fatigue, anorexia, nausea, polyuria, polydipsia, weakness, constipation, lethargy, and confusion. As serum calcium level increases, the patient may develop central nervous system symptoms including psychotic behavior, seizures, and coma. Multiple myeloma patients with extensive bone destruction often present with bone pain and pathologic fractures.

Symptom severity correlates directly with the magnitude of serum-ionized calcium concentration. Clinical manifestations of hypercalcemia of malignancy are summarized in Table 3.1.

Table 3.1 Clinical manifestations of hypercalcemia of malignancy

Non-specific symptoms
Fatigue
Anorexia

Neurologic manifestations
Muscle weakness
Diminished deep tendon reflexes
Increased intracranial tension
Delirium with personality change
Cognitive dysfunction
Disorientation
Incoherent speech
Hallucinations and delusions
Obtundation
Coma

Cardiovascular manifestations
Prolonged P-R interval,
Widened QRS complex
Shortened Q-T interval.
S-T segments may be shortened or absent
Bradyarrhythmias
Bundle branch block
Incomplete or complete AV block
Asystole.

Gastrointestinal manifestations
Increased gastric acid secretion
Anorexia
Nausea and vomiting
Constipation

Renal manifestations
Polyuria
Decreased proximal reabsorption of sodium, magnesium, and potassium
Hypotension
Renal insufficiency

Bone manifestations
Fractures
Skeletal deformities
Bone pain

An accurate history and physical examination are the most helpful diagnostic tools to exclude correctable non-malignant causes of hypercalcemia. The presence of weight loss, fatigue, or muscle weakness should increase clinical suspicion of malignancy as the cause of hypercalcemia. Laboratory findings in patients with hypercalcemia of malignancy include extremely low or undetectable serum PTH, low or normal inorganic phosphorus; and low or normal 1,25-dihydroxy-vitamin D level. Use of additional tests to identify the underlying malignancy responsible for the hypercalcemia often depends on the history and physical findings.

3.1.3 Treatment

The treatment plan should aim to improve the mental status, renal function, and quality of life, allow effective antitumor therapy, shorten hospitalization, and prolong life (see Fig. 3.1). Treatment of hypercalcemia should include restoration of intravascular volume by saline infusion to correct dehydration and to increase urinary calcium excretion. Dietary restriction of calcium plays a minor role in those patients who have increased intestinal absorption. Calcium and vitamin D supplements should be discontinued, as should medication that interferes with urinary excretion of calcium such as thiazide diuretics. Specific measures including effective antitumor therapy should be started if available; however, most hypercalcemic patients require additional hypocalcemic agents until antitumor response is achieved.

Fluid replacement

Isotonic saline infusion is the most effective first step. Volume expansion and natiuresis increase renal blood flow and enhance calcium excretion secondary to the ionic exchange of calcium for sodium in the distal tubule. The volume required depends on the extent of hypovolemia, as well as the patient's cardiac and renal function. Although fewer than 30 percent of patients achieve normocalcemia with hydration alone, replenishing extracellular fluid (ECF), restoring intravascular volume, and saline diuresis are fundamental to initial therapy.

Diuretics

Thiazide diuretics increase renal tubular calcium absorption and may exacerbate hypercalcemia. Thus, thiazide diuretics are contraindicated in patients with hypercalcemia. Loop diuretics (e.g. frusemide, bumetanide, and ethacrynic acid) induce hypercalciuria by inhibiting calcium reabsorption in the ascending limb of the loop of Henle, but should not be administered until volume expansion is achieved as they can exacerbate fluid loss, further reducing calcium clearance. Sodium and calcium clearance are closely linked during osmotic diuresis, therefore loop diuretics will depress the proximal tubular resorptive mechanisms for calcium, increasing calcium excretion from 400 to 800 mg/day. Moderate doses of frusemide (20–40 mg every 12 hours) increase saline-induced urinary calcium excretion and are useful in preventing or managing fluid overload in adequately rehydrated patients. Aggressive treatment with frusemide (80–100 mg every 2–4 hours) is problematical because it requires concurrent administration of large volumes of saline to prevent intravascular dehydration. This in turn requires intensive hemodynamic monitoring to avoid volume overload and cardiac decompensation as well as frequent serial urinary volume and electrolytes measurements to prevent life-threatening hypophosphatemia, hypokalemia, and hypomagnesemia.

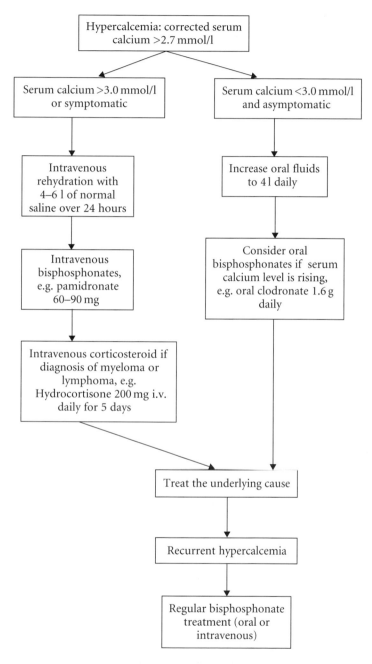

Fig. 3.1 Treatment of hypercalcemia.

Bisphosphonates

Bisphosphonates represent one of the most significant advances over the last 10 years in the field of supportive care and cancer. They now constitute the standard treatment of tumor-induced hypercalcemia. Bisphosphonates bind avidly to hydroxyapatite crystals and inhibit bone resorption. Their anti-resorptive effects may be mediated by inhibition of osteoclasts and activation by cytokines. Bisphosphonates also inhibit recruitment and differentiation of osteoclast precursors. They are poorly absorbed from the GI tract, have a very long half-life in bone, and appear to accumulate at sites of active bone turnover. Numerous bisphosphonates are available or are undergoing clinical investigation, including etidronate, clodronate, pamidronate, alendronate, tiludronate, ibandronate, and risedronate.

Pamidronate is the most commonly used bisphosphonate. It has been shown to be effective in restoring normocalcemia in 60–100 percent of patients with tumor-induced hypercalcemia. This drug is usually tolerated well and its side effects are usually limited to infusion site irritation, fever, and flu like symptoms that occur after the first infusion in approximately 20 percent of patients. Pamidronate is most often given in doses of 60 or 90 mg infused over 2–4 hours.

Zoledronate is a new heterocyclic imidazole bisphosphonate that is the most potent bisphosphonate administered in humans. It is 100–850 times more potent than pamidronate. Very low doses of zoledronate administered by a short-term infusion are effective in treating patients with tumor-induced hypercalcemia. The fall in serum calcium is rapid, and normocalcemia is often maintained for several weeks. Zoledronate is generally well tolerated. The main side effects include transient hypophosphatemia, transient hypocalcemia and an increase in body temperature, occurring in 30 percent of treated patients.

Ibandronate is a third generation bisphosphonate, which inhibits bone resorption. Ibandronate is more potent than clodronate, pamidronate and alendronate in inhibiting induced hypercalcemia and bone resorption. Adverse events associated with the use of ibandronate in the management of hypercalcemia of malignancy include increased body temperature, hypocalcemia and hypophosphatemia. Less commonly, flu-like symptoms and gastrointestinal intolerance may occur.

In conclusion, a single 90-mg pamidronate infusion normalizes serum calcium levels in more than 90 percent of patients with tumor-induced hypercalcemia. Newer, more potent bisphosphonates, such as ibandronate and zoledronate, may improve these results, especially in patients with severe hypercalcemia and they may simplify the therapeutic regimens.

Corticosteroids

Steroids decrease intestinal calcium absorption and inhibit osteoclast-mediated bone resorption. In certain malignancies including lymphomas, myeloma and hormone-sensitive breast cancers steroids may be of some value in producing a direct antitumor effect. They are also active when hypercalcemia is associated with vitamin D synthesis or intake. In the majority of solid tumors, however, steroids are of limited or no value.

The onset of action is 3–5 days. Doses of hydrocortisone (or its equivalent) may range from 100 to 200 mg/day. The main side effects include hyperglycemia, gastrointestinal bleeding, osteoporosis, myopathy, hypertension, and opportunistic infections. Steroids should be used for a short time only to avoid these side effects.

Calcitonin

Calcitonin is a peptide hormone secreted by specialized cells in the thyroid and parathyroid. Its synthesis and secretion normally increase in response to high serum-ionized calcium concentrations. Calcitonin opposes physiologic effects of PTH on bone and renal tubular calcium resorption. Calcitonin rapidly inhibits calcium and phosphate resorption from bone and decreases renal calcium reabsorption. It is thought to inhibit bone degradation by binding directly to receptors on the osteoclast. Calcitonin derived from salmon is much more potent and has a longer duration of activity than the human hormone. Initial dose schedule is 5 IU/kg body weight, administered subcutaneously or intramuscularly every 12 hours. Dose and schedule may be escalated after 1 or 2 days to 10 IU/kg every 12 hours and finally to IU/kg every 6 hours if the response to lower doses is unsatisfactory. Unfortunately, tachyphylaxis commonly occurs. Calcitonin in combination with bisphosphonates may hasten the onset and duration of a hypocalcemic response due to calcitonin's rapid onset of action.

Calcitonin is usually well-tolerated and can be given to patients with organ failure; adverse effects include mild nausea, transient cramping abdominal pain, and cutaneous flushing. Rarely, hypersensitivity reactions are seen. The formation of antibodies against heterologous calcitonins like salmon calcitonin is common and occurs in 40–70 percent of patients treated for more than 4 months.

Plicamycin

Plicamycin (mithramycin) is an inhibitor of osteoclast RNA synthesis and may also block the effects of vitamin D or PTH. It is effective in ~80 percent of patients with tumor-induced hypercalcemia. Onset of response occurs within 12 hours of a single intravenous dose of 25–30 μg/kg of body weight given as a short infusion for 30 min or longer. Maximum response, however, does not occur until approximately 48 hours after administration and may persist for 3–7 days or more after administration. Repeated doses may be given to maintain plicamycin's hypocalcemic effect but should not be given more frequently than every 48 hours. Multiple doses may control hypercalcemia for several weeks, but rebound hypercalcemia usually occurs without definitive treatment of the underlying malignancy. Although single dose treatment of hypercalcemia is generally well tolerated with few adverse effects, dysfibrinogenemia and nephrotoxicity have been reported after single doses (20–25 μg/kg). Rapid intravenous administration is associated with nausea and vomiting. High and repeated doses predispose the patient to thrombocytopenia, qualitative platelet dysfunction that may be associated with bleeding diatheses, transient increases in hepatic transaminases, nephrotoxicity, hypophosphatemia, flu-like syndrome, dermatologic reactions, and stomatitis.

Gallium nitrate

Gallium nitrate was originally developed as an antineoplastic agent that was coincidentally found to produce an hypocalcemic effect. However, further studies have revealed that this drug has extremely potent effects on turnover of bone, and that low doses can be used to reduce bone resorption.

Elemental gallium is a potent inhibitor of bone resorption. It directly inhibits osteoclasts and increases bone calcium without producing cytotoxic effects on bone cells. Low doses of gallium nitrate reduce biochemical parameters of accelerated bone turnover, including urinary excretion of calcium, hydroxyproline, and urinary collagen cross-linked N-telopeptides. It successfully restores normocalcemia in 75–85 percent of patients.

The results of randomized double blind studies have suggested that gallium nitrate has superior clinical efficacy relative to etidronate, calcitonin, and pamidronate for the acute control of tumor-induced hypercalcemia. Gallium therapy has several disadvantages, including the need for inpatient care and daily IV infusions. Also, nephrotoxicity is a major side effect of this drug. It is recommended that the drug not be used in patients with creatinine levels >200 mmol/l. Gallium's onset of action is 24–48 hours. The dose range is 100–200 mg/m^2 given by continuous IV infusion for 5 days. It should not be used with other potentially nephrotoxic drugs (e.g. aminoglycosides and amphotericin B).

Phosphates

An increase in serum phosphate concentration decreases osteoclastic activity, inhibits bone resorption, and decreases urinary calcium excretion. Phosphate offers a minimally effective chronic oral treatment for mild to moderate hypercalcemia. It should probably be reserved for patients who are both hypercalcemic and hypophosphatemic. The usual treatment is 250–375 mg four times daily to minimize the potential for developing hyperphosphatemia. Supranormal phosphate administration may result in decreased renal calcium clearance and presumably decreases serum calcium concentrations by precipitating calcium into bone and soft tissues. Extraskeletal calcification in vital organs may have adverse consequences and is especially significant after intravenous administration of phosphate. Intravenous administration of phosphate produces a rapid decline in serum calcium concentrations but is rarely used for the treatment of hypercalcemia because there are safer and more effective anti-resorptive agents for life-threatening hypercalcemia (calcitonin and plicamycin). Hypotension, oliguria, left ventricular failure, and sudden death can occur as a result of rapid intravenous administration. Contraindications for phosphate include normophosphatemia, hyperphosphatemia, and renal insufficiency. Oral phosphate induced diarrhea may be initially advantageous in patients who have experienced constipation secondary to hypercalcemia.

Dialysis

Dialysis is indicated in patients with hypercalcemia complicated by renal failure. Peritoneal dialysis with calcium-free dialysate fluid can remove 200–2000 mg of calcium in 24–48 hours. Hemodialysis is equally effective. Because large quantities of phosphate are lost during dialysis and phosphate loss aggravates hypercalcemia, serum inorganic phosphate should be measured after each dialysis session, and phosphate should be added to the dialysate during the next fluid exchange or to the patient's diet.

3.1.4 Recent advances

Several groups are working on several new inhibitors of bone resorption. Osteoprotegerin probably will be the first available for clinical use. Osteoprotegerin recently was shown to specifically inhibit osteoclast differentiation by acting as a decoy receptor for osteoprotegerin ligand, which is also known as osteoclast differentiation factor. The bone-resorbing effects of osteoprotegerin ligand are physiologically counterbalanced by the endogenous, naturally occurring soluble receptor osteoprotegerin. A single intraperitoneal injection of osteoprotegerin exerts potent hypocalcemic effects in both normal animals and in a nude mouse model of human xenografts associated with tumor-induced hypercalcemia. Recent data obtained in a murine model of tumor-induced hypercalcemia suggest that osteoprotegerin may act more rapidly than pamidronate.

3.2 Hyponatremia

Hyponatremia is a common electrolyte abnormality in patients with malignancy. It can be caused by the primary tumor, metastases, diagnostic or therapeutic interventions or from a secondary complication of cancer.

3.2.1 Etiology and pathophysiology

Common causes of hyponatremia in cancer patients may be classified as follows:

Hyponatremia associated with extra cellular fluid (ECF) volume depletion

This may result from renal loss of sodium as in excessive diuretic use, mineralocorticoid deficiency, salt-wasting nephropathy secondary to chemotherapeutic agents such as cisplatin, cerebral salt wasting following intracranial surgery or subarachnoid hemorrhage and renal tubular acidosis. ECF volume depletion may also be due to extrarenal sodium loss as in vomiting, diarrhea, and drainage of ascites or pleural effusion or in third space loss as in peritonitis, ileus, or pancreatitis. Also, patients with external biliary drainage can lose significant amounts of sodium daily.

The pathogenesis of hyponatremia associated with ECF volume depletion is due to a decreased effective arterial volume, which stimulates antidiuretic hormone (ADH) secretion, which in turn impairs the capacity to excrete dilute urine.

Hyponatremia associated with ECF volume excess

This is usually a consequence of edematous states, such as congestive heart failure, hepatic cirrhosis, and the nephrotic syndrome. These disorders all have in common a decreased effective circulating arterial volume, leading to increased ADH levels.

Hyponatremia associated with a normal ECF volume

This is mostly seen in the syndrome of inappropriate antidiuretic hormone secretion (SIADH). This syndrome is due to the release of ADH from either the posterior pituitary gland or an ectopic source as in tumors, such as small cell lung cancer (SCLC). It occurs in 15 percent of cases of SCLC, 3 percent of patients with head and neck cancer, and 0.7 per-cent of patients with non-small cell lung cancer. The syndrome has also been described in a variety of other malignant tumors, including primary brain tumors, hematologic malignancies, intrathoracic non-pulmonary cancers, skin tumors, gastrointestinal can-cers, gynecologic cancers, breast cancer, prostate cancer, and sarcomas. It may also be caused by various other conditions other than cancer, such as disorders involving the central nervous system, intrathoracic disorders such as infections, positive pressure ven-tilation and conditions with decrease in left atrial pressure. A large number of pharma-ceutical agents have been shown to produce SIADH, including a number of cytotoxic drugs such as vincristine, vinblastine, cisplatin, cyclophosphamide, and melphalan. It is also associated with the use of immunomodulators as interferon, interleukin-2 and levamisole and monoclonal antibodies. Hyponatremia due to enhanced ADH release or effect can also occur with medications such as morphine, carbamazepine, and selective serotonin re-uptake inhibitors.

3.2.2 **Clinical manifestations**

Clinical features of acute hyponatremia are related to osmotic water shift that leads to increased intracellular fluid volume, specifically brain cell swelling. Therefore, the symptoms are primarily neurologic, and their severity depends on the rapidity of onset and absolute decrease in plasma sodium. Patients may be asymptomatic or may com-plain of nausea and malaise. As the plasma sodium falls, the symptoms progress to include headache, lethargy, confusion, stupor, seizures, and coma. In chronic hypo-natremia, adaptive mechanisms tend to minimize the increase in increased intracellular fluid volume and its symptoms. Other manifestations depend on ECF volume status as follows:

1. Patients with hyponatremia associated with ECF volume depletion due to renal salt losses typically are non-oliguric and the urine contains high levels of sodium although patients with extrarenal losses tend to be oliguric and the urine contains little sodium. Patients with ECF volume depletion are clinically hypovolemic with orthostatic hypotension, tachycardia, and rapid weight loss.

2. Patients with hyponatremia associated with ECF volume excess are usually oliguric and gaining weight. The urinary findings typically show concentrated urine with

low sodium levels (<20 mmol/l) and/or low fractional sodium excretion. The increase in total body sodium is exceeded by the rise in total body water.

3. Patients with normal ECF volume as in SIADH usually have hyponatremia with corresponding hypo-osmolality of the serum and ECF, continued renal excretion of sodium, absence of clinical evidence of fluid volume depletion, osmolality of the urine greater than that appropriate for the concomitant osmolality of the plasma and normal function of kidneys, suprarenal glands and thyroid glands. Patients with SIADH appear clinically normovolemic. They have no edema; nonetheless, there is a modest expansion of the intravascular volume, and this is reflected in a low BUN, low serum uric acid level, and urine that, despite being inappropriately concentrated, has large amounts of sodium.

3.2.3 Treatment

The therapeutic goal is to restore normovolemia and normal sodium level. Thus, in patients with hyponatremia and ECF volume depletion replacing sodium and volume deficit is usually sufficient while patients with ECF volume excess are usually treated with water restriction (see Fig. 3.2).

The goal of therapy for SIADH is to treat the underlying malignant disease. If this is not possible, or if the disease has become refractory, other treatment methods are available such as water restriction and demeclocycline therapy. In patients who do not respond to water restriction, the administration of demeclocycline in doses of 300–600 mg twice a day may be used to create a state of drug-induced nephrogenic diabetes insipidus, which will allow for continuing water intake and improvement in the hyponatremia. It may take up to 2 weeks to have its full effect. The side effects are photosensitive rashes and liver toxicity. An alternative is administration of fludrocortisone, which in doses of 0.1–0.3 mg/day will correct hyponatremia partially, but at the risk of developing edema and congestive heart failure. In severe acute, symptomatic hyponatremia, the therapeutic options are infusion of hypertonic saline (3–5 percent saline) or administration of saline and frusemide with careful monitoring. The latter regimen has the advantage of not rapidly expanding ECF volume in an already volume-expanded patient. The goal of acute treatment is to raise the serum sodium above 125 mmol/l. Such an increase will take the patient out of immediate danger, and further correction can be accomplished in a more leisurely fashion. Rapid correction of hyponatremia can predispose to central pontine myelinolysis and other neurologic sequelae.

In the future, effective vasopressin V2 antagonists will become available for clinical use in the treatment of hyponatremia, and are expected to improve the management of hyponatremia.

3.3 Hypokalemia

Hypokalemia has been estimated to occur in approximately 75 percent of all patients with malignancy at some time during their illness.

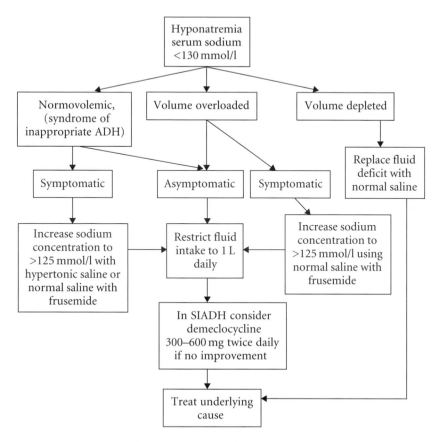

Fig. 3.2 Treatment of hyponatremia.

3.3.1 **Etiology and pathophysiology**

The most common causes of hypokalemia in patients with malignancy are the following:

Inadequate dietary intake

Inadequate dietary intake usually due to anorexia secondary to tumor, chemotherapy or radiotherapy.

Gastrointestinal losses

Gastrointestinal losses usually due to vomiting, gastric suction, or diarrhea; vomiting may occur as a side effect of chemotherapy or radiotherapy, or it may be associated with complications of malignancy. Vomiting also causes metabolic alkalosis, which increases urinary potassium excretion in an attempt to conserve hydrogen ions. Diarrhea may be associated with malignancy such as villous adenoma of the colon, pancreatic carcinoma, carcinoid syndrome, medullary carcinoma of the thyroid, tumors producing vasoactive intestinal peptide, and the Zollinger–Ellison syndrome. Diarrhea may also result from infectious agents or antibiotic therapy or be a side effect of chemotherapeutic agents and radiotherapy.

Redistribution

Hypokalemia may result from an intracellular shift of potassium due to insulin, which is frequently given with total parenteral nutrition. Metabolic alkalosis, which is commonly associated with vomiting or gastric suction, may also cause hypokalemia owing to redistribution.

Renal losses

Renal loss of potassium may result from either the tumor or therapeutic agents. Magnesium depletion causes potassium loss by the kidney as seen in patients treated with cisplatin. Tumors such as SCLC, bronchial adenoma, thymoma, islet cell pancreatic cancer, and bowel carcinoid may secrete ectopic adrenocorticotropic hormone. Tumors of the adrenal cortex may secrete steroids possessing mineralocorticoid activity. Renin-secreting tumors may increase aldosterone production. Steroids used in the treatment of hematologic malignancy may increase renal potassium excretion. Excessive endogenous production or exogenous administration of mineralocorticoids enhances renal potassium excretion. Diuretic therapy or renal tubular damage as a result of antibiotics or chemotherapeutic agents may lead to increased urinary potassium loss.

3.3.2 **Treatment**

Treatment of hypokalemia includes potassium replacement by using a potassium-rich diet, oral supplementation, or intravenous administration of potassium depending on the clinical setting, severity of the hypokalemia, and the degree of urgency to correct the deficit (see Fig. 3.3). The treatment should aim at correction of the underlying cause of hypokalemia if possible.

3.4 **Hypomagnesemia**

Less is known about the physiologic and pathophysiologic importance of magnesium compared to sodium, potassium, and calcium. Intracellular magnesium is commonly ascribed to a role as a cofactor for about 300 cellular enzymes participating in reactions concerning cellular energy metabolism. Extracellular magnesium takes part in regulation of muscle and nerve conduction. Malignant cells have an increased requirement for substances involved in cell multiplication and are able to take magnesium from the extracellular compartment. Moreover, malignant cells have higher intracellular magnesium content than normal tissues. It is reported that erythrocyte magnesium is higher and serum magnesium is lower in patients with malignancy as compared with normal

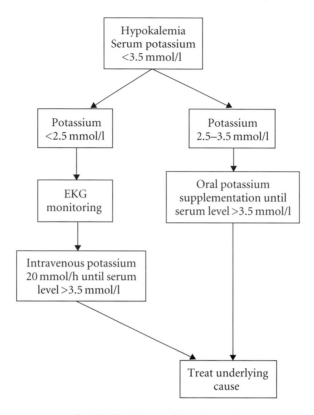

Fig. 3.3 Treatment of hypokalemia.

controls. The extent to which erythrocyte magnesium is increased and serum magnesium is decreased is positively correlated with advancement of the stage of malignancy. Studies also suggest that hypomagnesemia in patients with malignancy results from the increase in intracellular content of the rapidly proliferating neoplastic cells.

3.4.1 **Etiology and pathophysiology**

Hypomagnesemia may result from toxic renal tubular damage due to medications such as cisplatin or antibiotics such as aminoglycosides. Cisplatin induces hypomagnesemia through its renal toxicity possibly through direct injury to mechanisms of the reabsorption in the ascending limb of loop of Henle as well as the distal renal tubule.

3.4.2 **Clinical manifestations**

Hypomagnesemia leads to impairment in magnesium-dependent sodium magnesium ATPase resulting in increased serum potassium loss with decrease in renal potassium conservation which leads to hypokalemia. Hypomagnesemia may also lead to secondary hypocalcemia due to end organ insensitivity to PTH. This secondary hypocalcemia

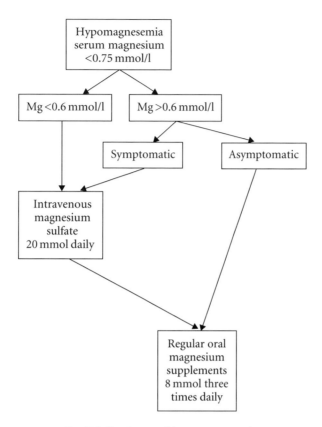

Fig. 3.4 Treatment of hypomagnesemia.

may result in muscular cramps, tetany and muscle weakness accompanied by hyper-reflexia and positive Chvostek's and Trousseau's signs. Low serum magnesium is also associated with prolonged QT interval, ventricular and supraventricular arrhythmias and Torsade de pointes.

3.4.3 Treatment

Adding magnesium to pre- and post-hydration fluids may prevent cisplatin-induced hypomagnesemia. Oral supplements with magnesium are used in patients with chronic hypomagnesemia following treatment with cisplatin (see Fig. 3.4).

3.5 **Hyperviscosity syndromes**

Marked elevations in paraproteins, marked leucocytosis or erythrocytosis in some cancer patients can result in elevated serum viscosity and the development of significant sludging, decreased perfusion of the microcirculation and vascular stasis with the development of the hyperviscosity syndrome.

3.5.1 **Etiology and pathophysiology**

Common causes of the hyperviscosity syndrome include dysproteinemias such as Waldenstrom macroglobulinemia, which accounts for 85–90 percent of all cases. Multiple myeloma is responsible for 5–10 percent of cases. Other etiologies include cryoglobulinemia and leukemias. The blastic phase of chronic myelogenous leukemia, chronic granulocytic leukemia, and the blast cell crisis of acute lymphoblastic and non-lymphoblastic leukemias are less common causes of the hyperviscosity syndrome.

3.5.2 **Clinical manifestations**

Clinical manifestations of the hyperviscosity syndrome become most apparent when the serum viscosity is greater than 4 to 5 (relative viscosity of normal serum ranges between 1.4 and 1.8). They include a triad of bleeding, visual disturbances, and neurologic manifestations.

Occlusive changes occur in small vessels, and may lead to progressive peripheral neuropathies and myelopathies. Hyperviscosity may also precipitate or aggravate heart failure in elderly patients. Circulatory disturbances can be appreciated most readily on examination of the fundi, where characteristic "link-sausage effects," consisting of alternating bulges and constrictions, are seen within the retinal veins. Neurologic manifestations, ranging from headaches, dizziness, and vertigo to somnolence, dementia, stupor, and even coma, are the result of intracerebral vascular occlusions. Some patients may also develop palsies of varying severity as well as Jacksonian or generalized seizures. Bleeding manifestations include chronic nasal bleeding, oozing from the gums, postsurgical or gastrointestinal bleeding. Retinal hemorrhages are common and may lead to serious visual disturbances. Dermatologic complications include Raynaud's phenomenon, livedo reticularis, palpable purpura, eruptive spider nevus-like lesions, digital infarcts, and peripheral gangrene.

3.5.3 **Treatment**

Management of hyperviscosity should aim at urgent reduction of serum viscosity in symptomatic patients by leucopheresis or plasmapheresis. This should be followed by specific chemotherapeutic agents to treat the underlying disease after relief of symptoms.

Temporary measures should focus on adequate rehydration and, in patients with coma and established dysproteinemia, a two-unit phlebotomy with replacement of the patient's red cells with physiologic saline should be performed.

3.6 **Syndrome of acute tumor lysis**

This is a group of metabolic complications that commonly occurs in cancer patients with rapidly proliferating large tumors that undergo rapid cell lysis and acute release of intracellular products into the circulation. It can occur spontaneously or after chemotherapy or radiation therapy of certain hematologic neoplasms and less commonly in chemosensitive or radiosensitive solid tumors.

3.6.1 Etiology and pathophysiology

Most commonly, tumor lysis syndrome is associated with treatment of hematologic malignancies such as non-Hodgkin's lymphoma (especially Burkitt's lymphoma) and acute or chronic leukemia. Less commonly, solid tumors such as breast carcinoma, small cell lung carcinoma and others have been associated with this syndrome. Although usually associated with agents that have potent cytotoxic activity, acute tumor lysis syndrome is occasionally seen following treatment with drugs such as interferon alpha, tamoxifen, cladribine, intrathecal methotrexate, and rituximab. It has also been described in patients with hepatocellular carcinoma after treatment with transcatheter chemo-embolization. Risk factors for development of acute tumor lysis syndrome include bulky abdominal disease, elevated pre-treatment serum uric acid or lactate dehydrogenase levels and poor urine output.

3.6.2 Clinical manifestations

The syndrome of acute tumor lysis is characterized by hyperuricemia, hyperkalemia, hyperphosphatemia, hypocalcemia and, often oliguric renal failure. The release of intracellular purines from fragmented tumor nuclei increases serum uric acid. Uric acid, with a pH of 5.4, exists in a soluble form at physiologic pH, however in the acidic environment of the kidney collecting ducts uric acid may crystallize in the collecting ducts and ureters. This may lead to an obstructive nephropathy and subsequent renal failure. In addition, purine precursors including adenosine triphosphate, adenosine diphosphate, and adenosine regulate vascular tone. With elevation of angiotensin II, adenosine may lead to pre-glomerular vasoconstriction and post-glomerular vasodilatation with the resultant reduction in filtration and renal failure.

The risk of renal failure may be increased in the setting of renal parenchymal tumor infiltration or ureteral or venous obstruction from tumor compression.

Hyperkalemia associated with tumor lysis syndrome may be accentuated by associated renal insufficiency and may cause electrocardiographic alterations and potentially fatal cardiac arrhythmia.

The major manifestation of hyperphosphatemia is secondary hypocalcemia caused by precipitation of calcium phosphate in the soft tissues, which may present as renal failure, pruritic or gangrenous changes in the skin, or inflammation of the eyes or joints. Signs and symptoms of hypocalcemia include anorexia, vomiting, cramps, carpopedal spasms, tetany, seizures, alterations in consciousness, cardiac dysrhythmia and occasionally cardiac arrest.

The severity of the metabolic alterations in acute tumor lysis syndrome is variable and influenced by the dose of chemotherapy, the size of the tumor mass, the number of cells lysed as well as the patient's state of hydration and renal function.

3.6.3 Treatment

The main goal of therapy is to identify those patients at risk of developing acute tumor lysis and to treat them prophylactically with allopurinol and vigorous intravenous hydration to prevent electrolyte disturbances (Fig. 3.5). Patients who are at risk should

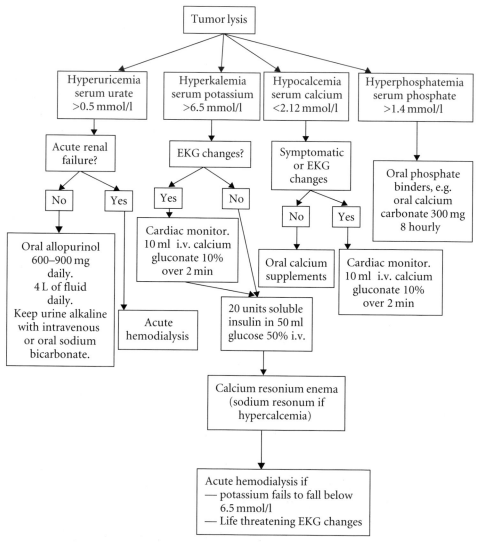

Fig. 3.5 Treatment of tumor lysis syndrome.

be hospitalized and fully hydrated, with ongoing diuresis before, during, and after chemotherapy treatment. These patients should also undergo frequent electrolyte monitoring. Diuresis serves to minimize the renal sludging from high urinary loads of uric acid, xanthine, and phosphate. Frusemide can safely be used to maintain satisfactory urine output so long as fluid status and serum electrolytes are monitored and replaced. Drugs that may interfere with uric acid excretion such as thiazide diuretics or drugs which produce acidic urine such as salicylates should be discontinued.

Alkalization of urine by adding sodium bicarbonate to intravenous fluids to keep urine pH greater than 7 is initiated to prevent precipitation of urate crystals in renal tubules. Acetazolamide, given orally or intravenously, may also be used to alkalinize the urine, especially in patients with metabolic alkalosis and/or with decreased renal function. Careful monitoring is critical as excess vigorous urinary alkalinization may increase the likelihood of calcium phosphate precipitation in the renal tubules.

Allopurinol is given orally once or twice daily at a dose of 300–900 mg to maintain the serum uric acid level below 0.5 mmol/l. It is readily absorbed after oral administration with peak levels reached within two hours of administration. Allopurinol is rapidly converted to its major active metabolite, oxyputinol. Oxyputinol is an inhibitor of xanthine oxidase, an enzyme that catalyzes the conversion of hypoxanthine and xanthine to uric acid. Oral allopurinol has been shown to be efficacious and safe with very few toxicities. Uncommon adverse effects that are attributable to oral allopurinol consist of the syndrome of fever, hepatitis, skin rash and eosinophilia. Intravenous allopurinol has recently been found to be as efficacious and safe as oral allopurinol and can be used in patients unable to take oral medication.

Urate oxidase, an enzyme extracted from Aspergillus flavus, converts uric acid to the water-soluble allantoin, thereby promoting uric acid excretion. It does not affect the metabolism of xanthine or hypoxanthine. Although available in Europe, it is only available for investigational use in United States.

Hyperkalemia is treated with oral sodium–potassium exchange resin or combined insulin/glucose therapy. Symptomatic hypocalcemia can be corrected by administration of calcium gluconate. Further treatment with calcitriol is only indicated if hypocalcemia persists.

Early renal dialysis should be started to correct hyperkalemia, hyperphosphatemia and hyperuricemia in patients with overt renal failure to prevent lethal complications.

Although conventional hemodialysis is most efficient at correcting the metabolic abnormalities (particularly hyperphosphatemia), continuous hemofiltration may benefit those critically ill patients who cannot tolerate the osmotic shifts associated with hemodialysis. Peritoneal dialysis clears uric acid with only 10 percent of the efficiency of hemodialysis and is ineffective in removing phosphates. It is contraindicated in patients with abdominal tumors.

Hyperphosphatemia can be managed by giving phosphate binders orally such as calcium carbonate and calcium acetate or by the administration of glucose and insulin.

Calcium should not be administered for hypocalcemia unless there is evidence of neuromuscular irritability such as a positive Chvostek or Trousseau sign, as it may precipitate metastatic calcification.

3.7 **Hypoglycemia**

Fasting hypoglycemia is a rare metabolic disorder that is usually caused by an underlying malignancy. Although insulin-secreting islet-cell tumors are the most common cause of this condition, the association between fasting hypoglycemia and non-insulin-secreting tumors is also well established.

3.7.1 **Etiology and pathophysiology**

About 80 percent of patients with insulin-secreting islet-cell tumors have intermittent, transient central nervous dysfunction secondary to hypoglycemia. An increase of serum levels of both insulin and C-peptide are usually diagnostic of this disease.

Non-islet-cell tumors associated with hypoglycemia are typically large and slow growing and can either be benign or malignant. Approximately 50 percent of the reported patients have mesenchymal tumors, including solitary fibrous tumors, fibrosarcomas, leiomyomas, liposarcomas, mesotheliomas and hemangiopericytomas. Tumors of epithelial origin, including hepatomas, carcinomas of the stomach, large intestine and others are found in about one-third of patients. In rare cases, hematopoietic tumors such as lymphomas, leukemias, and myelomas can cause hypoglycemia. In contrast to insulinomas, patients with non-islet-cell tumors frequently experience weight loss rather than weight gain. They may have other paraneoplastic manifestations such as seborrheic warts and skin tags. Serum insulin levels are typically low or undetectable. Growth hormone, which is typically elevated in patients with hypoglycemia, is suppressed in these patients. These tumors are believed to cause hypoglycemia by increasing the insulin-like activity of the circulating insulin-like growth factor (IGF) system. The critical elements that regulate IGF system include ligands, receptors and IGF-binding proteins (IGFBPs). To date, this family comprises three ligands (insulin, IGF-I and IGF-II), three cell-surface receptors (the insulin, IGF-I and IGF-II mannose-6-phosphate receptors) and at least six IGFBPs, which bind circulating IGFs and modulate their function.

In addition, non-islet-cell tumor-induced hypoglycemia is characterized by major changes in the composition of the circulating IGFBPs with a shift in the circulating IGF-II from ternary 150 kDa to binary 40-kDa complex. In these patients, the levels of serum total IGF-II are often within the normal range, or only modestly elevated. Therefore, it appears more likely that changes in the bioavailability rather than in the absolute levels of IGF-II are of importance in the induction of hypoglycemia.

Non-islet-cell tumors can also cause hypoglycemia either through excessive glucose utilization by the bulky tumor or failure of counter-regulatory mechanisms that usually prevent hypoglycemia.

3.7.2 **Clinical features**

Classic symptoms of hypoglycemia are usually non-specific and may develop slowly. Symptoms such as weakness, dizziness, diaphoresis and nausea are thought to be symptoms of the cancer or its treatment. However, in the initial phases, symptoms tend to be worse in the early morning after overnight fasting and improve after a meal. However, patients may also present acutely with seizures, coma, and focal or diffuse neurologic deficits.

3.7.3 **Treatment**

The management of patients with tumor-induced hypoglycemia consists of symptomatic treatment of the low blood glucose levels and measures to reduce the tumor bulk. Symptomatic treatment should include frequent meals during the day and intravenous glucose infusions during the night. Several pharmacologic interventions may also increase blood glucose level. Glucocorticoids or administration of growth hormone has also been reported to alleviate or even abolish hypoglycemia in these patients. Growth hormone is thought to suppress production of IGFBP-3 and acid labile glycoprotein, which are necessary for the assembly of the 150-kDa complex.

   The most effective therapeutic approach in these patients is resection or debulking of the tumor, which may lead to resolution of the hypoglycemia, reduction in IGF-II levels, and increases in the levels of IGF-I and GH. In some patients with large unresectable tumors, other procedures may be tried to decrease the bulk of the disease such as embolization of the tumor blood supply by use of polyvinyl alcohol foam particles. Chemotherapy or radiation may be helpful in specific situations.

3.8 **Paraneoplastic syndromes**

Paraneoplastic syndromes may be defined as effects of cancer which occur at sites remote from both the primary tumor and its metastases. They are estimated to occur in less than 15 percent of malignancies. However their exact frequency seems to be underestimated as their manifestations might be overlooked. Paraneoplastic syndromes are most commonly associated with cancers of the lung, stomach, and breast. Although uncommon, their effects are often dramatic and sometimes more disabling than the tumor itself. They may precede, co-exist or follow the primary tumor by months or years and have an unpredictable course. Their clinical recognition is of great importance as they can be the first sign of malignancy. They also can be used as tumor markers as the severity of the syndrome may parallel the activity of the associated tumor and in some instances can be used to follow the clinical course of the disease. Their manifestations may be confused with those of the accompanying tumor and may lead to an erroneous diagnosis of the anatomical location or tumor type. Table 3.2 focuses on the four most commonly involved: the endocrine, nervous, hematologic, and dermatologic systems.

Table 3.2 Manifestation of paraneoplastic syndromes

Metabolic manifestations
Hypercalcemia
Ectopic Cushing's syndrome
Syndrome of inappropriate antidiuretic hormone (SIADH)
Cancer related cachexia

Neuromuscular manifestations
Cerebellar degeneration
Encephalomyelitis
Opsoclonus-myoclonus
Cancer-associated retinopathy
Subacute sensory neuronopathy
Polyradiculopathy (Guillian Barré Syndrome)
Eaton-Lambert myasthenic syndrome
Myasthenia gravis
Polymyositis and dermatomyositis

Hematologic manifestations
Anemia of chronic disease
Autoimmune hemolytic anemia
Neutropenia
Thrombocytopenia
Erythrocytosis
Leukemoid reaction in the absence of infection
Thrombocytosis
Hypercoagulable state
Disseminated intravascular coagulation

Dermatologic manifestations
Acanthosis nigrans
Tripe palms (cutaneous keratoderma)
Erythema gyratum repens (a slowly expanding, mildly scaling
  dermatosis with a "wood-grain" pattern)
Necrolytic migratory erythema
Exfoliative dermatitis
Sweet's syndrome

Suggested reading

Agarwala, S.S. (1996) Paraneoplastic syndromes. *Med Clin North Am*, **80**(1), 173–84.

Barri, Y. and Knochel, J.P. (1996) Hypercalcemia and electrolyte disturbance in malignancy. *Hematol Oncol Clin North Am*, **10**(4), 775–90.

Body, J.J. (2000) Current and future directions in medical therapy. *Cancer*, **88**(S12), 3054–8.

Flombaum, C.D. (2000) Metabolic emergencies in the cancer patient. *Semin Oncol*, **27**(3), 322–34.

Frystyk, *et al.* (1998) Increased levels of circulating free insulin like growth factors in patients with non-islet cell tumor hypoglycemia. *Diabetologia*, **41**, 589–94.

Gross, P. and Palm, C. (2000) The treatment of hyponatremia using vasopressin antagonists. *Exp Physiol*, **85** Spec No: 253–257S.

Kelly, *et al.* (1997) Metabolic emergencies. *Pediatr Clin North Am*, **44**(4), 809–30.

Lajer, H. and Daugaard, G. (1999) Cisplatin and hypomagnesemia. *Cancer Treat Rev*, 25, 47–58.

Rabbani, S.A. (2000) Molecular mechanism of action of parathyroid hormone related peptide in hypercalcemia of malignancy: therapeutic strategies. *Int J Oncol*, 16(1), 197–206.

Rose, M.G. (1999) Malignant hypoglycemia associated with a large mesenchymal tumor. *Cancer J Sci Am*, 5(1), 48–51.

Smally, R.V. (2000) Allopurinol: intravenous use for prevention and treatment of hypercalcemia. *J Clin Oncol*, 18(8), 1758–63.

Werner, H. and Dileroith (2000) New concepts in regulation and function of insulin-like growth factors: implications for understanding normal growth and neoplasia. *Cell Mol Life Sci*, 57, 932–42.

Yang, H. (1999) Tumor lysis syndrome occurring after the administration of rituximab in lymphoproliferative disorders. *Am J Hematol*, 62(4), 247–50.

Chapter 4

Respiratory Emergencies

Tracey Evans and Thomas Lynch

Shortness of breath is an ominous symptom in cancer patients, and its presence in patients with end-stage malignancy is associated with poor short-term prognosis. The differential diagnosis of shortness of breath in the patient with cancer is broad (Table 4.1). In most cancer patients, new onset of shortness of breath is a complication of the underlying malignancy or its treatment. However, respiratory complaints secondary to disorders unrelated to cancer become increasingly relevant as cancer treatments improve and more patients survive longer or are cured.

Disorders of the lungs and breathing are a common cause of death of cancer patients. In an autopsy series comprised of patients with solid tumors, 41 percent died as a result of pulmonary complications (pneumonia, respiratory failure, pulmonary embolism, and pulmonary hemorrhage). Patients with hematologic malignancies also have a high incidence of pulmonary complications: 98 percent of leukemia patients who came to autopsy in one series had pulmonary pathology. In patients with solid tumors, neoplastic disease within the lung is the most common cause of pulmonary complications. Patients with hematologic malignancies are more likely to experience pulmonary complications as a result of their immunocompromised status or antineoplastic treatment.

An analysis of cancer patients presenting to the emergency department of the M.D. Anderson Cancer Center found dyspnea to be the fourth most common presenting complaint. Of the patients with dyspnea, 37 percent had lung cancer and 30 percent had breast cancer. Half of the patients had more than one factor contributing to their dyspnea. In patients with lung cancer, tumor within the chest was the most common cause of shortness of breath followed by chronic obstructive pulmonary disease. In breast cancer patients, pleural effusion was the most common etiology followed by congestive heart failure. Metastatic disease to the lung was the most common cause of shortness of breath in patients with other malignancies. The median survival for all cancer patients presenting to the emergency department with dyspnea was 12 weeks, and the lung cancer patients experienced the shortest median survival at 4 weeks. Nineteen percent of the patients presenting to the emergency room with dypsnea were admitted and died during that hospitalization.

Shortness of breath is the most common presenting complaint of patients with respiratory complications. Other potential symptoms include fever, chest pain, cough, and hemoptysis. An approach to the cancer patient with shortness of breath is outlined

Table 4.1 Differential diagnosis of dyspnea in the cancer patient

Malignancy-associated
Widespread malignancy of the lung
    Multiple pulmonary masses/nodules
    Lymphangitic carcinomatosis
    Leukemic lung involvement (leukostasis)
Pleural effusion
Airway obstruction
SVC syndrome
Pericardial tamponade
Ascites

Treatment-associated
Diffuse alveolar hemorrhage
Bronchiolitis obliterans
Idiopathic pneumonia syndrome
Radiation fibrosis
Pulmonary drug toxicity
Pneumothorax
Congestive heart failure
Transfusion reaction

Resulting from both underlying malignancy and treatment
Pulmonary infection
    Bacterial pneumonia
    Fungal pneumonia
    Pneumocytis carinii pneumonia
    Viral pneumonia/pneumonitis (CMV, RSV)
    Mycobacterial disease
Pulmonary embolism
Anemia
Metabolic acidosis

Co-morbid illness in the cancer patient
Coronary artery disease
Cardiac valvular disease
Cardiac arrythmia
Chronic obstructive pulmonary disease
Asthma
Anxiety

CMV = cytomegalovirus
RSV = respiratory syncitial virus

in Fig. 4.1. Chest X-ray can immediately establish the etiology of dyspnea for patients who have a significant pleural effusion, pneumothorax, lobar atelectasis, or newly discovered widespread pulmonary metastases. Massive pleural effusion can be distinguished from total lung collapse by deviation of the trachea. A pleural effusion increases the volume of the involved hemithorax thereby deviating the trachea away from the involved lung. With complete atelectasis, the trachea deviates toward the involved hemithorax. Diffuse and localized pulmonary infiltrates seen on chest X-ray

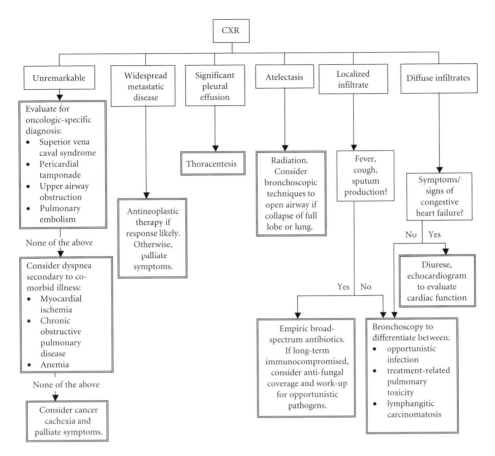

Fig. 4.1 Approach to the cancer patient presenting with dyspnea.

have an extensive differential diagnosis (Table 4.2). Sometimes the clinical scenario points to a likely diagnosis as in bacterial pneumonia. Chest computed tomography may help to suggest a particular diagnosis. Invasive diagnostic procedures are sometimes necessary. In these cases, bronchoscopy with or without transbronchial lung biopsy is frequently sufficient, but occasionally open lung biopsy is required.

While a chest X-ray is the most important test in any patient with dyspnea, four diagnoses for which chest X-ray is frequently not definitive are essential to bear in mind during the initial history and physical of the cancer patient with shortness of breath. These are SVC syndrome, pericardial tamponade, upper airway obstruction, and pulmonary embolism. To the appropriately receptive examiner, the diagnoses of SVC syndrome and pericardial tamponade (discussed in Chapter 1) are frequently apparent on history and physical alone. Computed tomography scan can confirm the diagnosis of SVC syndrome while cardiac ultrasound verifies the presence of pericardial tamponade. Stridor in the cancer patient with dyspnea suggests upper airway

Table 4.2 Differential diagnosis of infiltrates on chest X-ray

Localized	Diffuse
Hemorrhage	Opportunistic infection
Bacterial pneumonia	Congestive heart failure
Tumor	Lymphangitic carcinomatosis
Pulmonary embolism	Drug toxicity
	Transfusion-related lung injury
	Bronchiolitis obliterans

obstruction. Flow-volume loops can establish the diagnosis. Because progressive upper airway obstruction can rapidly lead to respiratory failure, urgent evaluation by bronchoscopy or laryngoscopy is frequently necessary.

The most common cause of dyspnea in the cancer patient presenting with an unchanged plain chest X-ray is pulmonary embolism (discussed in Chapter 1). One autopsy series found pulmonary embolism in 17 percent of cancer patients. Pulmonary embolism can be quite challenging to diagnose; presenting symptoms are frequently non-specific, and objective findings on examination or chest X-ray may be minimal. Pulmonary embolism can also mimic many other respiratory complications of cancer by causing fever, hemoptysis, pleural effusion, and infiltrates on chest X-ray. To make the diagnosis, the clinician must have a high index of suspicion. Unfortunately, once considered, the diagnosis of pulmonary embolism is difficult to rule-out with absolute certainty.

Respiratory emergencies are a common concern for the practicing cancer physician. The most important first step is to accurately determine the underlying cause of the breathing disorder. Superior vena caval syndrome and pulmonary embolism are two of the most crucial diagnoses to make in this setting and are covered extensively in Chapter 1. This chapter will consider the remaining causes of respiratory emergencies of the cancer patient including pneumonia, airway obstruction and compression, hemoptysis, malignant pleural effusion, lymphangitic carcinomatosis, and, finally, causes of disordered breathing related to cancer treatments.

4.1 **Pneumonia**

Pneumonia is the leading cause of death in cancer patients. In the Pneumonia Patient Outcomes Research Team (PORT) cohort study, the presence of neoplastic disease was the variable (other than age) most predictive of 30-day hospital mortality in patients with community acquired pneumonia. Clearly the patient with cancer is more susceptible to pneumonia, and the cancer patient with pneumonia has a worse outcome. The causes for this are multifactorial and are related to both the underlying neoplastic process and its treatments. The debilitated patient with advanced cancer generally has an increased risk of aspiration and decreased effective pulmonary toilet. Tumor within the lungs and therapy-induced breakdown of mucosal barriers cause mechanical derangement of normal respiratory clearance. Cellular and humoral immunosuppression result through poor nutritional status, underlying neoplastic disease (as with many hematologic malignancies), and treatment (including cytotoxic chemotherapy, radiation, and steroids).

In managing the patient with malignancy and pneumonia, admission to the hospital and early administration of broad-spectrum antibiotics is critical. This may be sufficient in the patient with a typical infiltrate and clinical course. Empiric anti-fungal treatment is reasonable in patients with impaired cellular immunity secondary to hematologic malignancies or following bone marrow transplant. If the patient fails to improve on standard antibiotics or has diffuse infiltrates on chest X-ray, bronchoscopy is often required to differentiate between an atypical pneumonia, treatment-related pulmonary toxicity, or neoplastic lung involvement. Pneumocytis carinii, fungal pneumonia, Legionella, and mycobacterial disease are atypical pulmonary infections to which the cancer patient is particularly susceptible.

4.2 Airway obstruction

Airway obstruction secondary to malignancy can occur anywhere from the base of the tongue to the terminal bronchioles. Patients may experience sudden respiratory failure and death or no symptoms at all depending upon the location and degree of obstruction. Shortness of breath is the most common presenting symptom.

Upper airway obstruction due to tumor is rare, but can rapidly lead to respiratory failure. Patients presenting with true stridor require emergent surgical evaluation. Stridor indicates extrathoracic obstruction and can be distinguished from wheezing by a more prominent inspiratory rather than expiratory phase that is best heard without a stethoscope near the patient's open mouth during forced inspiration. Extrathoracic obstruction produces a plateau of inspiratory phase on flow-volume loops because the rate of airflow on inspiration is fixed.

Approximately 5 percent of laryngeal cancers present with impending respiratory obstruction. Airway maintenance is obviously the chief concern in these cases, but ideally the acute treatment should not jeopardize potential for cure and long-term survival. Some experts recommend laryngectomy when airway obstruction is an issue as patients who undergo tracheostomy prior to laryngectomy have worse long-term survival than patients who do not, and stomal recurrences are common. Certainly selection bias confounds these data; patients requiring emergency tracheotomy are likely to have more advanced and aggressive tumors. Emergency laryngectomy, defined as one performed within 24 hours of presentation, is logistically difficult to perform, and it may prevent a thorough evaluation of the patient presenting with a new laryngeal mass. It also eliminates the possibility of a larynx-sparing approach that may offer similar survival from a cancer standpoint. A very small retrospective comparison of patients treated with emergency laryngectomy versus tracheostomy followed by laryngectomy failed to show a survival advantage to either method. An alternative method for supporting the patient with an obstructing upper airway tumor is through mechanical or laser debulking.

Neoplasms may obstruct the trachea and bronchi by occurrence within the airways, invasion from adjacent structures, or extrinsic compression. Tumors originating within the trachea are rare and are usually of adenoid cystic or squamous-cell histology. Primary tumors of the esophagus, thyroid, thymus, and lung can progress to invade the trachea and large airways. External tracheal compression is common in children with mediastinal masses, especially non-Hodgkin's lymphoma. Tracheal compression in the pediatric population is often coupled with superior vena caval obstruction.

Primary lung cancers are overwhelmingly the most frequent endobronchial tumors. While patients with solid tumors other than lung have pulmonary metastases in about 50 percent of cases, clinically significant endobronchial lesions in major airways are found in fewer than 5 percent. Carcinoma of the kidney is the most common cause of central airway metastasis. Bronchial carcinoids (formerly bronchial adenomas) can also present as obstructing lesions and are usually not metastatic at presentation. Extrinsic obstruction of the airways occurs most commonly by pathologic enlargement of intrathoracic lymph nodes. This is usually secondary to lung cancer although other possibilities include esophageal cancer, thyroid cancer, and lymphoma.

4.2.1 Approach to the patient with airway obstruction

Bronchoscopy is the preferred initial approach to most patients with airway obstruction as it can be both diagnostic and therapeutic (Fig. 4.2). A histologic diagnosis can be obtained via direct biopsy, bronchial–alveolar lavage, and endobronchial brushing. Lesions causing extrinsic compression of the airways can be diagnosed with excellent success via transbronchial needle aspiration. If life-threatening airway obstruction is not imminent, treatment should be tailored to the underlying disease following biopsy and appropriate staging. If the obstruction is caused by a malignancy with the potential for surgical cure, such as a localized non-small cell lung cancer (NSCLC), the optimal treatment for both the underlying disease and the airway obstruction is surgical excision and airway reconstruction. If the etiology of the airway obstruction is a chemotherapy-sensitive tumor such as small cell lung cancer (SCLC) or lymphoma, chemotherapy can rapidly relieve symptoms of airway obstruction as well as potentially cure the underlying malignancy.

More than half of lung cancer patients present with advanced disease and therefore are not candidates for curative surgery. In addition, except for patients with lymphoma, germ cell tumors, and the rare solid tumor patient with a single pulmonary metastasis, patients with intrathoracic metastases are not candidates for surgery and are unlikely to respond rapidly to chemotherapy. Therefore, palliative maneuvers to

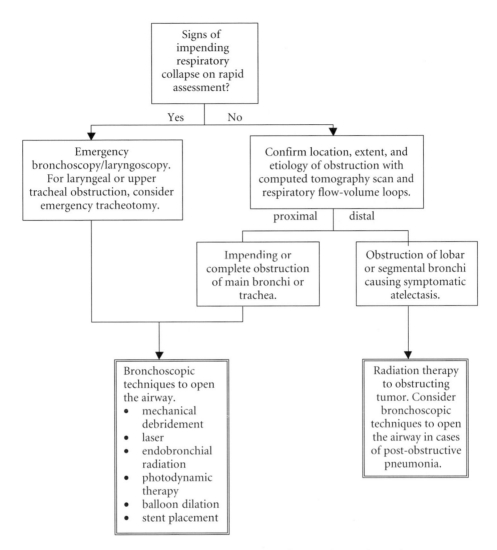

Fig. 4.2 Approach to the patient with malignant airway obstruction.

alleviate symptomatic airway obstruction are necessary. Non-life-threatening airway obstruction by tumor causing atelectasis is commonly managed with external beam radiation therapy. Up to 60 percent of patients with NSCLC have improvement of atelectasis by chest X-ray criteria when treated with radiation therapy.

A variety of bronchoscopic maneuvers can alleviate airway obstruction. These include mechanical debridement, laser treatment, photodynamic therapy, stent placement, and endobronchial radiotherapy (Table 4.3). The location of the obstructing lesion, available equipment, and expertise of the operator determine the optimal treatment. A rigid bronchoscope allows for better control of the airway, but a flexible bronchoscope can

Table 4.3 Methods to alleviate airway obstruction

Intrinsic	Extrinsic
Mechanical debridement	EBB
Laser treatment	Stent placement
EBB	Balloon dilation
Photodynamic therapy	
Stent placement	

EBB – endobronchial brachytherapy

more easily reach the distal airways. Palliation of symptoms from airway obstruction is more successful when the obstructing lesion is located in the larger, more central airways. Bronchoscopic treatment of obstruction in lobar and segmental airways are useful only in cases of post-obstructive pneumonia.

Mechanical debridement may be the least elegant of the available options, but it is nonetheless effective. A series of 56 patients with malignant airway obstruction at the Massachusetts General Hospital underwent mechanical 'core out' of tumor using biopsy forceps and the tip of a rigid bronchoscope. Ninety percent of patients had immediate improvement in obstructive symptoms, and in 96 percent only a single bronchoscopic procedure was necessary. There were no procedure-related deaths, and major complications were rare. Minor bleeding was common but was easily controlled with irrigation, tamponade, and topical epinephrine. Mechanical debridement is only possible for lesions intrinsic to the trachea and proximal bronchi.

Endobronchial laser treatments allow for immediate relief of airway obstruction in over 90 percent of cases. In one series, there was a longer interval to recurrence than with mechanical debridement. Laser therapy is more successful in producing symptomatic relief in central airway obstruction than in those of the lobar or segmental bronchi, and airway patency is less likely to be re-established if the obstruction has been long-standing. The most common type of laser used in the treatment of endobronchial obstruction is the Neodymium : yttrium–aluminum–garnet (Nd : YAG) laser. The wavelength used by this laser is near infrared and can penetrate from several millimeters up to several centimeters. Massive hemorrhage from tumor necrosis or blood vessel perforation is the most serious potential complication of laser therapy. Additional complications include pneumothorax and pneumo-mediastinum. To preserve the integrity of the wall of the airway, the laser operator must direct the beam parallel to the wall and thus avoid perforation. For this reason, lesions extrinsic to the bronchial wall and lesions causing complete obstruction are not amenable to laser treatment. As a general rule, the bronchoscopist must be able to see past the lesion to apply successful laser therapy. Laser therapy requires special training, and the equipment is expensive. Because of the risk of fire, it is recommended that patients be maintained on oxygen concentrations under 50 percent.

Endobronchial brachytherapy (EBB) is also quite effective at palliating symptoms due to endobronchial tumors. This procedure involves delivering a single high dose of radiation through the use of high-energy seeds applied in close proximity to the obstructing tumor in the airway. A prospective, randomized study of external beam radiation with or without EBB as definitive treatment for inoperable NSCLC found improved local control for the combined modality, but, as expected, no significant effect on overall survival. In a study of palliative EBB, out of 175 patients who received high dose rate EBB, 115 (66 percent) had symptomatic improvement. In 32 percent the improvement was considerable and in 34 percent slight. There was a significant association between patients who experienced symptom palliation and those who had an objective response (defined as at least 50 percent of the normal lumen reopened). The overall objective response rate was 78 percent. In malignant airway obstruction specifically, endobronchial brachytherapy in 56 patients followed by bronchoscopic surveillance documented an improved airway lumen and symptom palliation in 64 percent. Approximately half of the responding patients had a recurrence of obstructive symptoms at a median of 8 months.

Fatal hemoptysis is the most serious complication of EBB. There is an element of selection bias affecting this conclusion as the centrally located tumors most amenable to EBB are also those most likely to cause massive hemoptysis. A retrospective analysis of 938 patients with inoperable NSCLC referred for radiation therapy sought to determine the true contribution of EBB to fatal hemoptysis. The authors compared patients who received EBB with patients who had similar endobronchial tumors in the central airways and therefore would have been EBB eligible, but were treated before the technology was available. Out of all patients referred for radiation, 11 percent died of massive hemoptysis. This included 4 percent of the patients who received only external beam radiation and would not have been considered "EBB eligible," 13 percent of the patients who were eligible for EBB but did not receive it, and 26 percent of the patients who did receive EBB. The differences between these groups are statistically significant. Therefore, while the type of tumors amenable to EBB do indeed increase the risk of fatal hemoptysis, EBB may further increase the risk. A dose–response relationship was also suggested; 46.2 percent of patients who received a single dose of EBB at 15 Gy at 1 cm distance in addition to external beam radiation died of massive hemoptysis. (Doses given in a single fraction for EBB have typically ranged from 10 to 20 Gy at 1 cm.)

Photodynamic therapy (PDT) has gained popularity in the last decade for the treatment of malignant obstruction of the esophagus and airways. In PDT, a photosensitizing agent given intravenously leads to a cytotoxic response when exposed to light of the appropriate wavelength via generation of oxygen singlets. Hematoporphyrin derivatives are the most commonly used photosensitizers because they are preferentially taken up by neoplastic tissue. The oxygen singlets have a radius of action of less than 0.02 μm, so the effect on adjacent normal tissue is negligible. In the treatment of endobronchial lesions, the light source is delivered by bronchoscope. A prospective, randomized trial comparing PDT and Nd–YAG laser treatment of partially obstructing advanced non-small cell lung cancer found that PDT was superior for palliation of dyspnea, cough, and hemoptysis, and the complications were similar. Complications of phototherapy include hemoptysis, expectoration of necrotic tumor, and skin photosensitivity.

Endobronchial stent placement is also useful for relieving airway obstruction, particularly that caused by extrinsic compression. Stents placed within the airway can also help maintain airway patency following balloon dilation or one of the above debulking techniques. Unfortunately, the ideal stent is yet to be invented. Current stents are typically either silicone or metal. The Dumon stent is the most commonly used silicone stent. General anesthesia and rigid bronchoscopy are required for its deployment. Silicone stents have the potential to migrate, and inspissated secretions are common secondary to a relatively small lumen and the inability of the mucociliary system to clear secretions. Wire stents have several advantages in that they can be placed via flexible bronchoscopy and without general anesthesia. Uncovered metallic stents allow for some maintenance of mucociliary clearance and will not obstruct branching airways. However, tumor growth can occur in between the wire struts, making uncovered metallic stents inappropriate for patients with malignant airway obstruction. Covered metallic stents can limit this complication. Once placed, metallic stents are difficult to remove secondary to granuloma formation. Granulomata themselves may lead to airway occlusion and occur primarily at the stent ends, especially with covered metallic stents.

The optimal management of the patient with central airway obstruction utilizes a combination of the above approaches tailored to the individual patient by a team experienced in the techniques. In a series of 97 patients with central airway obstruction (49 patients with malignancy) the endoscopic and surgical airway practice of the University of Washington used multiple treatment modalities to successfully relieve the obstruction in 94 percent of patients. Forty-two percent of patients required more than one procedure to maintain patency of the airway.

4.2.2 Airway compression by mediastinal mass

While bronchoscopy forms the cornerstone of diagnosis and treatment of airway obstruction, an important exception to this is the patient with extrinsic tracheal compression from an anterior mediastinal mass. Anesthetic agents in these patients can relax the bronchial smooth muscle and exacerbate the airway obstruction. Intubation and mechanical ventilation eliminates the negative intrathoracic pressure provided by spontaneous respiration, thereby further increasing the effect of extrinsic compression. Ventilation in this setting can become impossible. Ideally, a tissue diagnosis can be obtained prior to initiating antineoplastic therapy. However, if the patient with an anterior mediastinal mass shows evidence of significant airway obstruction on examination, imaging, or flow-volume loops, general anesthesia becomes significantly more dangerous. General anesthesia is not required for bone marrow or lymph node biopsy which may be able to make the diagnosis. Many anterior mediastinal masses are lymphomas and germ cell tumors and are, therefore, very sensitive to radiation and chemotherapy.

4.3 **Hemoptysis**

Hemoptysis is a frightening event for the patient and can be the presenting sign of a new malignancy or a life-threatening complication. Cancer patients can experience hemoptysis as a result of an endobronchial tumor oozing blood, tumor invading the bronchial or pulmonary vasculature, damage to the lung from infection or drug toxicity, or as a result of pulmonary infarction from a thromboembolism. A recent retrospective series of Israeli patients with hemoptysis found malignancy to be the underlying cause in 19 percent. Bronchiectasis was the most common cause of hemoptysis accounting for 20 percent of the cases, and bronchitis and pneumonia accounted for 18 percent and 16 percent of the cases respectively. Tuberculosis was a rare cause of hemoptysis accounting for 1.4 percent of cases. Of the patients with malignancy, 52 percent had a primary lung cancer whereas 46 percent had disease metastatic to the lung. The most common of these were breast cancer, laryngeal carcinoma, melanoma, and lymphoma. Only 10 percent of cases of hemoptysis secondary to malignancy were characterized as massive (>500 ml in 24 hours). A recent US series performed in a Veteran's Hospital found bronchogenic carcinoma was the leading cause of hemoptysis and was present in 29 percent of the cases of hemoptysis. Bronchitis accounted for 23 percent of the hemoptysis cases, tuberculosis 6 percent, bronchiectasis 2 percent, and in 22 percent no cause could be found. In general, more recent series report a smaller percentage of hemoptysis cases secondary to bronchiectasis and tuberculosis than previous series. This is likely due to improved antibiotic therapy and access to health care.

Approximately 30 percent of lung cancer patients experience some degree of hemoptysis as an initial symptom of disease, and about half will experience hemoptysis during their disease course. Predicting which patients will develop life-threatening hemoptysis can be difficult. Massive hemoptysis and malignancy are a lethal combination; the in-hospital mortality rate for patients with malignancy and hemoptysis of at least 200 ml in 24 hours is 59 percent. If the rate of bleeding is over 1000 ml in 24 hours, the in-hospital mortality rate for patients with malignancy is 80 percent (Fig. 4.3).

Fortunately, fatal hemoptysis is rare. A retrospective analysis by Miller of 877 autopsy reports of patients with lung cancer found massive hemoptysis as the cause of death in 3 percent. The incidence of non-fatal hemoptysis in that same series was approximately 15 percent and was similar across all histologic subtypes. However, the incidence of massive hemoptysis varied significantly depending on the histologic subtype. Out of the 877 patients, 36 percent had squamous cell histology, but this subtype was present in 83 percent of the patients with fatal hemoptysis. Of all patients with squamous cell lung cancer, 7.4 percent died from massive hemoptysis. In contrast, fatal hemoptysis occurred in 2 percent of large cell cases and less than 1 percent of adenocarcinoma and small cell carcinoma. Approximately half of all cases of fatal hemoptysis had cavitary

Life-threatening hemoptysis	Minor hemoptysis
• Strict attention to maintenance of secure airway.	• Evaluate for pneumonia, pulmonary embolism.
• Attempt to localize bleeding with CXR, chest CT, and bronchoscopy.	• Chest computed tomography to assess for intrathoracic tumor.
• Position bleeding lung down.	
• Correct low platelets/coagulopathy.	• Correct low platelets/coagulopathy.
• Consider surgery if appropriate candidate.	• Appropriate treatment for underlying malignancy (surgery if curable, chemotherapy if disease sensitive, otherwise palliative radiation).
• Consider selective intubation.	
• Consider infusion of pitressin.	
• Consider topical bronchoscopic therapies (tamponade, fibrin precursors, laser photocoagulation, iced saline lavage).	• Consider bronchoscopy if risk factors for life-threatening hemoptysis (central squamous cell carcinomas).
• Consider bronchial artery embolization.	

Fig. 4.3 Approach to the patient with malignancy and hemoptysis.

lesions, although cavitation was present in only 7 percent of all cases. A tumor in either main stem bronchus was also associated with fatal hemoptysis. Antecedent bleeding occurred in most (79 percent) cases of fatal hemoptysis, but in six cases, the event of fatal hemoptysis was the very first time the patient expectorated blood. Of note, approximately one-third of patients with squamous cell carcinoma identified in this analysis as having submassive hemoptysis went on to develop fatal hemoptysis. However, this method of autopsy report review was unlikely to identify all patients with squamous cell carcinoma and minor hemoptysis who did not go on to develop lethal hemoptysis. This strong association between fatal hemoptysis and squamous cell carcinoma has been confirmed in other series.

The relationship between central squamous cell carcinomas and hemoptysis has become of great interest in the development of the anti-vascular endothelial growth factor (VEGF) monoclonal antibody. This novel agent appears to have antitumor activity based on its anti-angiogenic properties. In a randomized phase II trial, six patients with NSCLC treated anti-VEGF monoclonal antibody along with standard chemotherapy developed massive hemoptysis, and four patients died. Nineteen percent of the 67 patients treated with anti-VGEF had squamous cell carcinoma, but this histology was present in four out of the six with life-threatening hemoptysis. Treatment with anti-VEGF and chemotherapy was also associated with significant tumor cavitation. Because of this association between squamous cell and massive hemoptysis, the planned randomized phase III trial of the anti-VGEF monoclonal antibody will exclude patients with squamous cell histology.

The Miller autopsy series discussed previously also noted a statistically significant association between fatal hemoptysis and the receipt of external beam radiation. However, submassive bleeding often preceded radiation, so Miller concluded that radiation was an innocent bystander and not the cause of hemoptysis. Indeed, external beam radiation therapy is an effective treatment for submassive hemoptysis secondary to tumor. About 80 percent of lung cancer patients will have palliation of low-grade hemoptysis with external beam radiation. Therefore, because most patients who develop fatal hemoptysis have had antecedent bleeding, and because radiation is a treatment for submassive hemoptysis, most patients who develop massive hemoptysis have had radiation. Overall, the percentage of lung cancer patients in thoracic radiation series who develop fatal hemoptysis is around 10 percent.

There is also a relationship between hemoptysis and EBB. As discussed above, EBB has been shown to be a contributing factor in massive hemoptysis and the effect may be dose-related. In multivariate analysis, tumor extension into the main bronchus, hemoptysis prior to receipt of radiation, localization to the upper bronchus, and fraction size of EBB were associated with massive hemoptysis. However, EBB can also be used to treat minor hemoptysis resulting in palliation in over 90 percent of patients.

Does radiation contribute to hemoptysis, or does it help to prevent hemoptysis? This apparent paradox arises from the different types of vessels causing minor versus massive bleeding in solid tumor patients. Oozing capillaries of endobronchial tumors give rise to minor hemoptysis. Radiation administered externally or endobronchially can ameliorate this. In contrast, tumor invasion into the bronchial arteries or large central pulmonary vessels leads to massive hemoptysis. Radiation to the tumor can prevent massive hemoptysis by halting the local progression of a tumor that would have otherwise invaded the vasculature. However, radiation theoretically can also contribute to the development of massive hemoptysis by causing a bronchovascular fistula. This can occur by radiation-induced regression of a bronchial tumor already extending into a vessel wall, or by direct radiation-induced necrosis of the bronchial mucosa and vessel walls.

Patients with hematologic malignancies are also at risk for hemoptysis during episodes of pulmonary infection and low platelets. A retrospective review of 24 patients with hematologic malignancy and hemoptysis found hemoptysis proved fatal in 10 patients. Fungal pneumonia was strongly associated with fatal hemoptysis and accounted for 60 percent of the fatal cases.

4.3.1 Treatment of massive hemoptysis

Treatment for the patient with massive hemoptysis secondary to malignancy is difficult because most patients (72 percent in one series) die suddenly at home where rapid medical intervention is not possible. Mortality rates increase with the quantity of hemoptysis. Definitions of massive hemoptysis differ, and randomized data for the treatment of massive hemoptysis is lacking. Institutional bias often determines whether patients with massive hemoptysis are treated with surgery or with conservative management. Advanced malignancy is invariably considered a contraindication to surgery in even the most aggressive series. An exception to this is the patient with hematologic malignancy and massive hemoptysis secondary to invasive *Aspergillis;* successful surgical outcomes have been reported in such patients.

Patients with massive hemoptysis die from asphyxiation rather than blood loss. Airway control and adequate ventilation are of utmost importance. Once the site of bleeding is localized, positioning the patient with the bleeding lung in the dependent position will help to avoid aspiration of blood into the unaffected lung. Chest X-ray, computed tomography, and bronchoscopy may help to localize the site of the bleed. Correction of a coagulopathy or thrombocytopenia is especially relevant in cancer patients who may be nutritionally deficient, on anticoagulant therapy, or receiving chemotherapy.

In addition to helping to localize the site of bleeding, bronchoscopy can be therapeutic. Local maneuvers to arrest bleeding include tamponade with a balloon catheter, application of fibrin precursors, laser photocoagulation, and iced-saline lavage. All of these methods require localization of the site of bleeding by bronchoscopy which can be quite challenging in the briskly bleeding patient. Double lumen endotracheal tubes or selective intubation of one lung can protect the uninvolved lung from aspirated blood but require expertise for placement.

Bronchial artery embolization (BAE) is a relatively new treatment for massive hemoptysis. In a recent intention-to-treat analysis of BAE by Mal *et al.* in 1999 and performed in 56 patients with life-threatening hemoptysis, BAE controlled bleeding immediately in 77 percent of patients. Long-term control of bleeding was achieved in 45 percent of patients. Seventeen percent of patients could not have the procedure because the vessel could not be successfully cannulated or because angiography revealed an anterior spinal artery arising from the offending bronchial artery. Spinal cord injury from the embolization of spinal arteries anastomotic with the bronchial circulation is the most serious complication of BAE. The study by Mal *et al.* is promising, but the series included only three patients with underlying lung cancer. Tuberculosis and idiopathic hemoptysis were the most common diagnoses. In the patients with lung cancer, one could not undergo BAE for technical reasons, in another BAE was unsuccessful at initially controlling the bleeding, and the third developed recurrent bleeding within 30 days and repeat BAE was unsuccessful. An earlier series of BAE in 209 cases of massive hemoptysis reported a 96 percent rate of cessation of bleeding. Only 4 percent of patients studied had lung cancer, and their outcome was not specifically addressed. The authors did conclude, "This procedure should not be performed in patients with lung cancer characterized by rapid reformation of neovascular circulations and the slight possibility of surgical intervention in [bleeding] free intervals." While BAE appears to be promising in patients with massive hemoptysis of other etiologies, it may have limited use in the patient with hemoptysis secondary to lung cancer.

Anecdotal reports exist of successful control of massive hemoptysis with intravenous pitressin. Serious side effects include vasoconstriction and hyponatremia.

Given the poor survival of cancer patients once massive hemoptysis develops, is there a way to prevent a patient with an upper lobe, cavity, squamous cell carcinoma and submassive hemoptysis from developing massive hemoptysis? Most likely this would require being able to halt the progression of intrathoracic tumor which is not yet in our capability. External beam thoracic radiation is the standard of care to palliate patients with submassive hemoptysis and may help prevent the development of massive hemoptysis as previously discussed. Chemotherapy may further assist in local tumor control. In high-risk patients who develop hemoptysis in excess of minimal blood-tinged sputum, early bronchoscopy may allow for laser photocoagulation or topical therapies.

4.4 Malignant pleural effusion

Pleural effusions are not as dramatic or immediately life-threatening as massive hemoptysis or central airway occlusion, but they are very common in patients with malignancy and portend a grave prognosis. The average survival of patients with malignancy and pleural effusion is about 6 months. In lung cancer, patients with pleural effusions and no other evidence of distant metastases nonetheless have a prognosis that is statistically indistinguishable from patients with stage IV disease. If the effusion is secondary to malignancy, whether the cytology is positive for malignant cells makes little difference in long-term survival. Patients with negative cytology have an average survival 2 months longer than those with positive cytology. Malignancy accounts for up to 50 percent of cases of pleural effusions in some series. Lung cancer is the most common cause followed by breast cancer and lymphoma. In about 10 percent of cases of malignant pleural effusions, a primary site cannot be identified. The causes of malignant pleural effusion in 811 patients compiled by Hausheer and Yarbro from six series is shown in Table 4.4.

Malignant pleural effusions are the result of both overproduction and underabsorption of fluid. The parietal pleura is responsible for the production and re-uptake of pleural fluid. Decreased reabsorption secondary to lymphatic obstruction has long been considered the cause of malignant pleural effusions. However, there is recent evidence that increased fluid production secondary to factors produced by the tumor may contribute. Cheng *et al.* in 1999 demonstrated increased VEGF in malignant pleural effusions. Tumors may involve the pleural space through direct chest wall invasion, hematogenous spread to the parietal pleura, and through metastatic embolization to the visceral pleura via the bronchial arteries, followed by seeding of the parietal pleura. Direct chest wall invasion is most commonly seen in lung and breast cancer. Cancer patients may also have pleural effusions resulting from the underlying malignancy

Table 4.4 Etiologies of malignant pleural effusions

	Percent
Lung cancer	35
Breast cancer	23
Adenocarcinoma of unknown primary	12
Lymphoma/leukemia	10
Reproductive tract	6
Gastrointestinal	5
Genito-urinary	3
Primary unknown	3
Other cancers	5

but without tumor involvement of the pleural space. These are called "paramalignant effusions," an example of which is a tumor causing a post-obstructive pneumonia and a parapneumonic effusion. Pulmonary embolism is also a potential cause of a paramalignant pleural effusion.

4.4.1 Treatment of malignant pleural effusions

Asymptomatic patients with malignant pleural effusions require no specific treatment. The most frequent symptom of malignant pleural effusion is shortness of breath, and many patients complain of a feeling of "fullness" on the affected side of their chest, especially when the effusion is large. Patients with advanced malignancy often have other reasons to be dyspneic, and it is important to establish that drainage of the effusion relieves shortness of breath prior to ruling out other causes and attempting definitive treatment of the pleural effusion (Fig. 4.4).

If thoracentesis relieves dyspnea, but the patient has limited anticipated survival, repeated thoracentesis as palliation is appropriate. A patient who has a good performance status and reasonable survival requires therapy to prevent reaccumulation of the pleural effusion. Chemotherapy can prevent the development of pleural effusion in sensitive tumors such as lymphoma, germ cell, SCLC, and sometimes breast carcinoma. If the effusion reaccumulates despite treatment with chemotherapy, or if chemotherapy is unlikely to be effective in preventing reaccumulation as is the case in NSCLC, sclerosis is the favored treatment. The success of sclerosis depends upon full expansion of the lung, thereby allowing apposition of the visceral and parietal pleura. Drainage of the effusion is accomplished by insertion of a chest tube into the pleural space or by evacuation during a video-assisted thoracoscopic surgery (VATS) procedure. A sclerosing agent can then be administered either directly via poudrage during VATS or via a chest tube. A sclerosant causes an inflammatory reaction that adheres the visceral pleura

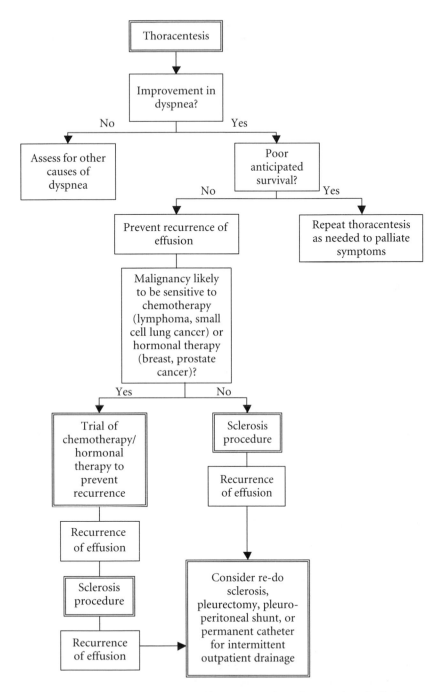

Fig. 4.4 Approach to the patient with symptomatic malignant pleural effusion.

to the parietal pleura, obliterates the pleural space, and prevents reaccumulation of pleural fluid.

Many different agents have been used as sclerosants, and availability, cost, and efficacy determines the optimum agent. Sterile talc is the most efficacious with reported success rates up to 93 percent. It can be instilled as a slurry mixed with normal saline and administered by chest tube at the bedside, or it can be insufflated into the pleural space during thoracoscopy or thoracotomy. A large randomized trial by Dresler in 2000 examined the difference between talc insufflation and chest-tube slurry in producing successful pleurodesis at 30 days. The success rate for talc administered via slurry was 70 percent, and via insufflation 79 percent; this was not a statistically significant difference. Toxicity rates were also similar. Side effects of talc sclerosis include pain, fever, and, rarely, the adult respiratory distress syndrome.

Bleomycin is the most commonly used antineoplastic agent for sclerosis, but its efficacy is more likely due to its ability to generate inflammation rather than due to an antitumor effect. The success rate with bleomycin sclerosis is 54 percent. A disadvantage of bleomycin is the high cost for a single intrapleural administration. A potential advantage is that it can be delivered via a small-bore catheter in the outpatient setting.

Tetracycline was the most commonly used agent for sclerosis until its production was discontinued in the United States in 1991 and in 1998 in the United Kingdom. It had a success rate of 67 percent. Doxycycline was frequently used once tetracycline became unavailable. While its success rate was 72 percent, multiple doses were required to achieve this level of success, and only 10 percent of patients have a successful pleurodesis following a single dose of doxycycline.

A major disadvantage of the above treatments is the requirement for a large bore chest tube which can be uncomfortable for the patient and dictates admission to the hospital. Recent studies have shown that drainage and sclerosis through small-bore catheters can be just as successful. Small-bore chest tube catheters connected to a one-way drainage system allow for outpatient therapy of malignant pleural effusions. A pilot study of 19 patients with malignant effusions treated as outpatients had a complete response rate of 53 percent and a partial response rate of 26 percent using bleomycin as the sclerosant.

For patients in whom sclerosis is not successful, reaccumulation of pleural fluid can be prevented by pleurectomy, though this is a very morbid procedure and should only be considered for the patient with an excellent performance status. In cases where simple drainage does not result in re-expansion of the lung, thoracoscopy with lysis of adhesions may allow for full expansion and successful sclerosis. For the patient who is not a surgical candidate or for whom no other treatment of a symptomatic pleural effusion has proved effective, a pleuro-peritoneal shunt can provide palliation, though shunt occlusion is common.

The latest advance in the treatment of malignant pleural effusions is a tunnelled pleural catheter recently approved for intermittent outpatient drainage of malignant pleural effusions. A randomized phase III comparison of the tunnelled pleural catheter with doxycycline pleurodesis found comparable symptomatic relief, and the catheter group had fewer recurrences and fewer days spent in the hospital. A significant number of patients with the pleural catheter will achieve successful pleurodesis without a sclerosant as a result of repeated drainage. The tunnelled pleural catheter can be used successfully as first-line treatment of malignant pleural effusions and in patients who have failed attempts at sclerosis. Some recommend that the tunnelled pleural catheter should become the new standard of care in the management of malignant pleural effusions.

4.5 **Lymphangitic carcinomatosis**

Lymphangitic carcinomatosis is a rare form of pulmonary metastases, and is defined pathologically by diffuse infiltration of the pulmonary lymphatics with metastatic tumor. About 6–8 percent of pulmonary metastases take the form of lymphangitic carcinomatosis. Adenocarcinoma is the usual histology, and the most common primary malignancies are lung, gastric, and breast cancer. The most common findings on chest X-ray are diffuse reticulonodular infiltrates, though the patient's symptoms frequently appear out of proportion to the X-ray abnormalities. Lymphangitic carcinomatosis is the most common cause of unilateral diffuse lung opacity. A CT exam demonstrates thickening of the bronchovascular bundle and many patients have hilar lymphadenopathy. Transbronchial or open lung biopsy can confirm the diagnosis. Lymphangitic carcinomatosis results in respiratory dysfunction by causing restrictive ventilation defects and a widened alveolar–arterial oxygen gradient. The treatment of lymphangitic carcinomatosis is antineoplastic therapy appropriate for the causative malignancy.

4.6 **Treatment-related lung complications**

Antineoplastic therapies contribute to many of the pulmonary complications seen in cancer patients. Chemotherapy aggravates hypercoagulability as do the implantable catheters used for its infusion, thereby increasing the risk of pulmonary embolism. Chemotherapy and steroids contribute to immunosuppression increasing the risk of pulmonary infections. Diagnostic procedures and placement of intravenous catheters can cause pneumothoraces. Certain chemotherapeutic agents and thoracic radiation can depress cardiac function thereby contributing to congestive heart failure.

Radiation and chemotherapeutic agents also have their own unique pulmonary toxicities. Radiation pneumonitis is discussed in Chapter 15. Bleomycin is the chemotherapeutic agent most commonly associated with respiratory dysfunction, and it is used to treat two of the most curable malignancies: Hodgkin's disease and germ cell tumors. Pulmonary toxicity is its most serious adverse effect and is dose-limiting. Bleomycin initially causes an interstitial pneumonitis that may progress to pulmonary fibrosis. Studies report a wide range of toxicity rates depending on patient population, dose of drug, use of other cytotoxic agents and radiation, and criteria used to define toxicity. A cumulative dose over 400 units results in a dose-dependent toxicity, though pulmonary

Table 4.5 Chemotherapeutic agents associated with pulmonary toxicity

Alkylating agents	**Nitrosoureas**
Cyclophosphamide	Carmustine (BCNU)
Ifosfamide	Lomustine (CCNU)
Busulfan	Semustine (Methyl-CCNU)
Chlorambucil	
Melphalan	**Vinca alkaloids**
	Vinblastine
Antimetabolites	Vindesine
Methotrexate	
Cytosine arabinoside	**Taxanes**
Azathioprine	Paclitaxel
6-Mercaptopurine	Docetaxel
Gemcitabine	
	Miscellaneous
Antibiotics	Procarbazine
Bleomycin	Teniposide (VM-26)
Mitomycin-C	Retinoic acid

dysfunction can occur sporadically at lower doses. Thoracic radiation, renal dysfunction, and age over 70 years appear to increase the risk of pulmonary toxicity. High inspired concentrations of oxygen also appear to increase the toxic effect of bleomycin on the lungs. The most common presenting symptoms of bleomycin-induced interstitial fibrosis are dyspnea and cough. Other chemotherapeutic agents reported to cause toxic injury to the lung are listed in Table 4.5.

Any chemotherapeutic agent can theoretically lead to a hypersensitivity reaction leading to shortness of breath via bronchospasm. However, this is most commonly seen with paclitaxel. Patients receiving paclitaxel are treated prophylactically with glucocorticoids and anti-histamines, and with this pre-treatment the rate of hypersensitivity is less than 10 percent. Reactions generally occur within minutes of starting the infusion, and bronchospasm can be quite severe. Treatment consists of stopping the infusion and administering additional anti-histamines and steroids.

4.6.1 Pulmonary complications of bone marrow transplant

Bone marrow transplant patients experience a complex variety of pulmonary complications resulting from high doses of chemotherapy and radiation, immunosuppression, and, in allogeneic recipients, the effects of the donor's immune system on the host's lungs. Approximately 50 percent of bone marrow transplant patients experience pulmonary complications. Infectious etiologies are the most common and include bacterial pneumonias as well as opportunistic infections.

Pulmonary edema is common early in the transplant course. This occurs secondary to the administration of large volumes of fluid, increased capillary permeability, and cardiac dysfunction. Diffuse alveolar hemorrhage (DAH) is a potentially rapidly fatal complication of bone marrow transplant occurring in the first couple of weeks following the transplant. Presenting symptoms and signs include shortness of breath, hypoxia, and diffuse infiltrates on chest X-ray; hemoptysis is rare. The diagnosis is established via bronchoscopy which classically demonstrates a bloody return on bronchial alveolar lavage that does not clear. Early diagnosis is critical as rapid administration of high dose corticosteroids has been shown to improve survival. Idiopathic pneumonia syndrome clinically resembles pneumonia and pathologically demonstrates diffuse alveolar damage; however, no infectious agent is demonstrated and antibiotic therapy is ineffective. Steroids are sometimes used but are of no proven benefit. Bronchiolitis obliterans occurs later in the transplant course. Patients experience progressive pulmonary deterioration, and the diagnosis is established via lung biopsy. Because patients following bone marrow transplant experience such a wide range of pulmonary complications with very different treatments and often similar chest X-ray findings, early bronchoscopy is crucial.

4.7 **Respiratory failure in cancer patients**

Respiratory failure is the ultimate endpoint of many pulmonary complications. It occurs when the patient can no longer maintain 'without mechanical assistance' the oxygenation and ventilation necessary to survive. The management of respiratory failure in cancer patients is controversial. A number of studies have pointed out the futility and expense of mechanical ventilation in patients with cancer. A series by Groeger *et al.* in 1999 summarized these. The in-hospital mortality rate for patients with solid tumors undergoing mechanical ventilation is 70–90 percent, for hematologic malignancies 75–90 percent, and for bone marrow transplant patients 95 percent. The overall in-hospital mortality rate for the 782 cancer patients requiring mechanical ventilation was 76 percent. Multivariate analysis revealed eight variables that were independent predictors of increased relative risk of death and were available prior to, or within, an hour of the initiation of mechanical ventilation. These included: diagnosis of leukemia, receipt of bone marrow transplant, presence of cardiac arrhythmias, need for vasopressors, intubation more than 24 hours following admission, and progressive or recurrent malignancy. All of these factors approximately doubled the relative risk of death. The presence of disseminated intravascular coagulation coupled with mechanical ventilation increased the mortality rate by a factor of four. Prior surgery with curative intent was protective and cut the relative risk of death by half.

The chance for meaningful survival following mechanical ventilation in the patient with cancer is very small, which certainly calls in to question the wisdom of using such an expensive resource in this near-futile pursuit. Physicians should discuss with their patients the poor outcomes of cancer patients requiring mechanical ventilation prior to pursuing this course. Preferably this discussion can take place before the patient develops a respiratory complication. However, the stakes are high. In patients with hematologic malignancies, cure of the underlying disease is often possible, and respiratory failure is usually a sequel of immunosuppression or treatment rather than of an untreatable malignancy. This is less likely to be the case for patients with solid tumors. Nevertheless, respiratory complications frequently develop suddenly, and in many cases neither the patient nor the physician anticipates imminent death. Most of the patients in the Groeger series had an ECOG performance status of 0–1 one week prior to their hospitalization.

4.8 Conclusion

Fifty percent of patients with advanced cancer experience dyspnea. Sometimes, this signifies a reversible complication that 'can and should be' treated. Other times, dyspnea represents the terminal phase of malignancy. In an evaluation of symptoms in patients with terminal cancer, 24 percent of the patients with dyspnea had no obvious underlying cardiac or pulmonary disease. Narcotic agents can alleviate this sensation of dyspnea as can oxygen therapy. While the appropriate treatment of oncologic patients with respiratory emergencies is critical, equally important is the appropriate palliation of symptomatic dyspnea when treatment is no longer possible.

Suggested reading

Braman, S. and Whitcomb, M. (1975) Endobronchial metastasis. *Arch Intern Med*, **135**, 543–7.

Cavaliere, S., *et al.* (1996) Endoscopic treatment of malignant airway obstructions in 2,008 patients. Chest, **110**, 1536–42.

Cheng, D., Rodriguez, R.M., Perkett, E.A., Rogers, J., Bienvenu, G., Lappalainen, U., and Light, R.W. (1999) Vascular endothelial growth factor in pleural fluid. *Chest*, **116**(3), 760–5.

Collins, T., *et al.* (1988) An evaluation of the palliative role of radiotherapy in inoperable carcinoma of the bronchus. *Clin Radiol*, **39**, 284–6.

Corey, G. and Hla, K. (1987) Major and massive hemoptysis: reassessment of conservative management. *Am J Med Sci*, **294**, 301–9.

Dougherty, T., *et al.* (1998) Photodynamic therapy. *J Natl Cancer Inst*, **90**(12), 889–905.

Escalante, C., *et al.* (1996) Dyspnea in cancer patients: etiology, resource utilization, and survival—implications in a managed care world. *Cancer*, **78**(6), 1314–19.

Fine, M., *et al.* (1997) A prediction rule to identify low-risk patients with community-acquired pneumonia. *New Engl J Med*, **336**(4), 243–50.

Groeger, J., *et al.* (1999) Outcome for cancer patients requiring mechanical ventilation. *J Clin Oncol*, **17**(3), 991–7.

Hausheer, F. and Yarbro, J. (1985) Diagnosis and treatment of malignant pleural effusion. *Semin Oncol*, **12**, 54–75.

Jules-Elysee, K. and White, D. (1990) Bleomycin-induced pulmonary toxicity. *Clin Chest Med*, **11**(1), 1–20.

Kelly, J., *et al.* (2000) High-dose-rate endobronchial brachytherapy effectively palliates symptoms due to airway tumors: the 10-year M.D. Anderson Cancer Center Experience. *Int J Radiat Oncol Biol Phys*, **48**(3), 697–702.

Mal, H., Rullon, I., Mellot, F., Brugière, O., Sleiman, C., Menu, Y., and Fourier, M. (1999) Immediate and long-term results of bronchial artery embolization for life-threatening hemoptysis. *Chest*, **115**(4), 996–1001.

Maltoni, M., *et al.* (1995) Prediction of survival of patients terminally ill with cancer. *Cancer*, 75(10), 2613–22.

Mathisen, D. and Grillo, H. (1989) Endoscopic relief of malignant airway obstruction. *Ann Thorac Surg*, 48, 469–75.

Mazzocato, C., Buclin, T., and Rapin, C. (1999) The effects of morphine on dyspnea and ventilatory function in elderly patients with advanced cancer: a randomized double-blind trial. *Ann Oncol*, 10, 1511–14.

Putnam, J., Light, R., and Rodriguez, R. (1999) A randomized comparison of indwelling pleural catheter and doxycycline pleurodesis in the management of malignant pleural effusions. *Cancer*, 86, 1992–9.

Shen, V. and Pollak, E. (1980) Fatal pulmonary embolism in cancer patients: is heparin prophylaxis justified? *South Med J*, 73(7), 841–3.

Twohig, K. and Matthay, R. (1990) Pulmonary effects of cytotoxic agents other than bleomycin. *Clin Chest Med*, 11(1), 31–54.

van de Molengraft, F. and Vooijs, G. (1989) Survival of patients with malignancy-associated effusions. *Acta Cytologica*, 33(6), 911–16.

Walker-Renard, P., Vaughan, L., and Sahn, S. (1994) Chemical pleurodesis for malignant pleural effusions. *Ann Intern Med*, 120, 56–64.

Chapter 5

Urologic Emergencies

Patrick F. Keane and Chris Hagan

5.1 Introduction

Urologic emergencies are common in cancer patients. They can be the presenting features of a new malignancy, or as complications of cancer treatment. The majority of these emergencies relate to urinary tract infection, hematuria, renal failure and upper urinary tract obstruction, urinary retention and priapism. Prompt diagnosis and early treatment reduces the complication rate and long-term morbidity.

5.2 Urinary tract infection

5.2.1 Pathogenesis

Disruption of normal defence barriers coupled with reduced immunity lead to urinary tract infection (UTI) in the cancer patient. The defence barriers consist of an anatomically intact and functionally normal urinary tract, and normal perineal flora (lactobacilli, streptococci, and coagulase-negative staphylococci). Foreign bodies in the urinary tract, for example, catheters, nephrostomy tubes and ureteric stents are the main disrupters of these barriers. Bladder catheterization leads to a 5 percent incidence of ascending UTI in neutropenic and bone marrow transplant patients that is directly related to the frequency and duration of catheterization. Bladder infection is caused by an initial periurethral colonization of the urethra followed by pathogenic bacteria tracking along the catheter. Bacteria adhere to mucosal and catheter surfaces in a glycocalyx biofilm (Fig. 5.1) which protects them from the flow of urine, inflammatory defences, and antibiotics. Ciprofloxacin demonstrates activity against bacteria in biofilm if given within the first 48 hours. The risk of bacteriuria increases by 5 percent for each subsequent day of catheterization. Broad-spectrum antibiotic treatment alters periurethral flora and increases the risk of infection with enteric organisms and candida. *E. Coli* can bind to receptors on vaginal squamous cells and are thus present in the vagina to cause infection. Thus, antibiotic therapy should be as specific as possible and given for as short a time as possible.

Bladder infection leads to acute or chronic bacterial cystitis, which is commonly associated with suprapubic pain and temperature. Bacteria may then ascend the ureters and invade the renal epithelium, resulting in acute pyelonephritis, characterized by fever, flank pain, bacteremia, and leucocytosis. Pyelonephritis may also be

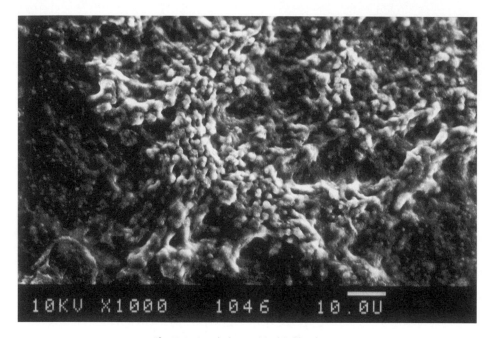

Fig. 5.1 Staphylococci in biofilm form.

caused by blood-borne infection from other sites. Gram-negative bacteria such as *E. Coli* are the commonest pathogens and are responsible for up to 75 percent of all cases of pyelonephritis. Continued upper tract infection may lead to stone formation due to alkalization of urine by urease-splitting organisms (e.g. *Proteus mirablis*).

Renal cortical abscess, perinephric abscess, renal carbuncle, and xanthogranulomatous pyelonephritis are complications of upper tract infection which may be life-threatening. Failure to get an early response to treatment should lead to further investigations and immediate treatment. The presence of urinary tract obstruction and infection represents a true emergency and the obstruction should be relieved immediately.

5.2.2 **Diagnosis**

Urinary tract infection is defined as the presence of 10^5 organisms/ml and bacteriuria is present when there are 10^2 per ml. In neutropenic patients treatment may have to be started regardless of colony counts, or if patients are symptomatic or at high risk of developing a UTI. The method of collection of the urine sample is critical and clean catch mid-stream urine is essential for a confident diagnosis of UTI to be made. In infants suprapubic aspiration of the bladder is the most reliable method of diagnosis. The presence of pus cells in the urine helps to confirm the diagnosis and patients with sterile pyuria should have cultures sent for the tuberculosis organism (TB).

Urine and blood cultures (when the patient is toxic) are mandatory to characterize the pathogen prior to institution of treatment. If pyelonephritis is suspected, then the patient requires a plain abdominal film to detect calculi, and an ultrasound or intravenous pyelogram (IVP) to exclude upper tract obstruction. Ultrasound has the additional benefit of demonstrating an abscess, but may not be a reliable indicator of obstruction in the absence of hydronephrosis.

5.2.3 Treatment

An algorithm for the management of UTI is shown in Fig. 5.2.

Acute cystitis rarely presents as an emergency. However, infections of the upper urinary tract usually present as emergencies with the patient having a high temperature, nausea, vomiting and flank pain. If obstruction is demonstrated with concomitant infection (pyonephrosis), then urgent upper tract drainage is required if life-threatening septicemia is to be avoided. This is best achieved with a percutaneous nephrostomy rather than cystoscopic placement of a ureteric stent. Insertion of a nephrostomy tube

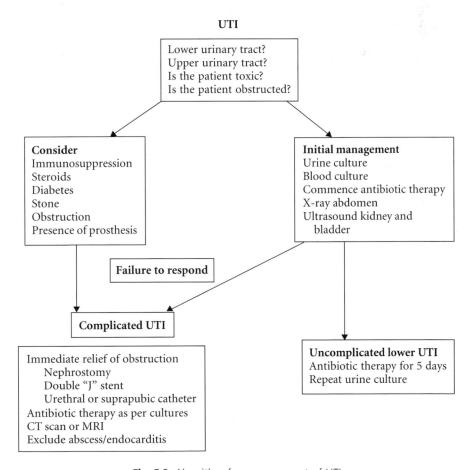

Fig. 5.2 Algorithm for management of UTI.

is straightforward, obviates the need for general anesthesia in a sick patient, and ultimately achieves superior drainage due to the larger caliber drain (9f vs 6f).

The initial choice of antibiotics in both pyonephrosis and pyelonephritis initially should be broad spectrum before cultures of blood and urine are available; typically a combination of a parenteral aminoglycoside to cover gram negative rods and *Pseudomonas*, and ampicillin to cover *Enterococcus* should be started. Fluroquinolones orally (ciprofloxacin, ofloxacin) provide excellent cover against these bacteria but are expensive when used parenterally. These can be changed according to the appropriate antibiotic sensitivities. Antibiotics should be maintained for 10 days.

If the patient's condition fails to improve after 48 hours of appropriate antibiotics, then the possibility of unsuspected ureteric obstruction or renal or cortical abscess should be considered. A repeat ultrasound scan or contrast-enhanced CT scan of the kidney should be performed. If an abscess is diagnosed, then the kidney should be drained by either percutaneous or open surgical means. Occasionally, the combination of obstruction and infection, or abscess formation, renders the kidney non-functioning and nephrectomy becomes the best treatment option.

A common complication of long-term catheterization in the presence of systemic antibiotics is candiduria. This is usually asymptomatic and resolves after catheter removal. Persistent candiduria should be treated with amphotericin B (50 mg/l water) bladder irrigation via a three-way catheter. If budding yeast forms are identified in the urine, then fungal balls must be excluded by IVP and cystoscopy.

5.2.4 Fournier's gangrene

Fournier's gangrene is an infective necrotizing fasciitis of the perineal, perianal or genital region. Diabetes, alcoholism and immunosuppression are commonly associated with the condition. Immunosuppression following chemotherapy, organ transplantation or AIDS particularly when associated with malnutrition and low socio-economic status is a frequent association. The urologic and colorectal conditions associated with Fournier's gangrene are shown in Table 5.1.

Fournier's gangrene is a polymicrobial infection and both aerobes and anaerobes are invariably present. *E. Coli*, Bacteroides and Streptococci are the most frequent organisms cultured. Fournier's gangrene begins as an area of infection close to the site of the

Table 5.1 Conditions associated with Fournier's gangrene

Urologic	Colorectal
Urethral stricture	Rectal biopsy and anal dilatation
Indwelling catheters	Banding of hemorrhoids
Traumatic catheterization	Carcinoma rectum and sigmoid
Urethral calculi	Appendicitis
Prostate biopsy	Rectal foreign bodies

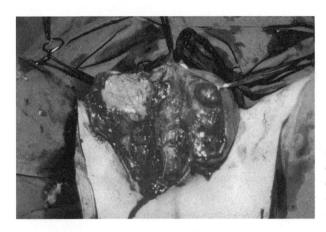

Fig. 5.3 Surgical debridement of Fournier's gangrene with extensive loss of scrotal skin. (Please see color section between pages 116 and 117.)

primary pathology. An obliterative endarteritis causes cutaneous vascular thrombosis and necrosis. Tissue destruction occurs rapidly due to the synergistic action of the various bacteria. The spread of Fournier's gangrene is defined by Colles' fascia in the perineum. In colorectal cases the infection has to reach Colles' fascia through the sphincteric muscle and the perianal margin is usually involved.

Pain, erythema, and swelling of the scrotum are early features, cyanosis, bronzing, and blistering of the skin suggest a deep infection. Crepitus may be felt in up to 60 percent of cases. Once gangrene is established then the patient becomes very ill. Shock, ileus, and delirium are common.

Treatment is based on rapid resuscitation, broad spectrum antibiotics, and emergency surgical debridement (Fig. 5.3). Wide local excision of the genital skin with removal of all devitalized tissue is essential. The testes are usually spared and can be placed in the inguinal region and replaced in the scrotum later. Urinary and fecal diversion may be necessary.

5.2.5 Prevention of urinary tract infection

The selective and limited use of urethral catheterization is the most effective means of preventing UTI in the cancer patient. Long-term catheters should be avoided, and the patient instructed in clean intermittent self-catheterization (CISC) if persistent urinary retention is a problem. Catheter care is important and an aseptic technique for insertion and handling of catheters and drains is essential if infection is to be avoided. Patients in whom a period of catheter drainage is unavoidable should have urine cultures and antibiotics prior to catheter removal, as there is an increased incidence of bacteremia on catheter withdrawal.

5.2.6 Antibiotic prophylaxis prior to genito-urinary procedures

It is recommended that only patients with a prosthetic heart valve or who have had endocarditis require antibiotic prophylaxis. This should be with I.V. amoxycillin 1 g and I.V. gentamicin 120 mg at induction of anesthesia, or 15 min prior to commencement of the procedure. Patients who are allergic to penicillin, or who have received more than a single dose of penicillin in the previous month should have either (a) I.V. vancomycin 1 g given over at least 100 min then I.V. gentamicin 120 mg or (b) I.V. teicoplanin 400 mg and I.V. gentamicin 120 mg. If urine is infected, then prophylaxis should also cover the infecting organism.

There is little evidence to support the use of routine prophylactic antibiotics in immunosuppressed patients prior to genito-urinary procedures (or any other procedures, including dental), unless the patient has a prosthetic heart valve or has had endocarditis. It is unacceptable to expose patients to the adverse effects of antibiotics, but those who develop intercurrent infection require prompt treatment with the antibiotics to which the infecting organisms are sensitive.

5.3 **Urinary tract hemorrhage**

Gross hematuria can be the presenting feature of benign or malignant urologic tumors, or as a result of direct invasion of another tumor into the urinary tract. Cancer treatment with radiotherapy or cyclophosphamide may induce hemorrhagic cystitis. Coagulopathies due to the systemic manifestation of a cancer or as a result of treatment may also produce significant urinary tract hemorrhage (Table 5.2).

5.3.1 **Hemorrhagic cystitis**

Hemorrhagic cystitis is an acute or chronic diffuse bladder inflammation with hemorrhage. It is caused by toxic agents, such as metabolites of chemotherapeutic agents, radiation therapy, and viral infection.

Drug-induced hemorrhagic cystitis

The first use of cyclophosphamide as a chemotherapeutic agent, or in preparation for bone marrow transplantation, produced a 40–68 percent incidence of hemorrhagic cystitis with an associated cystectomy rate of 9 percent due to uncontrollable bleeding. Mortality rates up to 75 percent occur when associated with massive hemorrhage. The

Table 5.2 Causes of urinary tract hemorrhage

Cause	Example
Urological malignancy	Transitional/squamous cell carcinoma, renal cell cancer
Invasion of urinary tract	Colonic and gynecological malignancy, pelvic sarcomas
Treatment-related	Radiotherapy, cyclophosphamide, ifosfamide
Infective	BK virus
Other	Thrombocytopenia, disseminated intravascular coagulation

incidence of bladder hemorrhage is unrelated to cyclophosphamide dose or frequency of administration. Acute hemorrhage usually occurs during or shortly after completing chemotherapy. Patients on long-term low-dose oral cyclophosphamide are at risk of delayed hemorrhage. Clinical symptoms include urinary frequency and dysuria. Cystoscopy reveals an ulcerated, edematous and hyperemic bladder mucosa.

Cyclophosphamide and its analogue, ifosfamide are metabolized in the liver to phospharamide mustard and acrolein. Acrolein is believed to be a urotoxic substance, but the exact mechanism by which urothelial injury occurs is unclear. Ifosfamide is associated with a greater incidence of hemorrhagic cystitis and this may be due to the release of a further metabolite, chloroacetaldehyde which is also believed to be urotoxic. Furthermore, chloroacetaldehyde is nephrotoxic and causes proximal and distal tubular damage.

Sodium 2-mercaptoethane-sulfonate (mesna) is a highly effective urothelial protector that does not interfere with the chemotherapeutic efficacy of cyclophosphamide or ifosfamide. Mesna is excreted by the kidney and binds urinary acrolein to form an inert thioether that is harmless to the urothelium. Mesna also detoxifies chloroacetaldehyde, but its concentration in the tubules may be insufficient to completely prevent nephrotoxicity. The serum half-life of mesna is 90 min, and that of cyclophosphamide 6 hours; to be effective, mesna must be in the urine *before* acrolein comes in contact with the urothelium. Mesna is administered before the first dose of cyclophosphamide and continued after the last dose employing either a continuous intravenous infusion or bolus doses. This is combined with overhydration which dilutes urinary acrolein. Mesna has reduced the incidence of cyclophosphamide-induced hemorrhagic cystitis to less than 5 percent, and obviated the need for chemotherapy dose reductions.

Radiation-induced hemorrhagic cystitis

Bladder problems occur in approximately 20 percent of patients receiving pelvic radiotherapy. Severe bladder hemorrhage is rare, and patients usually complain of irritative or obstructive urinary symptoms. Radiation produces small vessel injury that leads to interstitial bladder wall fibrosis, reduced bladder capacity, and the formation of friable, telangiectatic blood vessels that can rupture, leading to hemorrhage.

The irritative symptoms of radiation cystitis are best managed with an anticholinergic such as oxybutynin (5–15 mg daily) or tolterodine 2 mg twice a day. A period of bladder catheterization may also help. Agents such as sodium pentosulfanpolysulphate, conjugated estrogen, or the use of hyperbaric oxygen, may promote urothelial healing and have been used with some success in the treatment of radiation-induced bladder hemorrhage.

Viral-induced hemorrhagic cystitis

Late onset hemorrhagic cystitis in bone marrow transplant patients has led researchers to suspect a possible viral cause. The BK virus, which is ubiquitous in healthy individuals, is activated in the immunosuppressed and is recoverable in the urine. Fifty percent of patients with persistent BK viruria who receive a bone marrow transplant develop hemorrhagic cystitis. The cause of BK virus-mediated urothelial damage remains uncertain.

5.3.2 Treatment of hemorrhagic cystitis

An algorithm for the management of hemorrhagic cystitis is shown in Fig. 5.4.

Massive bladder hemorrhage may lead to the development of clot and urinary retention. A urologist should be contacted, and a three-way large bore (20 French or larger) irrigating catheter should be passed. The bladder should be lavaged to wash out clots and continuous irrigation with saline commenced. If urine flow cannot be established, then the patient should be taken to the operating theatre for endoscopy and bladder lavage under anesthesia (Fig. 5.5a,b). Clots can be broken up under direct vision, and any obvious bleeding areas can be fulgarated with diathermy.

These simple measures are usually sufficient to deal with most bladder hemorrhage. Should hemorrhage persist, then instillation of an intravesical agent usually controls bleeding. Commonly used agents include formalin, alum, prostaglandins, silver nitrate,

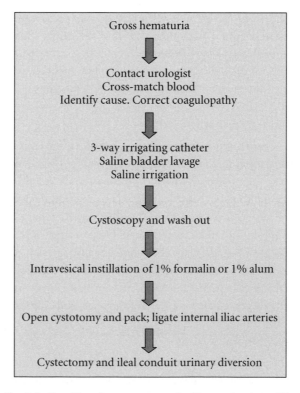

Fig. 5.4 Algorithm for management of hemorrhagic cystitis.

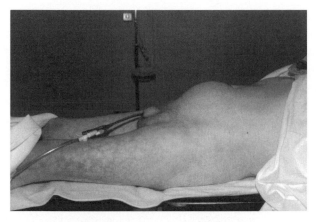

Fig. 5.5a Patient with hemorrhagic cystitis: note the suprapubic swelling, the presence of a 3-way irrigating catheter and the presence of poor peripheral circulation due to shock. (Please see color section between pages 116 and 117.)

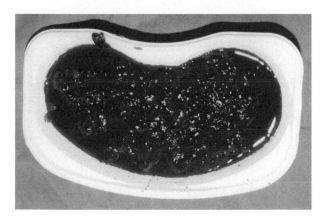

Fig. 5.5b Evacuation of clot from bladder. (Please see color section between pages 116 and 117.)

phenol and iced saline. Hydrostatic dilatation and parenteral aminocaproic acid have also been used with some success.

Intravesical formalin is highly effective and acts as a chemical cauterizing agent. Initial experience with 10 percent formalin solution produced significant complications including renal papillary necrosis, renal failure, ureteric strictures, bladder contracture, and fatal bladder rupture. The use of 1–2 percent solutions have been shown to be equally effective without the toxicity of 10 percent formalin, controlling bleeding in up to 75 percent of cases.

Formalin instillation is performed under general or regional anesthesia; preliminary cystoscopy allows clot evacuation and fulgaration of bleeding points. A cystogram is mandatory to exclude vesico-ureteric reflux (VUR). If reflux is present then the ureteric orifice(s) should be occluded with a Fogarty balloon catheter. If there is evidence of bladder perforation, then formalin instillation is contraindicated. Approximately 500 ml of 1 percent formalin solution is then instilled under gravity at no more than 15 cm above the pubis for 10–15 min. The catheter should not be clamped, as formalin-induced bladder contraction may be induced, leading to an increased risk of reflux or intravascular absorption. The female perineum and vagina should be protected with petroleum jelly in case of formalin leak. After instillation, the bladder should be lavaged with water and then continuous irrigation via a three-way catheter maintained for 24 hours. Re-treatment with 2 percent or 4 percent solutions may be required if hemorrhage continues, though an interval of 48 hours should be allowed to assess the full benefits of the formalin.

Intravesical 1 percent alum solution and prostaglandins E_2 and F_2 have also demonstrated some benefit in controlling hemorrhage, and have the advantage that neither general nor regional anesthesia is required. Alum solution is administered by continuous bladder irrigation at the bedside, causing vasoconstriction and decreased capillary permeability. Bladder spasm can be controlled with antispasmodics. The main disadvantage of alum is that 7 days treatment may be required before hemorrhage ceases. Rarely, aluminium-induced encephalopathy has been described, and aluminium levels should be monitored.

Prostaglandins E_2 and F_2 are administered in a similar manner to alum at the bedside. They act by protecting the microvasculature and epithelium, preventing the development of tissue edema. Success rates of up to 50 percent have been reported with carboprost tromethamine (Prostaglandin $F_{2-\alpha}$), though severe bladder spasm can occur.

A small proportion of patients who fail with conservative measures and continue to have life-threatening hemorrhage will require open surgery to control bleeding. Bladder preservation should be the initial aim, with cystotomy, packing, and ligation of the internal iliac arteries. Angiography may delineate bleeding from one side of the bladder and selective embolization may be attempted. Cystectomy and ileal conduit urinary diversion may be necessary if these measures fail, though the mortality in these already critically ill patients is extremely high.

5.4 Obstructive uropathy

5.4.1 Upper tract obstruction

Obstruction to the flow of urine produces upper tract dilatation and progressive renal damage. This may be caused by obstruction to bladder outflow, or to one or both ureters, and occurs commonly in genito-urinary malignancy (Table 5.3). Ureteric obstruction may be produced by intraluminal, intramural or extramural tumors. Retroperitoneal fibrosis and stricture caused by radiotherapy, chemotherapy, or surgery may also lead to progressive upper tract obstruction.

The risk of developing late ureteric obstruction following pelvic external beam radiotherapy is under-reported. Despite achieving disease-free status, patients require long-term surveillance of their upper tracts, with an actuarial risk of developing severe stricture of 0.15 percent per year.

Table 5.3 Malignant causes of urinary tract obstruction

Type	Cause
Bladder outlet obstruction	Carcinoma of prostate, transitional cell carcinoma of bladder and urethra, carcinoma of penis
Ureteric obstruction	
Intraluminal	Transitional cell carcinoma
Intramural	Transitional cell carcinoma
Extramural	Carcinoma prostate, cervix, uterus, colon, breast, testes, lymphoma
Retroperitoneal fibrosis and stricture	Radiotherapy, chemotherapy, surgery

5.4.2 Clinical features of upper tract obstruction

Patients commonly present with the insidious onset of uremia and reduced urine output. Pain is rarely a feature, unless there is acute obstruction of a ureter. If there is concomitant infection, then urosepsis may intervene unless prompt drainage is performed. Patients may present with acute renal failure and are at risk of sudden death from hyperkalemia because of the insidious clinical presentation.

There are several radiologic methods by which a diagnosis of upper tract urinary obstruction may be confirmed. These include intravenous urography (IVU) (Fig. 5.6), ultrasound scanning (US), renography and CT or MR scanning. Of these, diuretic renography is the most accurate in confirming obstruction.

Dilatation of the urinary tract does not always equate with obstruction and in the absence of complications, isotope renography and doppler ultrasound may be needed to define the clinical problem.

5.4.3 Treatment

The cause and site of the obstruction should be identified. If bilateral obstruction is present then the presence of chronic retention should be excluded and a urethral or suprapubic catheter should be passed. Chronic retention is seen commonly in patients with prostate cancer and catheterization may be all that is necessary to relieve it. Post-obstructive diuresis may occur and the patient should have their urinary output, blood pressure and weight monitored. Intravenous saline may be necessary to keep pace with the output due to the inability of the collecting tubules to concentrate sodium chloride. Bilateral ureteric obstruction is seen in prostate cancer and other pelvic malignancies due to invasion of the trigone. If the patient's renal function allows, then cystoscopic examination and biopsy should be performed. Retrograde pyelography should be performed and if possible the obstruction relieved by the placement of a ureteric stent (Fig. 5.7). Ureteric stents need to be replaced every 6 months in patients with cancer and longer lasting stents may provide better palliation. In patients with pelvic malignancy it is often impossible to cannulate the ureters and a nephrostomy should be inserted in these circumstances.

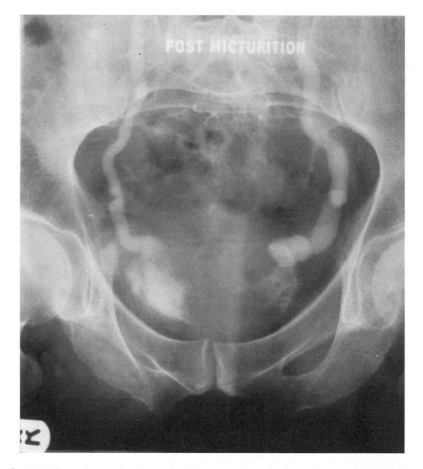

Fig. 5.6 Bilateral ureteric obstruction from transitional cell carcinoma of the bladder.

If there is hyperkalemia in association with uremia then it should be corrected by urgent placement of a nephrostomy under local anesthetic using ultrasound localization, as there is a risk of sudden death from cardiac arrhythmia. The emergency management of acute hyperkalemia is shown in Fig. 5.8.

The majority of patients presenting with hyperkalemia are in acute renal failure, which carries a mortality rate of up to 50 percent. Specific complications include:

(1) *Fluid overload*   The patient complains of dyspnea with clinical signs of fluid overload. Treatment is with diuretics or dialysis if there is little or no urinary output.

(2) *Hyperkalemia*   This is a true emergency. Untreated, it may lead to arrhythmias and cardiac arrest. If this is unsuccessful, then dialysis is required. There are three absolute indications for dialysis:

   (a) Increasing hyperkalemia
   (b) Fluid overload resistant to diuretics
   (c) Severe uremia and acidosis.

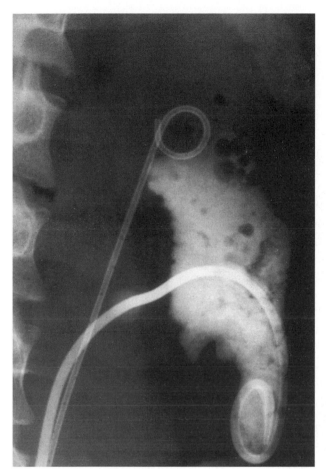

Fig. 5.7 X-ray showing a double "J" stent in a patient with obstruction and a "pig"-tail nephrostomy catheter draining an infected urinoma.

- Stop all potassium sparing drugs and NSAID's
- If EKG changes, give 10 ml calcium gluconate I.V. (10% over 2 min)
- Shift potassium into cells—give 20 units soluble insulin in 50 ml 50% dextrose I.V.
- Promote potassium loss
  Loop diuretic
  Calcium resonium (pr or po)
  Dialysis

Fig. 5.8 Emergency management of hyperkalemia.

(3) *Hypertension*   May be due to renal disease or hypertension, and will improve with fluid removal and/or anti-hypertensives.

(4) *Bleeding tendency*   This is primarily due to platelet dysfunction causing decreased endothelial adhesion. In very ill patients, this may also be associated with abnormal clotting and thrombocytopenia.

(5) *Infection*   Uremic patients are more susceptible to infection due to suppression of their immune system.

Upper tract decompression relieves obstruction and its complications. On occasion an ethical dilemma surrounds the decision to insert a nephrostomy in a patient who is dying of terminal cancer. Lau *et al.* followed 77 patients with pelvic malignant disease who developed upper tract obstruction. Overall median survival was 26 weeks. Patients were classified into four groups: Group 1 (primary untreated malignancy), Group 2 (recurrent malignancy with further treatment), Group 3 (recurrent malignancy with no further treatment), and Group 4 (benign disease as a consequence of previous treatment). Patients in Groups 1 and 2 had similar survival (median survival 27 and 20 weeks; 5-year survival 20 percent and 10 percent respectively). Patients in Group 3 had a poor prognosis with a median survival of 6.5 weeks and no patient surviving beyond one year. Group 4 patients fared best, with a 5-year survival of 64 percent. Thus if the patient has advanced pelvic malignancy for which there is no treatment, then quality of life and the patient's own wishes should determine whether to intervene or not.

5.5 Priapism

Priapism is a persistent erection of greater than 6 hours without sexual desire. It can occur at any age, but patients with hematologic malignancy may be as young as 5 to 10 years of age. Priapism commonly occurs at night or after prolonged sexual activity when the smooth muscle of the cavernosa is most relaxed.

Priapism may be classified as high or low flow. High flow priapism occurs following genital trauma or surgery. It is arterial and therefore non-ischemic. Conversely, low flow priapism, which occurs more commonly, is veno-occlusive and hypoxia leads to ischemic damage of the erectile mechanism. Low flow priapism can be seen in patients with cancer most commonly in patients with hematologic malignancy where altered viscosity of the blood contributes to stasis.

5.5.1 Etiology of low flow priapism

Priapism is idiopathic in 60 percent of cases, while the remaining 40 percent are associated with disease (Table 5.4). Intracavernosal injections of papavarine, before being superceded by prostaglandin E1 (PGE_1), were the commonest cause of priapism.

The patient with low flow priapism usually presents with several hours of painful erection. The glans penis and corpus spongiosum are soft and uninvolved. The corpora cavernosa are tense with congested blood and tender to palpation. The exact mechanism

Table 5.4 Etiology of low flow priapism

Primary	Idiopathic
Secondary	
Hematologic	Leukemia, lymphoma, myeloma, sickle cell disease, thalassemia
Neoplastic	Metastatic renal cell cancer, lung cancer and melanoma prostate cancer
Neurogenic	Spinal cord lesions, cauda equina compression, spinal cord injury
Iatrogenic	Intracavernosal papavarine (>5% incidence; PGE_1 <1%)
Trauma	Genital or perineal
Drugs	
Neuroleptics	Chlorpromazine, thioridazine, trifluoperazine, haloperidol
Antidepressants	Fluoxetine, sertraline, trazodone
Anticoagulants	Heparin
Recreational drugs	Cocaine, alcohol abuse
Total parenteral nutrition	Intralipid component

of priapism remains unclear, but it is believed to be secondary to prolonged veno-occlusion and possibly excessive neurotransmitter release. This causes anoxia of the cavernosal smooth muscle, which is then unable to contract and prevent further inflow of blood, leading to persistent erection. Anoxia therefore persists, and if the priapism is untreated, smooth muscle necrosis and cavernosal fibrosis occurs, leading to impotence in the long-term.

5.5.2 Treatment of priapism

It is important to distinguish low from high flow priapism, as low flow requires urgent treatment if erectile function is to be maintained, whereas treatment for high flow may be deferred. The diagnosis is usually apparent clinically but Doppler ultrasound will confirm the presence or absence of arterial flow. Most patients will regain potency if the priapism is aborted within 12–24 hours of onset. Priapism beyond 36 hours carries a dismal prognosis for future erections.

Blood should be aspirated immediately and sent for pO_2 estimation; low pO_2 with acidic pH indicates low flow priapism. Treatment for low flow priapism should follow the guidelines in Fig. 5.9.

The principle of shunt surgery is to create a fistula between the corpora and a venous structure. The cavernosal–spongiosal shunt at the base of the penis or in the perineum should be tried first if simple measures fail. This can be bilateral if necessary. The cavernosal–glandular fistula (Winter) is produced by pushing a tru-cut needle through the glans tissue and into the corporal tissue beneath. This has limited success and produces an ugly deformity of the glans. The cavernosal–saphenous shunt (Grayhack) is created by anastomosing the long saphenous vein to the corpora unilaterally. If shunt surgery is unsuccessful, then a decision should be made to insert a penile prosthesis at

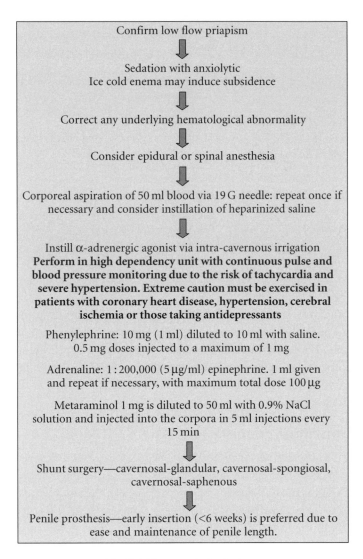

Confirm low flow priapism

⬇

Sedation with anxiolytic
Ice cold enema may induce subsidence

⬇

Correct any underlying hematological abnormality

⬇

Consider epidural or spinal anesthesia

⬇

Corporeal aspiration of 50 ml blood via 19 G needle: repeat once if
necessary and consider instillation of heparinized saline

⬇

Instill α-adrenergic agonist via intra-cavernous irrigation
**Perform in high dependency unit with continuous pulse and
blood pressure monitoring due to the risk of tachycardia and
severe hypertension. Extreme caution must be exercised in
patients with coronary heart disease, hypertension, cerebral
ischemia or those taking antidepressants**

Phenylephrine: 10 mg (1 ml) diluted to 10 ml with saline.
0.5 mg doses injected to a maximum of 1 mg

Adrenaline: 1 : 200,000 (5 μg/ml) epinephrine. 1 ml given
and repeat if necessary, with maximum total dose 100 μg

Metaraminol 1 mg is diluted to 50 ml with 0.9% NaCl
solution and injected into the corpora in 5 ml injections every
15 min

⬇

Shunt surgery—cavernosal-glandular, cavernosal-spongiosal,
cavernosal-saphenous

⬇

Penile prosthesis—early insertion (<6 weeks) is preferred due to
ease and maintenance of penile length.

Fig. 5.9 Treatment of priapism.

an early stage. This avoids the complication of a later difficult insertion due to penile fibrosis and shortening.

Suggested reading

Bedi, A., Miller, C.B., Hanson, J.L., *et al.* (1995) Association of BK virus with failure of prophylaxis against haemorrhagic cystitis following bone marrow transplantation. *J Clin Oncol,* **13,** 1103–9.

Choong, S.K.S., Walkden, M., and Kirby, R. (2000) The management of intractable haematuria. *BJU Int,* **86,** 951–9.

DeVries, C.R. and Freiha, F.S. (1990) Haemorrhagic cystitis—a review. *J Urol,* **143,** 1–9.

Friar, W.B. (1974) Formalin in the treatment of massive bladder haemorrhage. Techniques, results and complications. *Urology*, **3**, 573–6.

Korzeniowski, O.M. (1991) Urinary tract infection in the impaired host. *Med Clin North Am*, **75**, 391–404.

Lau, M.W., Temperley, S., Mehta, R., Johnson, R.J., Barnard, R.J., and Clarke, N.W. (1995) Urinary tract obstruction and nephrostomy drainage in pelvic malignant disease. *Br J Urol*, **76**, 565–9.

Levine, L.A. and Richie, J.P. (1989) Urologic complications of cyclophosphamide. *J Urol*, **141**, 1063–9.

Liu, Y.K., Harty, J.L., and Steinbock, G.S. (1990) Treatment of radiation or cyclophosphamide induced cystitis using conjugated oestrogen. *J Urol*, **144**, 41–3.

Matthews, R., Natarajan, R., *et al.* (1999) Hyperbaric oxygen therapy for radiation induced haemorrhagic cystitis. *J Urol*, **161**, 435–7.

McIntyre, J.F., Eifel, P.J., and Levenback, C. (1995) Ureteral stricture as a late complication of radiotherapy for stage 1B carcinoma of the uterine cervix. *Cancer*, **75**, 836–43.

Neild, G.H. (1999) Acute renal failure. In *Scientific basis of urology*. (ed. A.R. Mundy, J.M. Fitzpatrick, D.E. Neal, and N.J.R. George) pp. 193–204. Isis Medical Media.

O'Reilly, P.H., Testa, H.J., Lawson, R.S., Farrer, D.J., and Edwards, E.C. (1978) Diuresis renography in equivocal urinary tract obstruction. *Br J Urol*, **64**, 125–9.

Parsons, C.L. (1986) Successful management of radiation cystitis with sodium pentosulfanpolysulphate. *J Urol*, **136**, 813–14.

Platt, J.F., Rubin, J.M., Ellis, H.M., and DiPietro, M.A. (1989) Duplex Doppler US of the kidney: differentiation of obstructive from non-obstructive dilatation. *Radiology*, **17**, 515–7.

Platt, J.F., Rubin, J.M., Ellis, H.M., and DiPietro, M.A. (1989) Distinction between obstructive and non-obstructive pyelocaliectasis duplex Doppler sonography. *Am J Roentgen*, **153**, 997–1000.

Ralph, D. (2000) Priapism—Recent Advances in Urology. pp. 1–20. British Assoc. Urological Surgeons Meeting. Birmingham.

Sheenan, G., Harding, G.K., and Ronald, A.R. (1984) Advances in the treatment of urinary tract infection. *Am J Med,* **15**, 141–7.

Simmons, N.A. (1993) Recommendations for endocarditis prophylaxis. The endocarditis working Party for antimicrobial chemotherapy. *J Antimicrob Chemother*, **31**(3), 437–8.

Smith, G.I., Bunker, C.B., and Dineen, M.D. (1998) Fournier's gangrene. *Br J Urol*, **81**, 347–55.

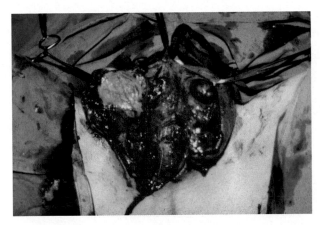

Fig. 5.3 Surgical debridement of Fournier's gangrene with extensive loss of scrotal skin.

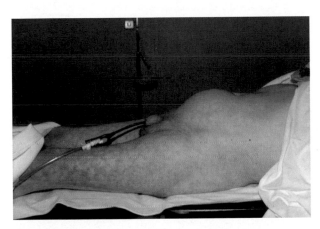

Fig. 5.5a Patient with hemorrhagic cystitis: note the suprapubic swelling, the presence of a 3-way irrigating catheter and the presence of poor peripheral circulation due to shock.

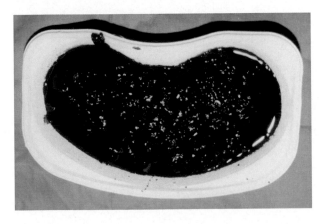

Fig. 5.5b Evacuation of clot from bladder.

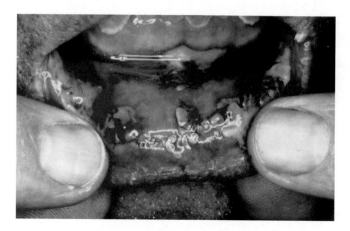

Fig. 14.2 Paraneoplastic pemphigus with marked labial ulceration and erosion.

(a)   (b)

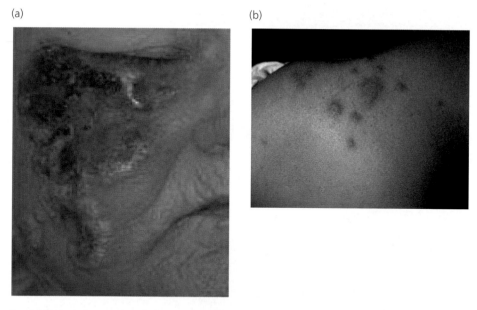

Fig. 14.3 Typical cutaneous features of Sweet's syndrome showing violaceous papules or plaques studded with pustules affecting the face (a) and torso (b).

Chapter 6

Gastrointestinal Emergencies

Richard Kennedy and Roy Spence

6.1 Introduction

Gastrointestinal complications are common in patients with a diagnosis of cancer and when assessing a cancer patient it is important to remember that not all emergencies will be due to the malignancy itself.

The most common gastrointestinal emergencies in cancer patients are:

1. Gastrointestinal bleeding
2. Gastrointestinal perforation
3. Nausea and vomiting
4. Diarrhea
5. Constipation
6. Gastrointestinal obstruction

These are discussed in more detail in the following sections (6.2–6.7)

As with any form of medical emergency it is important to take an adequate history and perform a proper examination before making a diagnosis and formulating a management plan. Table 6.1 gives some general guidelines to assessing a cancer patient with a gastrointestinal complication.

Table 6.1 Assessment of a cancer patient with a gastrointestinal complication

1. Does the patient require immediate resuscitation?
2. What factors have predisposed to the emergency?
(a) The underlying malignancy.
(b) Cancer treatment such as chemotherapy, radiotherapy or surgery.
(c) Other medications such as non-steroidal anti-inflammatory drugs, warfarin, or dexamethasone.
(d) Other medical conditions such as a previous history of peptic ulceration or inflammatory bowel disease.
3. Could this emergency be unconnected to cancer?
(a) Diarrhea may be due to food-borne bacterial or viral enteritis.
(b) Bowel perforation can be due to medication or preceded by other medical conditions such as diverticulitis or peptic ulceration.
(c) Acute abdominal pain can be due to other surgical emergencies such as cholecystitis or appendicitis.

Table 6.1 (continued)

4. What quality of life has the patient had prior to this emergency? In particular is this the terminal event of an advanced cancer or is there a possibility of returning the patient to a good quality of life? Patients with a potentially curable cancer should have aggressive management of their acute condition and be admitted to an intensive care unit if necessary.
5. What are the patient's wishes regarding medical or surgical intervention?

6.2 Gastrointestinal bleeding

This is one of the most common and dangerous gastrointestinal emergencies in cancer medicine. Only one-fifth of gastrointestinal bleeds are due to the malignancy itself, the majority being due to gastritis or benign gastrointestinal ulceration, particularly after the use of non-steroidal anti-inflammatory drugs or corticosteroids (see Table 6.2).

Table 6.2 Causes of gastrointestinal bleeding in cancer patients

Upper gastrointestinal tract
Gastritis and gastro-duodenal ulceration
   Non-steroidal anti-inflammatory drugs
   Corticosteroids
Bleeding from gastric or esophageal tumor
Esophagitis
Esophageal varices
Mallory–Weiss tear (after retching)
Post-operative complications of gastrointestinal surgery

Lower gastrointestinal tract
Bleeding from colonic tumor
Diverticular disease
Infective colitis
Post-chemotherapy colitis (especially paclitaxel or docetaxel)
Angiodysplasia

6.2.1 Clinical assessment

It is important to ask the patient or family if there are any symptoms of severe blood loss causing anemia or hypotension such as dizziness, shortness of breath or drowsiness. Also enquire about risk factors for gastro-duodenal bleeding such as the use of non-steroidal anti-inflammatory drugs, aspirin, steroids, alcohol, and smoking. If the patient is taking an anticoagulant such as warfarin the prothrombin time may require correction in order to stop the bleeding.

Ask the patients if they take beta-blocking drugs that may prevent a tachycardia and increase the risk of shock.

In patients with an upper gastrointestinal bleed the symptoms are:

1. Hematemesis that is either bright red if fresh, or dark brown if present in the stomach for more than a few minutes.

2. Melena, which may be the only symptom in some patients.

3. Epigastric or chest pain if the patient has had a Mallory–Weiss tear or peptic ulceration.

In patients with a lower gastrointestinal bleed the symptoms are:

1. Passage of dark or bright red blood per rectum depending on the site and severity of bleeding.

2. Occasionally dizziness after passing a stool.

The most sensitive indicators of significant blood loss are tachycardia and a postural fall in systolic blood pressure of greater than 20 mm Hg. Postural blood pressure can be measured from the supine to the seated position. A systolic blood pressure less than 90 mm Hg, especially with cold peripheries, suggests severe blood loss. Patients with severe bleeding may also be dyspneic due to anemia.

Abdominal tenderness in the epigastric region suggests an upper gastrointestinal source for bleeding. Rectal examination may reveal melena in upper gastrointestinal bleeding or fresh blood in lower gastrointestinal bleeds.

The patient may have pale conjunctiva due to anemia, especially when there has been chronic blood loss.

6.2.2 **Investigations**

1. *Hemoglobin* This may be low if the patient has previously had acute or chronic blood loss but can also be falsely elevated if taken too soon after hemorrhage to allow hemodilution.

2. *Platelet level* This should be checked to ensure thrombocytopenia is not contributing to bleeding.

3 *Coagulation screen* It is important to rule out an underlying coagulation abnormality that may make bleeding worse.

4. Send an urgent blood sample for blood grouping. Cross-match four units of packed red cells if significant blood loss is suspected.

Most patients will require endoscopy of either the upper or lower gastrointestinal tract as a diagnostic and often therapeutic intervention as discussed below.

6.2.3 **Management**

The principles are outlined in Fig. 6.1. Management of gastrointestinal bleeding requires a team approach involving oncologists, surgeons, physicians and the patients themselves. In some cases when the patient has advanced malignancy gastrointestinal bleeding may represent the terminal event and management may be aimed at preventing distress with analgesics and sedation as required. Patients with a reasonable expectation of good quality of life, particularly those who are potentially curable or have bled due to a side effect of medication will require active management of the bleeding. The priority is resuscitation before definitive treatment can be attempted.

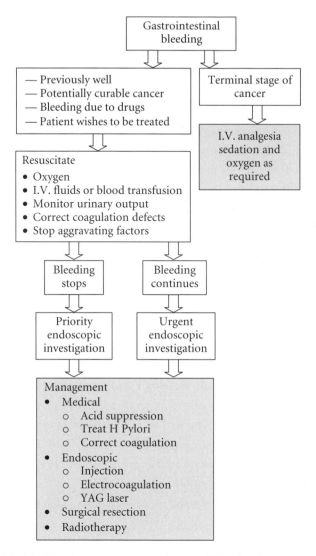

Fig. 6.1 Principles in managing gastrointestinal bleeding in a cancer patient.

Immediate management

(a) In patients with hypotension or dyspnea commence inspired oxygen via a mask.

(b) Insert a large intravenous cannula.

(c) If the patient has had severe blood loss commence transfusion of packed red cells (intravenous colloids can be used to maintain blood pressure until blood is available). The systolic blood pressure should be maintained above 90 mmHg and the pulse rate below 100 beats per minute.

(d) In hypotensive patients (where systolic blood pressure is less than 90 mmHg) insert a urinary catheter to measure urinary output. Urinary output should be kept above 0.5 ml kg^{-1} h^{-1} by maintaining the patient's blood pressure with intravenous colloid and packed red cell transfusion.

(e) In elderly patients or those with an adverse cardiovascular history a central venous line can be used to monitor intravascular blood volume.

(f) Ensure the platelet count is over 50×10^9 l^{-1} (transfuse donor platelets if less than this).

(g) Correct coagulation abnormalities with fresh frozen plasma (vitamin K, 10 mg slow I.V. may be used if immediate correction of a prolonged prothrombin time is not required). Remember to recheck the coagulation screen after transfusion of four or more units of packed red cells, as prolonged bleeding will exhaust the patient's clotting factors.

(h) Commence an acid suppressant for gastro-duodenal bleeds such as an H$_2$-antagonist or a proton pump inhibitor.

(i) Stop any medication that may contribute to bleeding such as non-steroidal anti-inflammatory drugs, aspirin, corticosteroids, warfarin, or heparin.

(j) If the patient has lower gastrointestinal bleeding and an elevated temperature suspect infective colitis and commence intravenous antibiotics that cover bowel flora, typically an intravenous cephalosporin and metronidazole.

(k) The majority of gastrointestinal bleeding will stop after the above measures. These patients should have upper or lower gastrointestinal endoscopy within 24 hours in order to identify the source of bleeding.

(l) Endoscopy needs to be performed urgently if:
  (i) The bleeding continues 12 hours post admission.
  (ii) There is continuing large volume of blood loss that fails to respond to resuscitative measures.
  (iii) The patient has a previous history of severe gastrointestinal bleeding.

(m) In patients with a known history of esophageal varices, severe hematemesis can be controlled with the insertion of a Sengstaken–Blakemore tube until resuscitation is completed and endoscopic management is available (injection or banding).

(n) Patients with inoperable, bleeding tumors may benefit from palliative radiotherapy to the affected site but this will take a few days before its maximal effect.

Medical management of gastrointestinal bleeding

(a) The majority of upper gastrointestinal bleeds are due to peptic ulceration, gastritis or esophagitis and will stop spontaneously without surgical intervention. Most of these can be managed by removing any aggravating factors such as non-steroidal anti-inflammatory drugs, alcohol or steroids and by prescribing an acid suppressing drug such as an H$_2$-receptor antagonist or proton pump inhibitor. Correction of coagulation or platelet abnormalities should also prevent further bleeding. Patients found to have a Helicobacter pylori infection on endoscopy should have appropriate antibiotic treatment. Bleeding from a tumor site may also respond to medical management but more commonly requires a surgical approach.

(b) Lower GI bleeding due to infective colitis or diverticulitis should stop with appropriate antibiotic treatment and correction of coagulation or platelet abnormalities. Lower GI tumor bleeding may respond to this treatment but usually will require a colonoscopic or surgical procedure.

Surgical management of gastrointestinal bleeding

Patients with severe ongoing blood loss (particularly when tumor site bleeding is suspected) should be considered for either an endoscopic or an open procedure (see Table 6.3).

(a) *Injection*   Seventy-eight percent of bleeding peptic ulcers can be stopped with injections of hypertonic saline and adrenaline at a concentration of 1 : 10 000 under endoscopic visualization. This method can also be successful in temporarily managing gastric or esophageal tumor bleeding.

(b) *Electrocoagulation*   This can control 70–80 percent of bleeding from peptic ulceration or upper gastrointestinal tumors. Electrodes are applied to the entry and exit points of a bleeding vessel causing thrombosis.

(c) *Laser therapy*   Nd : YAG (neodymium : yttrium–aluminum–garnet) lasers can successfully cause thrombosis in 70–80 percent of bleeding vessels in the upper or lower gastrointestinal tract.

(d) *Resection*   Severe bleeding from upper or lower gastrointestinal tumors or peptic ulceration can be controlled by local resection. Unfortunately many patients with advanced malignancy are poor surgical candidates (see Table 6.15) and 25 percent will die peri-operatively from thrombotic, hemorrhagic or infective complications.

Table 6.3 Surgical management of gastrointestinal bleeding

Source of bleeding	Treatment
Peptic ulceration or gastritis not controlled medically	Injection with adrenaline Electrocoagulation Surgical resection or undersewing
Mallory–Weiss tear	Injection with adrenaline Electrocoagulation
Esophageal varices	Sclerotherapy Banding
Gastric cancer	Injection with adrenaline Surgical resection
Colonic cancer	Surgical resection Endoscopic laser
Diverticular disease	Surgical resection

6.3 **Gastrointestinal perforation**

Gastrointestinal perforation, in the cancer patient, is most often due to weakening of the gut wall at the site of a tumor. Another important cause is tumor necrosis during radiotherapy or cytotoxic chemotherapy. Perforation due to peptic ulceration is also common and is often associated with the use of non-steroidal anti-inflammatory drugs or corticosteroids. Other causes for perforation are listed in Table 6.4.

Table 6.4 Causes for gastrointestinal perforation in oncologic patients

Malignant infiltration of gut wall
Non-malignant
Peptic ulceration (especially with the use of non-steroidal anti-inflammatory drugs and corticosteroids)
Surgical dehiscence
Colonoscopy
Radiation enteritis
Diverticulitis
Infective colitis
Typhlitis (particularly after paclitaxel therapy, see section on diarrhea)

6.3.1 **Clinical assessment**

Typically the patient with gastrointestinal perforation complains of a sudden onset of abdominal pain, nausea, vomiting and fever.

If the patient or relatives can give a history, inquire about non-steroidal anti-inflammatory drugs or corticosteroids that can predispose to perforation. Also ask if the patient has recently received chemotherapy as this may cause perforation by weakening the bowel wall at a site of tumor. Chemotherapy can also make the patient thrombocytopenic, anemic, or neutropenic, which will be important if surgery is being considered. Remember to specifically ask the patient if they have been receiving paclitaxel or docetaxel chemotherapy as these drugs can predispose to typhlitis leading to perforation (see Section 6.5). Consider radiation enteritis or local tumor necrosis as a cause for perforation if the patient has recently had radiotherapy involving bowel.

Ask if the patient was complaining of a fever or diarrhea prior to the perforation, which would suggest an infective cause for perforation.

Remember that if the patient has recently had a surgical procedure there may be a risk of dehiscence of anastomosis or wound.

Typically the patient presents with signs of peritonism including severe abdominal tenderness and guarding, abdominal distension, and absent bowel sounds. The patient may also have an elevated temperature and be hypotensive if there has been a large amount of spillage of gastrointestinal contents into the peritoneal cavity.

The symptoms and signs, however, may be reduced or absent if the patient is receiving corticosteroid treatment.

6.3.2 Investigations

The physical examination along with the history of the preceding condition, treatment and symptom onset are often most important guides to diagnosis. The following investigations may help confirm the clinician's suspicion and the patient's suitability for surgery.

1. White cell count may demonstrate a leukocytosis.

2. Platelet count and coagulation screen to ensure patient is safe for surgery.

3. An erect abdominal X-ray demonstrating free air under the diaphragm helps confirm gastrointestinal perforation but *50 percent of patients with perforation will not have this finding.*

6.3.3 Management

The principles are outlined in Fig. 6.2. Patients with a reasonable quality of life, particularly those with potentially curable disease, a low tumor burden or in whom perforation

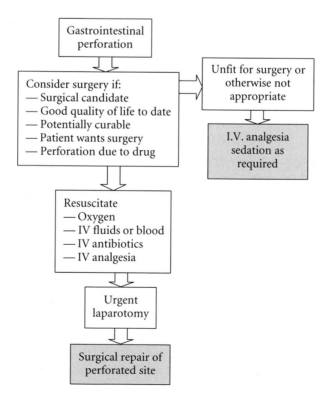

Fig. 6.2 Principles in management of gastrointestinal perforation.

Table 6.5 Surgical procedures for gastrointestinal perforation

Site of perforation	Procedure
Stomach	Oversew with omental patch
Small bowel	Resection and re-anastomosis or ileostomy
Large bowel	Resection and re-anastomosis or colostomy

is due to medication should be resuscitated with a view to surgery. It is important to discuss the situation fully with the patient (or their closest family if the patient is unable to communicate) to ensure that their wishes are adhered.

Despite surgery 40 percent of cancer patients with gut perforation will die in the peri-operative period, mostly from bacterial peritonitis.

Immediate management

(a) Insert a large gauge intravenous cannula.

(b) Supply oxygen via a mask.

(c) Use intravenous colloids if the patient is hypotensive. Maintain systolic blood pressure above 90 mmHg and a urinary output of at least 0.5 ml kg^{-1} h^{-1}.

(d) Insert a urinary catheter to monitor urinary output if the patient is hypotensive.

(e) Commence analgesia, typically intravenous morphine or diamorphine with a suitable anti-emetic such as cyclizine.

(f) Commence intravenous antibiotics, which cover bowel flora such as metronidazole and a cephalosporin.

(g) Refer urgently to a gastrointestinal surgeon for consideration of a laparotomy and definitive management (see Table 6.5).

(h) Patients with a poor performance status or advanced intra-abdominal disease may be too unwell to undergo anesthesia or the chances of recovery from surgery may be considered too small (see Table 6.15). This therefore represents the terminal phase of the disease in this group and symptoms should be managed with adequate analgesia (usually parenteral diamorphine) and sedation as required.

6.4 **Nausea and vomiting**

These symptoms are present in 50 percent of patients with advanced cancer and 70–80 percent of those receiving chemotherapy. Nausea and vomiting have one of the largest impacts on quality of life in patients undergoing care for cancer and can make other symptoms such as pain or fatigue worse. Cytotoxic drugs and opioids are the major causes of nausea and vomiting. Others are listed in Table 6.6.

The selection of appropriate prophylactic anti-emetics should prevent most cytotoxic related emesis (Table 6.7).

Table 6.6 Causes of nausea and vomiting in patients with cancer

Direct effect on chemoreceptor trigger zone
Cytotoxic chemotherapy
Opioid drugs
Antibiotics
Non-steroidal anti-inflammatory drugs
Electrolyte disturbance especially renal impairment and hypercalcemia
Infection

Gut irritation or disturbance in motility
Gastritis or ulceration (especially with NSAIDS or corticosteroids)
Cytotoxic chemotherapy
Constipation
Extrinsic pressure
Carcinoma of gastrointestinal tract
Gastric outlet obstruction
Duodenal ulceration
Small bowel obstruction
Abdominal/pelvic radiotherapy
Electrolyte disturbance

Cerebral causes
Anxiety
Anticipatory vomiting
Cerebral malignancy
Altered taste due to chemotherapy

Direct effect on vomiting center
Raised intracranial pressure

Vestibular disturbance due to cytotoxic chemotherapy

Cough-induced

Table 6.7 Examples of chemotherapy drugs causing nausea and vomiting along with appropriate prophylactic anti-emetics

Low risk
Dopamine antagonist, antihistamine or anticholinergic prior to and following treatment
    Vinca alkaloids
    Oral cyclophosphamide
    Oral chlorambucil
    Bleomycin
    5-fluorouracil
    Fludarabine

Moderate risk
Dopamine antagonist, antihistamine or anticholinergic with corticosteroid prior to and following treatment.
    Intravenous cyclophosphamide
    Taxanes
    Etoposide
    Gemcitabine
    Methotrexate

Table 6.7 (continued)

High risk
Oral or intravenous 5HT$_3$ antagonist prior to and following treatment which may be combined with corticosteroid, dopamine antagonist, antihistamine or anticholinergic if required.
  Cisplatin
  Carboplatin
  Dacarbazine
  Anthracyclines
  Ifosfamide
  High dose cyclophosphamide

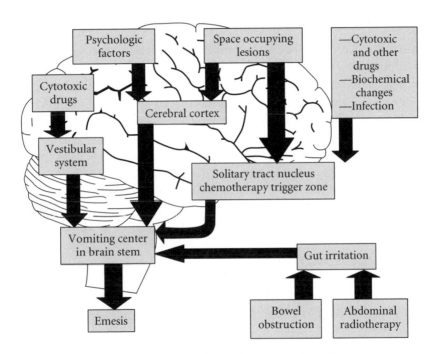

Fig. 6.3 Physiologic pathway of nausea and vomiting.

In order to assess the cause of nausea and vomiting an understanding of the emetic process is required (see Fig. 6.3). In most cases, especially in advanced cancer, the causes for vomiting are multifactorial. Consequently, no one anti-emetic treatment is effective for all patients.

An adequate history followed by a clinical examination will reveal most underlying causes for these symptoms.

6.4.1 Clinical assessment

Table 6.8 gives the National Cancer Institute grading for severity of vomiting. Vomiting which occurs six or more times per day (grade III or greater) is severe and usually requires admission to a hospital ward.

Table 6.8 National Cancer Institute grading for vomiting

Grade 1	Grade 2	Grade 3	Grade 4
1 episode in 24 hours over pre-treatment level of vomiting	2–5 episodes in 24 hours over pre-treatment level of vomiting	≥6 episodes in 24 hours over pre-treatment level of vomiting or need for intravenous fluids	Requiring parenteral nutrition or consequences requiring intensive care or hemodynamic collapse

Ask the patient about ongoing cancer treatment, specifically any emetogenic chemotherapy or radiotherapy which may have involved small bowel or brain.

Inquire about the content of vomitus. Recognizable food suggests upper gastrointestinal disease whereas lower gastrointestinal disease results in feculent vomiting. A large volume of vomit is consistent with a mechanical cause whereas retching with little or no vomit suggests a central cause. Early morning vomiting can be a sign of raised intracranial pressure especially if the patient complains of neurologic symptoms. If the patient is suffering from vertigo suspect vestibular disease.

Remember that if the patient has recently commenced an opioid about one-third will feel nauseated in the first week. This usually resolves spontaneously.

When examining the patient ensure that the temperature is not elevated indicating infection. Also look for signs of dehydration, particularly dry mucous membranes, poor skin turgor, concentrated urine or no urinary output.

Examine the abdomen to rule out gastrointestinal obstruction or tenderness due to peptic ulceration and perform a rectal examination if fecal impaction is a possibility.

Check for signs of central nervous system disease including fundoscopy if appropriate.

6.4.2 Investigations

These are largely governed by the history and examination. In most patients with nausea and vomiting it is appropriate to check:

1. *Serum urea and electrolytes* A raised creatinine and urea confirm dehydration. A low potassium confirms persistent vomiting. A raised calcium may confirm hypercalcemia as an underlying cause for the symptoms.

2. *Urinary specific gravity* This is a simple bedside urinary dipstick test which will confirm dehydration if the specific gravity is greater than 1.001. Urine can also be sent for microbiological analysis to rule out a urinary tract infection.

3. A plain abdominal X-ray is appropriate if small bowel obstruction is suspected.

6.4.3 **Management**

The principles of management of nausea and vomiting are summarized in Fig. 6.4.

1. If the patient is taking adequate oral fluids and the vomiting is less than 6 times per day it may be possible to manage their symptoms in the outpatient setting with oral fluids and anti-emetics.

2. Those with severe vomiting, dehydration, hypotension, or an inability to take adequate fluids should be admitted for resuscitation and appropriate treatment.

Table 6.9 gives the appropriate management for the most common causes of emesis in cancer patients.

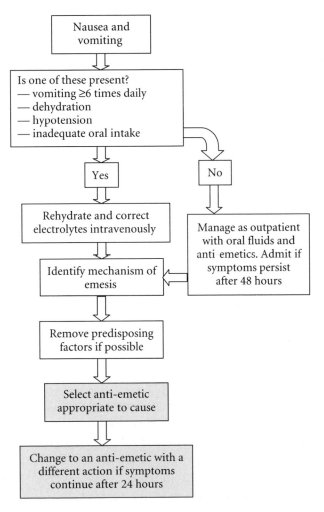

Fig. 6.4 Principles in managing nausea and vomiting.

Table 6.9 Management of nausea and vomiting

Cause and treatment	Examples
Cytotoxic chemotherapy Agents, which act on chemoreceptor, trigger zone	$5HT_3$ Antagonists ± corticosteroids ± antihistamines, anticholinergics, or dopamine antagonists
Radiotherapy Agents acting on chemoreceptor trigger zone, particularly $5HT_3$ antagonists	$5HT_3$ Antagonists ± antihistamines, anticholinergics, or dopamine antagonists,
Constipation Relieve constipation	Oral/rectal laxatives (see Section 6.6)
Gastritis/Peptic ulceration Reduce gastric acid secretion	Antihistamines, anticholinergics, or dopamine antagonists + proton pump inhibitor
Small bowel obstruction Relieve pressure in gastrointestinal system	See Section 6.7
Gastric Outlet Obstruction Improve peristalsis	Dopamine antagonists ± Surgical bypass or stenting
Infection Treat infection to relieve pyrexia	Antibiotics, + Paracetamol + Rehydration
Hypercalcemia Increase calcium excretion	Rehydration with intravenous fluids, + IV bisphosphonates
Renal impairment Reduce uremia Prevent chemotherapy trigger zone activation	Dopamine antagonist ± dialysis if appropriate
Intracranial metastases Reduce mass effect	Corticosteroids + cranial irradiation
Vestibular disease Reduce activity of vestibular system	Antihistamines/anticholinergics

Immediate management

(a) *Rehydration*   Patients who have become severely dehydrated particularly if they are anuric or hypotensive will require hospital admission for intravenous fluids. A urinary output of at least $1\ ml\ kg^{-1}\ h^{-1}$ with a fall in urine specific gravity indicates adequate rehydration.

(b) *Electrolyte correction*   Patients with severe vomiting will often require potassium supplementation.

(c) Identification and correction of the predisposing factors.

(d) *Anti-emetics*   The majority of patients will require anti-emetics to control their symptoms. Those with severe vomiting will require parenteral (subcutaneous, rectal or buccal) medication as opposed to the oral route. It is important to understand where these drugs act and their side effects in order to use them most effectively. As nausea and vomiting are often multifactorial a combination of drugs may be required but as more drugs are taken more side effects occur. A suggested method for introducing anti-emetics is given in Fig. 6.5 but patients with severe vomiting after chemotherapy will most likely require a $5HT_3$ antagonist early in their management.

The anti-emetics

Serotonin receptor antagonists ($5HT_3$ antagonists)   The serotonin type-3 receptors within the chemoreceptor trigger zone (CTZ) of the brain are particularly important

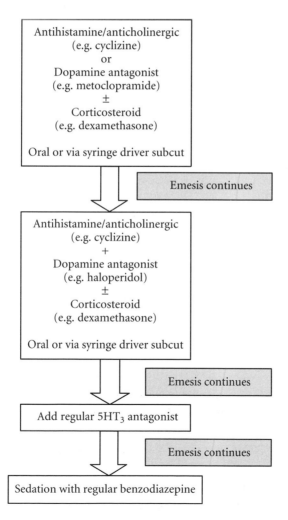

Fig. 6.5 Suggested pathway in the use of anti-emetic treatment.

in the mechanism of cytotoxic chemotherapy and radiotherapy-related nausea and vomiting. As well as a direct effect on the CTZ, both chemotherapy and radiotherapy cause a release of serotonin from the gut that acts on the receptors in the CTZ. Several $5HT_3$ antagonists are now used in the prevention and treatment of cytotoxic and radiotherapy-related emesis.

Side effects

- Constipation
- Headache

Examples

- Ondansetron 8 mg oral or intravenously twice daily
- Tropisetron 5 mg oral or intravenously once daily.

Corticosteroids   Corticosteroids have most of their effect on the CTZ. Their main use is in the prevention and treatment of cytotoxic emesis. Steroids are particularly useful in late emesis related to the use of platinum-based drugs. They can be safely combined with other anti-emetics such as $5HT_3$ antagonists or antihistamines.

Side effects

- Hyperglycemia in diabetic patients necessitating careful blood sugar monitoring.
- Psychiatric symptoms such as depression or elation during their usage.
- Peptic ulceration, particularly in those with a previous history.

Examples

- Dexamethasone 8 mg intravenously
- Dexamethasone 4 mg oral twice daily.

Antihistamines/anticholinergics   These drugs act directly at the levels of the vomiting center and vestibular centers of the brain stem. They are active against most causes of vomiting but are less effective than $5HT_3$ antagonists in cytotoxic or radiotherapy-related emesis.

Side effects

- Sedation
- Dry mouth
- Blurred vision
- Constipation

Examples

- *Antihistamine*   Cyclizine 50 mg oral or intravenously three times daily or 150 mg subcutaneously over 24 hours.
- Anticholinergic: Hyoscine hydrobromide oral 300 mg six hourly.

Dopamine antagonists These drugs act on dopamine receptors within the CTZ. Domperidone and metoclopramide also improve gut motility, which can be useful in gastric outlet or partial bowel obstruction. They are less effective than $5HT_3$ antagonists in cytotoxic or radiotherapy-related emesis but can be safely combined with them.

Side effects

- Extrapyramidal symptoms (especially in young adults and children). These side effects are less common with domperidone, which does not cross the blood–brain barrier as easily as the other dopamine antagonists.
- Abdominal cramps, particularly in gastrointestinal obstruction.
- Diarrhea.

Examples

- Metoclopramide 10 mg oral / intravenously three times daily or 40 mg subcutaneously over 24 hours.
- Domperidone 10 mg oral six times daily or 30 mg rectally six times daily.
- Haloperidol 1.5 mg oral three times daily.
- Prochlorperazine 10 mg oral three times daily or 3 mg twice daily buccally.

Benzodiazepines These drugs appear to work by their anxiolytic, sedative and amnesic properties. They are particularly useful in treating anticipatory nausea and vomiting and also are used to sedate patients where other methods of controlling cytotoxic emesis have failed.

Side effects

- Drowsiness
- Confusion
- Ataxia
- Respiratory depression

Example

- Lorazepam 1–2 mg oral or intravenously twice daily.

6.4.4 Problems with nausea and vomiting specific to chemotherapy

Platinum-based chemotherapy

Platinum-based chemotherapy (cisplatin or carboplatin) regimens are particularly emetogenic. Nausea and vomiting is best avoided in the first 48 hours by using a combination of a $5HT_3$ antagonist and dexamethasone. Twenty percent of patients suffer late emesis, which can last up to two weeks post-chemotherapy. This can often be controlled with a combination of oral dexamethasone and cyclizine.

It is important to remember that patients who are receiving cisplatin-based chemotherapy are at particular risk of renal tubular damage and subsequent renal impairment if they become dehydrated. Admit these patients early for intravenous fluids if vomiting is not controlled quickly by oral anti-emetics.

Anticipatory emesis

Anticipatory nausea and vomiting is a psychologic condition that may occur prior to chemotherapy in patients who expect to be unwell during treatment. This particularly affects those who have had severe nausea and vomiting during previous cycles of treatment. Symptoms may respond to supportive psychotherapy and light sedation with benzodiazepine drugs. It is best avoided by using adequate prophylactic anti-emetics along with cytotoxic treatment and ensuring that these drugs are changed in future cycles if they do not control vomiting.

6.5 Diarrhea

Diarrhea is defined as the frequent passage of unformed liquid stools. The cause in cancer patients is often multifactorial and can include direct cytotoxic damage to the intestinal epithelium, inflammation, infection and antibiotics. The major causes are listed in Table 6.10. One of the most common causes is the overuse of laxatives.

In assessing the patient with diarrhea a thorough history and examination will often reveal the underlying cause.

Table 6.10 Causes of diarrhea in cancer patients

Drugs
Laxatives
Cytotoxic chemotherapy
Antibiotics
Antacids

Abdominal or pelvic radiotherapy

Fecal impaction

Infection (including typhilitis)

Malabsorption
Bowel resection
Pancreatic carcinoma

Malignancy
Pelvic tumor
Carcinoid syndrome

6.5.1 Clinical assessment

It is important to record the frequency and consistency of stool passage. This will provide a guide to the success of treatment. Also, sometimes the patient's concept of

Table 6.11 NCI criteria for grading severity of diarrhea

	Grade 1	Grade 2	Grade 3	Grade 4
Without colostomy	Increase of <4 stools/day over pre-treatment	Increase of 4–6 stools per day or nocturnal stools	Increase of ≥7 stools or incontinence or dehydration	Consequences requiring intensive care or hemodynamic collapse
With colostomy	Mild increase in loose watery colostomy output compared to pre-treatment	Moderate increase in loose watery stools not interfering with normal daily activity	Severe increase in loose watery stools interfering with normal daily activity	Consequences requiring intensive care or hemodynamic collapse

diarrhea may be different to the physician's. It is useful to grade the severity of diarrhea using a recognized scale (see Table 6.11). Seven or more loose bowel motions per day is classified as severe diarrhea (grade III or above).

Inquire about blood in the diarrhea as this would suggest either an infective cause for the diarrhea or severe mucositis involving the gastrointestinal tract.

Ask about any medications that the patient is currently taking, particularly laxatives, antibiotics or antacids that can cause diarrhea. If the patient has recently completed a course of antibiotics this may predispose to a pseudomembranous colitis (Clostridium difficile infection).

If the patient was constipated prior to the onset of diarrhea consider a diagnosis of fecal impaction.

It is important to rule out an infective cause for the symptoms if the patient has had an elevated temperature, sweats or rigors, particularly if he/she has had any close contacts with other individuals with diarrhea.

If the patient has received recent chemotherapy specifically ask about:

1. *Irinotecan* (Campto©) Diarrhea associated with this drug has a specific management as discussed later in this section.

2. *Paclitaxel or docetaxel* These drugs have a rare but potentially life-threatening side effect that presents with diarrhea (see typhlitis discussed under management of specific causes of diarrhea).

3. Mouth ulceration, particularly in patients receiving 5-fluorouracil which can cause mucositis affecting the whole gastrointestinal tract.

Look for signs of dehydration due to severe diarrhea such as dry mucous membranes, poor skin turgor, low blood pressure or postural fall in systolic blood pressure >20 mmHg and poor (or no) urinary output.

An elevated temperature indicates an infective cause for the diarrhea. Examine the abdomen for tenderness suggesting intestinal inflammation. Remember to perform a rectal examination where fecal impaction may be a possible underlying cause for diarrhea.

6.5.2 **Investigations**

These will largely be guided by the history and investigation.

1. In patients where an infective cause is suspected, fecal samples should be sent for bacteriologic analysis. Inform the bacteriologist if the patient has recently received antibiotics so that toxin assays can be performed to exclude pseudomembranous colitis.
2. If the patient has had severe diarrhea (seven or more loose stools per day) or appears dehydrated send a blood sample for serum electrolytes.
    (a) A raised urea and creatinine confirms dehydration.
    (b) A low potassium is consistent with electrolyte loss in severe diarrhea.
3. Urinary specific gravity which will confirm dehydration if the specific gravity is elevated.
4. In patients receiving chemotherapy a full blood picture should be requested to rule out neutropenia.
5. If fecal impaction is suspected a plain abdominal film may confirm a full rectum and colon.

6.5.3 **Management**

The principles are outlined in Fig. 6.6.

1. Patients with mild to moderate diarrhea (six or less loose bowel motions daily) may maintain adequate hydration with oral fluids (4 L of fluid orally per day) and oral antidiarrheals. This group of patients can be managed in the outpatient setting but should be admitted for management if symptoms continue beyond 48 hours on oral treatment.
2. Those with severe diarrhea or signs of dehydration, hypotension, electrolyte imbalance or an inability to take adequate oral fluids will require immediate admission for resuscitation prior to definitive management of the diarrhea.

Immediate management

(a) Insert an intravenous cannula.

(b) Commence intravenous crystalloids with potassium supplementation as required.

(c) If the systolic blood pressure is less than 90 mm Hg give intravenous colloids with crystalloids and insert a urinary catheter to monitor urinary output. Consider the use of a central venous line to monitor the intravascular volume in the elderly or patients with an adverse cardiac history.

(d) Keep the urinary output above 0.5 ml $kg^{-1} h^{-1}$ with intravenous fluids.

(e) If the patient has an elevated temperature or is neutropenic commence intravenous antibiotics that cover bowel flora. For example, metronidazole with an aminoglycoside and a cephalosporin intravenously. The choice of antibiotics may be changed with advice from a microbiologist once fecal cultures are available.

(f) Commence an oral antidiarrheal (see below).

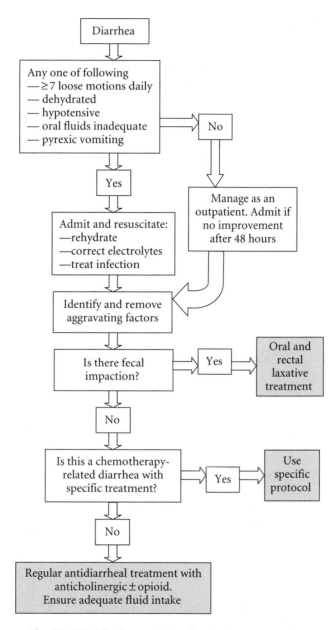

Fig. 6.6 Principles in managing diarrhea in cancer patient.

Antidiarrheal drugs

Most patients will require the use of an antidiarrheal agent along with rehydration in order to control their symptoms. These drugs can be divided into anticholinergics and opioid-based treatments.

Anticholinergic antidiarrheal drugs   These drugs block the action of cholinergic receptors in the gut wall. This results in a reduction in peristalsis and gut secretions. They are preferable to opioid-based antidiarrheals as a first line treatment since they cause less drowsiness or sedation. These drugs are particularly useful in managing diarrhea due to radiotherapy affecting the small bowel. Their use in managing irinotecan-related diarrhea is discussed below.

Side effects

- Abdominal cramps and bloating
- Urinary retention
- Dry mouth

Example

- Oral loperamide hydrochloride 4 mg initially then 2 mg after each loose stool to a maximum of 16 mg daily.

Opioid antidiarrheal drugs   These drugs work on opioid receptors in the gut wall resulting in increased intestinal smooth muscle tone, suppression of peristalsis, and increased anal sphincter tone. They can be combined with the anticholinergic drugs when diarrhea is difficult to control.

Side effects

- Drowsiness
- Nausea

Example

- Oral codeine phosphate 30 mg four times daily.

Management of specific causes of diarrhea

Once the patient has been resuscitated and the diarrhea controlled the underlying causative factors should be identified and managed. In the case of diarrhea related to known medications this may simply involve removing the offending drug. In patients who have been misusing laxatives explaining the correct usage may prevent further episodes of diarrhea. The managements of more specific causes of diarrhea are discussed below.

Infective diarrhea   Patients suspected of having infective diarrhea must have fecal samples sent to a bacteriology department in order to identify the organisms responsible. If the patient is relatively well an oral antibiotic that covers most bacteriological causes of infective colitis may be used initially (such as oral ciprofloxacin). In more severe infections or in patients with neutropenia a wider spectrum intravenous antibiotic regimen is required.

The management of Clostridium difficile infections will require advice from a bacteriologist. Typically this is managed with oral vancomycin or oral metronidazole.

There is some controversy over the use of antidiarrheal drugs in patients with an infective cause for their diarrhea as they may prolong symptoms by preventing the clearance of enterotoxins. Despite this antidiarrheals are still recommended in severe infective diarrhea as they improve patient comfort and reduce fluid and electrolyte loss.

Typhlitis　Typhlitis is a necrotizing infection of the cecum that is fatal in 30 percent of cases. The organisms involved are often gram-negative anaerobic bacteria. It is seen in chemotherapy-induced neutropenia, particularly when wide spectrum antibiotics have been used. The taxoid family of drugs (paclitaxel and docetaxel) are the cytotoxic drugs most commonly associated with this condition.

The patient with typhlitis may complain of:

● Right iliac fossa pain

● Diarrhea (may be bloody)

● Fever

A plain abdominal X-ray may demonstrate dilatation of the cecum or thickening of the cecal wall. This can be confirmed with an ultrasound scan.

If not managed quickly with intravenous fluids and antibiotics (to cover bowel flora) the patient will develop bowel necrosis, perforation and septicemia. In patients with severe bloody diarrhea, septic shock or perforation an urgent bowel resection may be required and the patient should be managed with a team approach including a physician, oncologist, and surgeon.

Fecal impaction　This may be a particular problem in the elderly or those receiving opioid-based drugs. Typically these patients initially develop constipation and then complain of frequent loose motions accompanied by colicky abdominal pain. There may also be a history of fecal incontinence. A rectal examination will demonstrate fecal loading. A plain abdominal X-ray showing feces in the rectum and ascending colon confirms the diagnosis. These patients, paradoxically, require oral and often rectal laxatives in order to relieve their symptoms (see Section 6.6).

Radiotherapy-related diarrhea　The majority of patients receiving pelvic or abdominal radiotherapy will develop diarrhea secondary to bowel irradiation. This symptom is more common when larger fractions of treatment are used and is due to direct damage to the replicating cells of the gut lining.

This is usually a self-limiting condition that will recover 1–3 months after completion of treatment. In the acute setting it can be controlled with regular oral loperamide with the addition of codeine phosphate if required. Occasionally some patients develop severe malabsorption due to small bowel irradiation and require total parenteral nutrition.

Cytotoxic chemotherapy-related diarrhea   The diarrhea caused by cytotoxic drugs, particularly irinotecan and 5-fluorouracil can significantly increase morbidity and mortality if not properly managed. Cytotoxic drugs can cause a loss of cells lining the absorptive surface of the small and large intestine. This results in an imbalance between secretion and absorption of fluid in the bowel leading to a loss of water and electrolytes as diarrhea. Irinotecan can also cause diarrhea due to a reduced gut transit time (a cholinergic effect) within the first 24 hours following administration. This form of diarrhea usually responds well to anticholinergic treatment and is distinct from diarrhea occurring after 24 hours which is more likely to be due to mucosal damage.

It is important to grade the severity of diarrhea (see Table 6.11) as this information will be required by the prescribing oncologist in order to adjust or perhaps omit the next dose of chemotherapy.

Management of irinotecan (Campto©)-related diarrhea

1. If diarrhea occurs within 24 hours of infusion give atropine 250 μg subcutaneously and premedicate with atropine in future cycles of treatment.

2. If diarrhea occurs after 24 hours commence oral ipratropium bromide 2 mg oral every 2 hours after each liquid stool until 12 hours after the last for a maximum of 48 hours. In this situation it is appropriate to exceed the usual limit of 16 mg of ipratropium bromide in a day.

3. Arrange admission to a hospital ward if:

    (a) Diarrhea continues after 48 hours of ipratropium bromide. The patient will usually require intravenous rehydration and investigation to rule out infection.
    (b) The patient has an elevated temperature. This may indicate infection and in the case of irinotecan the patient should be prescribed intravenous ciprofloxacin.
    (c) The patient is dehydrated and requires intravenous fluids.

Management of diarrhea due to other cytotoxic drugs

    (a) Ensure adequate rehydration, especially when treatment contains a platinum drug that may cause renal impairment if the patient becomes dehydrated.
    (b) Send fecal samples for bacteriological analysis.
    (c) Administer oral ipratropium bromide 4 mg then 2 mg after each loose bowel motion.
    (d) If diarrhea fails to be adequately controlled add oral codeine phosphate 30 mg four times daily (note that this may cause drowsiness, particularly in the elderly).
    (e) If diarrhea still persists attempt reduction of small bowel fluid secretion with octreotide 100–200 μg subcutaneously three times daily.

Remember that patients receiving chemotherapy are also at an increased risk from infective causes of diarrhea, particularly during the periods of neutropenia. Patients presenting with diarrhea along with pyrexia or a low neutrophil count should commence widespread antibiotics as discussed above under infective diarrhea. If the patient has acute abdominal pain, pyrexia or blood in the diarrhea suspect typhlitis, particularly if they are receiving paclitaxel or docetaxel chemotherapy (see above).

6.6 **Constipation**

This is defined as the passage of hard fecal material less frequently and with more difficulty than is normal for the patient.

The causes can be divided into the four main groups listed in Table 6.12 although it is important to realize that constipation is often multifactorial in origin. The most common factor in cancer patients is the use of opioid analgesics that have a direct inhibitory effect on gut motility. Oral laxatives should be routinely prescribed along with opioid drugs.

As there are many potential causes for constipation in a patient with cancer it is essential to perform a proper assessment prior to definitive treatment. This involves a detailed history to help identify the factors involved and a full examination including the anus and rectum. The temptation is often to skip the history and examination and treat

Table 6.12 Causes of constipation in cancer patients

Directly cancer-related
Constipation is a direct effect of the malignant disease and includes:
    Tumor invasion of bowel
        Advanced colonic malignancy
        Metastatic disease from elsewhere
    Extrinsic compression of bowel
        Advanced tumor within pelvis
        Diffuse intraperitoneal metastases
        Malignant ascites
    Hypercalcemia
    Neurologic
        Spinal cord compression
        Cauda equina syndrome
        Direct tumor invasion of autonomic nerves supplying bowel

---

Treatment-related
This may either be treatment for the cancer directly, managing side effects of treatment or analgesia:
    Cancer treatment
        Vincristine and vinorelbine autonomic neuropathy
    Anti-emetics
        Serotonin antagonists
        Cyclizine
    Anti-spasmodic
        Atropine salts
    Analgesics
        Morphine preparations
        Codeine preparations
        Non-steroidal anti-inflammatory drugs

Table 6.12 (continued)

Local anal/rectal pathology
Often the pain associated with defecation prevents normal bowel habit:
    Hemorrhoids
    Anal fissures
    Proctitis
    Anorectal abcess

Debilitation
The secondary effects of advanced disease or long periods of in-patient treatment for cancer can cause constipation due to:
    Poor dietary intake
    Poor fluid intake
    Weakness and immobility
    Inconvenient or unfamiliar toilet arrangements
    Depression
    Confusion
    Hypokalemia

---

immediately with laxatives. Although this approach is often successful there is a risk of neglecting simple factors that could be easily rectified such as inconvenient toilet facilities or inappropriate medication. It is also important to consider serious underlying conditions such as hypercalcemia, malignant bowel obstruction or spinal cord compression.

6.6.1 Clinical assessment

An accurate history is essential in the effective management of constipation.

Inquire about the frequency and consistency of stools. Remember that a diagnosis of constipation can only be made when the patient's bowel habit is significantly less frequent than is *normal for them*. Colicky left iliac fossa pain is typical in constipation.

Ask if the patient is complaining of nausea or vomiting as severe symptoms along with abdominal pain may suggest bowel obstruction.

If the patient is complaining of neurologic symptoms consider spinal cord compression or the cauda equina syndrome. A full neurologic examination must be carried out if there is a history of leg weakness, numbness in the lower limbs or perianal area or urinary dysfunction (but remember that severe constipation can also cause urinary retention or incontinence). Ask about the use of vinca alkaloid chemotherapy (such as vincristine or vindesine) as this family of drugs can cause an autonomic neuropathy leading to severe constipation.

Specifically ask about thirst and polyuria which may suggest a diagnosis of hypercalcemia underlying the constipation.

It is also important to distinguish true diarrhea from *constipation with fecal overflow*. The latter tends to follow a history of constipation, consists of thin watery fecal material and is usually associated with other symptoms of constipation such as cramping.

Enquire if the patient is taking opioid medication, as this is one of the most common predisposing factors of constipation in cancer patients.

When examining the patient remember that constipation may lead to confusion in the elderly. The patient may have malodorous breath and complain of fecal leakage due to severe constipation with overflow.

Examine the abdomen for an easily palpable colon with an indentable fecal mass. A fecal mass is usually mobile (unlike tumor masses which are fixed). Look for signs of bowel obstruction (see Section 6.7) that include general abdominal distension, resonance to percussion and high-pitched bowel sounds.

Ensure there are no neurologic signs in the lower limbs consistent with a spinal cord lesion.

Digital rectal examination

This is essential if constipation is suspected. The exception is in the case of patients receiving chemotherapy where there may be a risk of introducing infection during the period of neutropenia.

A rectal examination will allow identification of:

- Fecal impaction
- Tumor masses
- Painful anal fissuring or ulceration
- Painful hemorrhoids
- Loss of peri-anal sensation in spinal cord compression or cauda equina syndrome
- Empty rectum in bowel obstruction.

6.6.2 **Clinical investigations**

These are usually only required if constipation does not respond to laxatives or a serious underlying cause such as hypercalcemia, neurologic disease or bowel obstruction is suspected.

1. *Serum electrolytes*
    (a) A raised urea or creatinine suggests dehydration that can either be the cause for constipation or be due to poor fluid intake secondary to constipation.
    (b) A raised calcium (when corrected for the serum albumin level) indicates constipation due to hypercalcemia.

2. *Plain erect abdominal X-ray* (see Fig. 6.7)
    (a) This will demonstrate fecal matter in the colon and rectum in constipation.
    (b) Multiple fluid levels, dilated bowel or an empty rectum would be consistent with bowel obstruction (see Section 6.7).

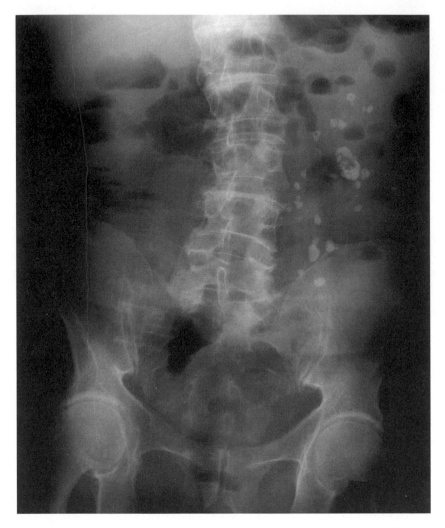

Fig. 6.7 Erect plain abdominal X-ray film demonstrating multiple fluid levels due to small bowel obstruction.

6.6.3 **Management**

This is guided by the history and physical findings. Before commencing treatment it is important to remove any underlying cause if possible. The principles are outlined in Fig. 6.8.

1. Ensure adequate diet and fluid intake.

2. Patients complaining of nausea and vomiting, especially when bowel obstruction is suspected should be admitted for treatment (see bowel obstruction, Section 6.7).

3. Commence an oral laxative (see below). This will take 1–2 days for full effect.

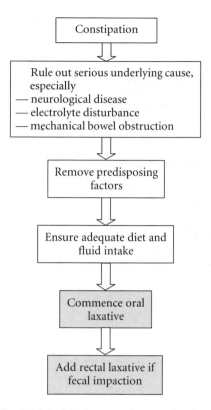

Fig. 6.8 Principles in managing constipation.

4. Rectal laxatives are useful for fecal impaction but must be combined with an oral laxative regimen,
   (a) For hard fecal material use a softening enema such as arachis oil overnight followed by a stimulant enema such as a phosphate.
   (b) For soft fecal material use a stimulant enema such as a phosphate.
   (c) When large amounts of fecal material are impacted high in the rectum enemas can be given via a Foley catheter.
   (d) In severe impaction fecal material may need to be removed manually.

Laxatives

The oral stimulant laxatives   These increase intestinal motility and are particularly useful in preventing and treating constipation associated with opioid use. They can be particularly effective when combined with a fecal softener such as poloxamer "188". Docusate has both a stimulant and softening action.

Their main side effect is crampy abdominal pain limiting their use in some patients, especially those developing bowel obstruction.

Dantron (danthron) is now only recommended for use in terminally ill patients, as it is a potential carcinogen in animal models.

Side effects

- Abdominal cramps
- Discoloration of urine (dantron)

Examples

- Oral docusate 25 mg three times daily
- Oral co-danthramer 25/200 (dantron 25 mg, poloxamer "188" 200 mg) capsules, 1 or 2 at bedtime
- Oral bisacodyl 10 mg once daily.

The oral osmotic laxatives   These osmotically draw fluid into the gut causing easier passage of fecal material. They cause an accumulation of fluid and gas when the gut transit time is reduced and therefore should be avoided in patients prone to bowel obstruction. To be effective the patient must have an adequate intake of oral fluid.

Side effects

- Abdominal cramps and bloating
- Flatulence

Examples

- Oral lactulose 15 ml twice daily
- Oral Movicol three sachets daily.

Rectal stimulant laxatives   These have both a local osmotic and irritant action that causes rectal stimulation and passage of feces. They are particularly effective for fecal impaction, especially when following a fecal softener.

Side effects

- Local rectal irritation
- Severe diarrhea, especially in elderly.

Examples

- Phosphate enema, once daily
- Sodium citrate enema once daily.

The rectal fecal softening laxatives   These cause local lubrication of fecal material helping its passage. They are well-tolerated and can be particularly useful in softening hard fecal material causing impaction.

Side effects

- Local irritation with prolonged use
- Allergy to peanut oil (arachis oil).

Examples

- Arachis oil enema 130 ml once daily
- Liquid paraffin enema 5 ml once daily.

6.7 **Gastrointestinal obstruction**

This affects 3 percent of all cancer patients and is one of the most common and serious gastrointestinal emergencies in oncologic practice. The most frequent cause for obstruction is the cancer itself that may:

- Invade the lumen of the bowel
- Extrinsically compress the bowel
- Disrupt the neurologic supply to the bowel wall muscle.

Advanced ovarian and colorectal cancers are particularly associated with bowel obstruction.

Although the cancer is often to blame it is important not to forget less common but easily reversible causes such as electrolyte disturbance, fecal impaction, herniae or post-operative adhesions. Causes for gastrointestinal obstruction are listed in Table 6.13.

Table 6.13 Causes of gastrointestinal obstruction in cancer patients

Tumor (particularly ovarian or colon cancer)
Involving bowel wall
Extrinsically compressing bowel
Neurologic involvement
Post-operative adhesions in small bowel
Fecal impaction
Hypercalcemia
Hypokalemia

6.7.1 **Clinical assessment**

The patient typically presents with nausea, vomiting, and constipation. The vomitus is frequent and in large volume if there is upper gastrointestinal obstruction and occasional and smaller volume if there is lower gut obstruction. Constipation is usually absolute with failure to pass flatus as well as feces although small amounts of flatus or fecal material may pass in subacute obstruction. The patient often complains of intermittent crampy abdominal pain. If pain becomes constant consider gut perforation.

Ask about previous recurrent episodes of obstruction especially after recent abdominal surgery as this may suggest post-operative adhesions. Also inquire about opioid medication as this may cause fecal impaction.

If the patient complains of excess thirst or polyuria, particularly if they are confused or dehydrated a diagnosis of hypercalcemia should be considered.

On general inspection the patient may be dehydrated and thin. The breath may smell of ketones due to poor calorific intake. In obstruction of the upper gastrointestinal tract the clinical findings are distension in the epigastric area, a succussion splash heard over stomach (gurgling noise when stethoscope held over stomach and patient gently moved from side to side). Profuse, large volume bilious or feculant vomiting occurs.

In lower gastrointestinal obstruction there is general abdominal distension, resonance to percussion, high-pitched bowel sounds and vomiting of feculant material that becomes less in volume and frequency the lower the obstruction in the bowel.

All patients with a diagnosis of gastrointestinal obstruction *must have a rectal examination* to ensure there is no fecal impaction.

If the patient is unwell or the bowel sounds absent and the abdomen is tender with peritonism then a diagnosis of gastrointestinal perforation must be ruled out (see Section 6.3).

6.7.2 Investigations

1. Check serum electrolytes to ensure potassium and calcium levels are normal. A raised urea and creatinine will confirm dehydration.

2. A plain erect abdominal X-ray will demonstrate multiple fluid levels (see Fig. 6.7 on p.144). This investigation will confirm fecal loading when the underlying cause is thought to be constipation. Air under the diaphragm suggests a diagnosis of bowel perforation.

3. Radio-opaque contrast small bowel series. This may be attempted to identify a level of obstruction when surgery is being considered to relieve the symptoms. Ten percent of patients will have both small and large bowel obstruction.

4. Endoscopy of the upper or lower gastrointestinal tract may also allow visualization of the area of obstruction.

5. Computed tomography of the abdomen will demonstrate any masses that may be infiltrating or compressing bowel.

6.7.3 Management

The principles of treatment are outlined in Fig. 6.9.

1. In 20 percent of patients, supportive care with intravenous fluids, analgesia and stopping oral intake will result in resolution of obstruction within 3–9 days.

2. Replacement of potassium loss in the intravenous fluids is essential. Serum electrolytes and urinary output should be measured daily to guide intravenous fluid and electrolyte replacement.

3. Commence a continuous subcutaneous analgesic and anti-emetic infusion. Typically diamorphine 10 mg with cyclizine 150 mg over 24 hours. A higher dose of

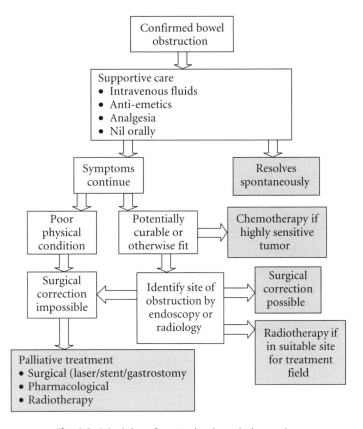

Fig. 6.9 Principles of managing bowel obstruction.

diamorphine will be required in those previously taking opioids. For example, a dose of diamorphine over 24 hours equals a total dose of morphine sulphate tablets in 24 hours divided by three.

4. If vomiting continues add haloperidol 5 mg to 24-hour subcutaneous infusion.

5. Prokinetic agents such as metoclopramide can occasionally help relieve bowel obstruction but more often aggravate symptoms such as colic and vomiting. These agents, therefore, should only be used in bowel obstruction by those experienced in palliative care.

6. In patients with large volume vomitus a subcutaneous octreotide infusion (300–600 μg) over 24 hours may reduce the frequency of vomiting.

7. In patients with upper gastrointestinal obstruction where anti-emetic medication and octreotide fails to control vomiting a nasogastric tube may relieve symptoms. If gastrointestinal secretions remain large consider insertion of a percutaneous venting gastrostomy which is more comfortable and less disfiguring for the patient.

8. All patients with malignant bowel obstruction who fail to recover bowel function with supportive care should be considered for surgical management (see Table 6.14). This will require the level of obstruction to be identified usually by endoscopy or radiologic contrast studies of the upper or lower gastrointestinal tract. Unfortunately many patients who present with advanced malignancy and obstruction are poor surgical candidates (see Table 6.15). Even in those assessed fit for surgery 25 percent will die perioperatively. Before proceeding to surgery a multi-disciplinary approach should be taken to decision-making involving surgeons, cancer physicians and palliative care physicians. It is also important to discuss the risks and benefits with the patients and ensure that their wishes are respected.

9. Where obstruction is due to highly chemosensitive tumors such as lymphoma, small cell or testicular cancer a trial of chemotherapy may be attempted. This can be potentially hazardous and the patient will require close monitoring by an experienced oncologist in the period following treatment.

10. Patients with esophageal obstruction or duodenal obstruction may benefit from local radiotherapy or stent insertion. As the maximum benefit from radiotherapy may not be seen for 6 weeks this is often preceded by stent insertion.

11. Feeding should be considered where the obstruction is expected to respond to treatment. This may be via a gastrostomy or duodenal feeding tube in upper gut obstruction or parenteral where the obstruction is lower in the digestive tract.

Table 6.14 Surgery for bowel obstruction

Level of obstruction	Procedures
Esophagus	Esophagectomy Stent insertion Laser treatment
Duodenum	Bypass surgery Stent insertion
Ileum	Resection of obstruction and re-anastomosis Division of adhesions Defunctioning ileostomy
Colon	Resection of obstruction and re-anastomosis Defunctioning colostomy

Table 6.15 Dangers in bowel surgery for patients with advanced cancer

Multiple levels of bowel obstruction due to intra-peritoneal tumor seeding
Poor anesthetic risk due to generalized debility
Poor surgical healing due to malnutrition or seeding of the surgical wound with tumor
High risk of thrombo-embolic episode
Large impact on remaining quality of life in those with a poor prognosis due to disseminated cancer

Table 6.16 Examples of palliative care for bowel obstruction

Symptom	Treatment
Colicky pain	Anti-spasmodic treatment. For example, hyoscine butylbromide 20–60 mg s/c over 24 hours Analgesic, for example, diamorphine 10 mg s/c over 24 hours
Nausea	Anti-emetic. For example, cyclizine 150 mg s/c or haloperidol 5 mg s/c over 24 hours
Vomiting	Octreotide 300–600 mg s/c over 24 hours Consider venting gastrostomy
Dehydration	1 L of normal saline subcutaneously overnight

Palliative care for bowel obstruction

Unfortunately in the majority of patients with advanced cancer the obstruction cannot be relieved. In this group eating and drinking may remain possible with nausea and vomiting largely controlled by medication. Self-administered subcutaneous fluids may provide adequate hydration. A specialist palliative care team is best suited to manage symptoms in these patients (see Table 6.16).

6.8 **Conclusion**

Gastrointestinal emergencies in the cancer patient can be due to several interacting etiologies including local or systemic effects of the tumor, side effects of medications and post-surgical complications. It is also important to consider coexisting conditions that are not related to the diagnosis of cancer.

A full history and clinical examination will avoid unnecessary investigations and will allow prompt, effective treatment.

Management of these often difficult conditions requires the input of a multi-disciplinary team and it is always important to ensure that the patients' and their family's wishes are adhered to.

Suggested reading

Anonymous (1997) NCCN antiemesis practice guidelines. *Oncology* (Huntington), **11**(11A), 57–89.

Chao, T.C., Jeng, L.B., Jan, Y.Y., *et al.* (1998) Spontaneous gastroduodenal perforation in cancer patients receiving chemotherapy. *Hepato-Gastroenterology*, **45**, 2157–60.

Chao, T.C., Wang, C.S., and Chen, M.F. (1999) Gastroduodenal perforation in cancer patients. *Hepato-Gastroenterology*, **46**, 2878–81.

Conlong, P.J. (1998) Practical advice on treating haematemesis. *Hosp Med*, **59**(11), 851–5.

Fallon, M. and O'Neill (1997) ABC of palliative care: constipation and diarrhoea. *Br Med J*, **315**, 1293–6.

Fallon, M.T. and Hanks, G.W. (1999) Morphine, constipation and performance status. *Palliat Med*, **13**, 159–60.

Hanks, G. (1997) Palliative care: clinical approach to chronic pain and intestinal obstruction. *Cleve Clin J Med*, **66**(8), 459–61.

Heys, S.D., Smith, I., and Eremin, O. (1997) The management of patients with advanced cancer (II). *Eur J Surg Oncol*, **23**, 257–69.

Ibrahim, N.K., Sahin, A.A., Dubrow, R.A., *et al.* (2000) Colitis associated with docetaxel-based chemotherapy in patients with metastatic breast cancer. *Lancet*, **355**(22), 281–3.

Kirby, D. and Teran, J.C. (1998) Enteral feeding in critical care, gastrointestinal diseases and cancer. *Gastrointest Endosc Clin N Am*, **8**(3), 623–43.

Kornblau, S., Benson, A.B., Catalano, R., *et al.* (2000) Management of cancer treatment-related diarrhoea: issues and therapeutic strategies. *J Pain Symptom Manage*, **19**(2), 118–29.

Kouroussis, C., Samonis, G., Androulakis, N., *et al.* (2000) Successful conservative treatment of neutropenic enterocolitis complicating taxane-based chemotherapy: a report of five cases. *Am J Clin Oncol*, **23**(3), 309–13.

Randall, T.C. and Rubin, S.C. (2000) Management of intestinal obstruction in the patient with ovarian cancer. *Oncology* (Huntington), **14**(8), 1159–63.

Scwartzentruber, D.J. (1997) Surgical emergencies. *Cancer principles and practice of oncology* (5th edn), pp. 2500–11, Lippincott-Raven publishers.

Veyrat-Follet, C., Farinotti, R., and Palmer, J.L. (1997) Physiology of chemotherapy-induced emesis and antiemetic therapy. Predictive models for evaluation of new compounds. *Drugs*, **53**(2), 206–34.

Chapter 7

Hepatic, Biliary, and Pancreatic Emergencies

Richard H. Wilson and Patrick G. Johnston

7.1 Introduction

There are a wide range of hepato-pancreaticobiliary problems and emergencies encountered in oncologic practice. They may be due to the tumor, therapy or non-related conditions common in the age-matched general population. Problems range from common ones, such as malignant jaundice or ascites to rare ones following allogeneic or autologous bone marrow transplantation such as graft-versus-host disease or hepatic veno-occlusive disease. The following chapter aims to aid the assessment and management of these problems in patients with cancer.

7.2 Jaundice

Jaundice results from increased production, or decreased hepatic uptake or excretion of bilirubin. Table 7.1 gives the main causes of jaundice in oncology patients. The development of jaundice is a common problem in oncologic practice, and requires urgent assessment and intervention (see Fig. 7.1).

In hemolytic anemias, erythrocytes are broken down in large numbers, resulting in excessive amounts of water-insoluble bilirubin which swamps the capacity of the liver to conjugate it to water-soluble bilirubin glucuronide. There is anemia, splenomegaly, and unconjugated hyperbilirubinemia without urinary bilirubin. Detailed studies such as red cell films and antibodies, and hemoglobin electrophoresis should be performed.

Mild unconjugated hyperbilirubinemia is also seen in Gilbert's syndrome (3–10 percent of population), in which there is a decreased ability to glucuronidate bilirubin. Fasting, tiredness, or illness result in mild jaundice, but investigation reveals normal liver function tests and reticulocyte counts.

Jaundice due to decreased excretion of bilirubin is usually divided into the two groups of hepatocellular and cholestatic jaundice. Hepatocellular jaundice is due to failure of secretion of conjugated bilirubin into biliary canaliculi, such as in parenchymal liver disease of infectious hepatitis, chronic active hepatitis, or cirrhosis of any cause. There is raised conjugated and unconjugated bilirubin, with normal urine and stools. Cholestatic jaundice is due to impaired biliary flow after conjugated bilirubin is secreted into the biliary canaliculi, such as in certain stages of infectious hepatitis,

Table 7.1 Causes of jaundice in oncology patients

Cause	Examples
Increased production of bilirubin	Hemolytic anemia
Decreased uptake of bilirubin	Gilbert's syndrome, severe congestive heart failure, drugs, portocaval shunts
Decreased excretion of bilirubin	Hepatotoxic drugs, viral hepatitis, malignant infiltration or replacement of liver, extra-hepatic biliary obstruction

- Full history—all drugs (including complementary and alternative), color of urine and stools, transfusions, operations, contact, itching, presence of fever, rigors, and systemic symptoms
- Examination—sclerae, buccal mucosa, scratching, signs of chronic liver disease, tenderness, size and consistency of liver, palpable masses including gallbladder, and spleen
- Urgent liver function tests, urinalysis for bilirubin, and urobilinogen
- Infectious hepatitis panel
- Red cell films, antibodies, and hemoglobin electrophoresis (if hemolytic type)
- Coagulation studies
- Serum immunoglobulins
- Autoantibodies including anti-mitochondrial, anti-smooth muscle, and anti-nuclear
- Ultrasound scan (ultrasound scan)—gallstones, intra- or extra-hepatic biliary dilatation, tumor masses and fluid collections but lower end common bile duct (CBD) not visualized well
- Computed tomography (CT)—hepatic texture, smaller hepatic, or pancreatic lesions, other masses
- Cholangiography—Endoscopic retrograde pancreaticocholangiography (ERCP), percutaneous transhepatic cholangiography (PTC), MRI
- Liver biopsy—percutaneous, ultrasound scan guided, laparoscopic, transjugular

Fig. 7.1 Assessment of the jaundiced oncology patient.

drugs, and malignant obstruction of the intra- or extra-hepatic biliary tree. This may be due to hepatocellular carcinoma, intra- or extra-hepatic cholangiocarcinoma, gallbladder cancer, enlarged metastatic nodes or a bulky tumor causing obstruction at the porta hepatis, peri-ampullary tumor, or pancreatic head cancer. Conjugated bilirubin is excreted renally, giving dark urine, while the stools are light due to the lack of bilirubin in the gut. Urobilinogen, formed by enteric bacterial degradation of conjugated bilirubin, is normally reabsorbed and then excreted in both urine and bile. No urinary urobilinogen is found on dipstick examination in cholestatic jaundice.

Management of malignant jaundice is summarized in an algorithm in Fig. 7.2. Non-operative palliation of obstructive jaundice with endoscopic stenting has been shown in randomized controlled trials to be as effective as surgical palliative bypass

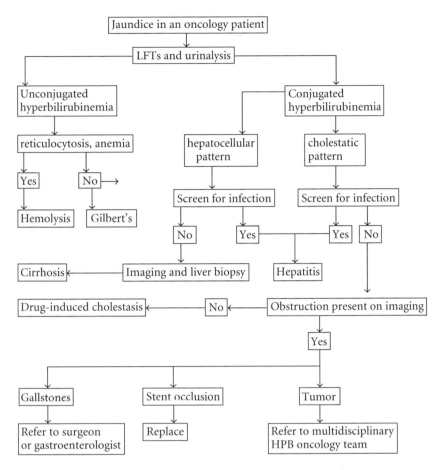

Fig. 7.2 Management of the jaundiced oncology patient.

and is associated with lower morbidity and mortality. Re-admission with recurrent jaundice following stent occlusion due to bacterial encrustation or tumor overgrowth is common. Technological advances in stent design have resulted in larger caliber plastic stents with improved patency rates, and expandable metal stents. These have decreased rates of bacterial colonization and potentially occlusive bio-film formation, but are much more expensive and are not removable.

In general, single plastic stents are used for patients with projected survival of 3–6 months, and expandable metal ones for those with better prognosis.

Surgical approaches for malignant causes of jaundice include complete resection of potentially curable tumors at any of the above sites, and palliative bypass procedures. The latter provide more durable relief of jaundice than endoscopic procedures, but have higher complication rates, and longer hospital stay and recovery time. In patients with projected survival of over one year, surgery may provide the best symptom control and quality of life.

In cases of irresectable tumor within the liver or at the hilum, biliary drainage may not be effective and may be associated with the introduction of sepsis. Careful consideration of the patient's symptoms, performance status and co-morbid conditions are required prior to biliary manipulation. If such intervention is appropriate, the best option is an interventional radiologic one with percutaneous transhepatic biliary drainage followed by placement of one or more expandable metal stents. In the future, stents that emit ionizing radiation or release cytotoxic drugs may provide a local anti-tumor effect in addition to their palliative benefits.

Irresectable disease causing biliary obstruction at any site may also be treated with palliative chemotherapy and/or radiotherapy. In view of the potential hepatotoxicity of these agents, stenting or bypass should be performed first in the jaundiced patient. For intrahepatic disease, chemotherapy may better be delivered as infusions via the hepatic artery rather than intravenously.

7.3 **Drug-induced hepatotoxicity**

Many drugs used as single agents or in combination in oncologic practice can cause hepatotoxicity, as can supportive therapies including analgesics, antibiotics, anti-emetics, immunosuppressants and total parenteral nutrition. Hepatotoxicity should be graded according to the National Cancer Institute Common Toxicity Criteria version 2.0 (see http://ctep.info.nih.gov/). In most cases, hepatotoxicity is fully reversible on cessation of the causative drug, and rechallenge at lower doses may be tolerated well, even though minor liver function test abnormalities may be seen. However, persistent hepatotoxicity and iatrogenic mortality have been reported, and each case must be carefully considered in the context of projected survival, response to therapy, co-morbid conditions, performance status and other relevant factors. There is no effective or specific treatment for drug-induced hepatotoxicity, other than discontinuation of the relevant drug. Management is principally supportive and symptomatic, with transplantation for severe and irreversible cases of hepatotoxicity in potentially curable patients. Corticosteroids and prostaglandins analogues are rarely beneficial, but ursodeoxycholic acid may be useful for pruritus.

Alkylating agents—Cyclophosphamide metabolism results in the production of acrolein. This causes profound glutathione depletion and death of sinusoidal epithelial cells. Hepatocellular necrosis and veno-occlusive disease are seen, usually after high doses prior to bone marrow transplantation. Melphalan and dacarbazine are also rare causes of hepatotoxicity in normal dosing, but in higher doses may cause raised transaminases or contribute to veno-occlusive disease.

Nitrosoureas—Carmustine and lomustine cause mild elevation of liver function tests in 25 percent of patients, but very rarely cause fatality. Streptozotocin causes deranged liver function tests in up to 70 percent of cases, but these rapidly normalize.

Platinums—Cisplatin and oxaliplatin are commonly associated with mild rises in liver function tests. In high-dose cisplatin and carboplatin regimens, cholestasis and hepatocyte necrosis have been reported.

Antimetabolites—Cytarabine may cause self-limiting abnormalities of liver function tests, often with a cholestatic pattern. Fluorodeoxyuridine may cause hepatocellular injury and sclerosing cholangitis (see below). Mercaptopurine is frequently associated with hepatocellular or cholestatic liver disease. Methotrexate commonly causes transaminase rises at high doses, and in prolonged low-dose oral therapy causes steatosis, fibrosis, and cirrhosis, with two reports of development of hepatocellular carcinoma in the fibrotic liver. Gemcitabine causes transaminase elevations in 65 percent of cases, with one report of fulminant hepatic failure.

Antitumor antibiotics—Mithramycin is rarely used because of ubiquitous hepatotoxicity with transaminase rises due to hepatocellular necrosis. Mitoxantrone may cause transient transaminase or bilirubin rises. Dactinomycin can cause transaminase rises, especially in children who have also had hepatic irradiation.

Taxanes—Paclitaxel has shown dose-dependent hepatotoxicity, occurring in 10 percent of patients below 200 mg/m^2 and 30 percent at doses above this.

Topoisomerase I and II inhibitors—Etoposide causes mild, transient liver function test rises occasionally, but higher doses can be associated with hepatocellular injury. Irinotecan causes transaminase and bilirubin elevations in 25 percent of cases, whereas topotecan causes transaminase rises in under 10 percent.

Biological therapies—Interferon use is often associated with transaminase rises, and at higher doses hepatotoxicity may become dose-limiting. Interleukin-2 causes intrahepatic cholestasis which reverses after stopping the drug.

Hormonal agents—Tamoxifen is associated with raised transaminases, fatty liver, and rarely cirrhosis. Cyproterone acetate causes altered liver function tests in 10–20 percent of cases, with rare reports of severe hepatitis which may be fatal. Flutamide may also cause increased bilirubin and transaminases, with reported cases of fatal hepatic necrosis.

Supportive therapies—Many antibiotics and anti-fungal agents in common use in oncologic practice cause hepatotoxicity. Paracetamol, even at normal dosages, should be carefully monitored in patients being treated with cytotoxics that decrease hepatic glutathione. Enteral feeding is often associated with a mild rise in transaminases which rarely requires cessation of therapy. Total parenteral nutrition causes transaminase rises in up to 90 percent of cases, associated with fatty infiltration and intrahepatic cholestasis. Rarely, this may progress to fibrosis and fatal liver failure.

7.4 **Malignant ascites**

Malignant ascites is usually caused by peritoneal metastases which increase secretion and decrease absorption of peritoneal fluid. Other causes of ascites include pseudomyxoma peritonei, hepatic dysfunction in advanced metastatic disease, portal hypertension, Budd–Chiari syndrome, inferior vena cava obstruction, hypoalbuminemia, and non-malignant causes such as congestive heart failure.

Clinical features are abdominal distension, anorexia, and weight gain. An ultrasound scan is important to confirm the diagnosis and mark a safe site for diagnostic or therapeutic peritoneocentesis. Aspirated fluid should be sent to exclude infection and to cytologically confirm the presence of malignant cells. Spontaneous bacterial peritonitis may occur, although less common with malignancy than with cirrhosis, and antibiotics should be given dependent upon bacteriology and sensitivity testing. The usual organisms are enteric bacteria such as *Escherichia coli* (50–60 percent), *S. fecalis*, Klebsiella, Bacteroides, Pnemococcus, and Hemophilus. After one attack, antibiotic prophylaxis should be considered due to the high risk of recurrence, again guided by bacteriological analysis.

The median survival for patients with malignant ascites is 8–12 weeks, with under 10 percent alive at one year. Management is therefore directed at palliation in most cases. A guideline for management of malignant ascites is summarized in an algorithm in Fig. 7.3. Appropriate systemic endocrine or cytotoxic therapy for the underlying malignancy may result in resolution of the ascites. Diuretic therapy with spironolactone (150–400 mg daily in divided doses) and/or frusemide (40–100 mg daily) plus salt and fluid restriction may aid control of ascites in some patients, but is much less effective than in non-malignant causes as sodium retention is rarely a feature. Intracavitary radioisotopes, cytotoxics, sclerosants and biological response modifiers are much less successful than in pleural effusions. Radioisotopes such as ^{198}Au or colloidal ^{32}CrPO$_4$; cytotoxics such as cisplatin, carboplatin, mitoxantrone, and etoposide; and biological agents such as interferon, tumor necrosis factor, interleukin-2, and granulocyte macrophage colony-stimulating factor have all been tried. Paracentesis, repeated as necessary, is useful in palliation but rapid refilling, development of loculi, protein loss, and potential introduction of infection or visceral injury limit its effectiveness.

Peritoneovenous shunts may be considered in selected patients with refractory malignant ascites, life expectancy of >12 weeks and reasonable performance status and organ function. Shunts comprise a proximal catheter in the superior vena cava, one-way compressible chamber and valve and a distal perforated catheter in the peritoneal cavity. Complications include fever, shunt failure, spread of metastases, disseminated intravascular coagulation, and sepsis. Peritoneogastric shunts in which the fluid is returned to the gastric lumen have been used in an attempt to avoid these complications and those of intermittent paracentesis.

An aggressive surgical approach for ascites due to peritoneal tumor involving radical peritonectomy followed by intraperitoneal chemotherapy has been attempted, but the excellent results in highly selected patients from single institutions have not yet been confirmed in large prospective controlled trials.

7.5 Hepatorenal syndrome

Hepatorenal syndrome is an acute oliguric renal failure occurring without intrinsic renal disease in the presence of liver disease such as cirrhosis, portal hypertension, or liver failure. There is intense renal cortical vasoconstriction with increased renal vascular resistance, decreased glomerular filtration rate, peripheral vasodilatation, and avid

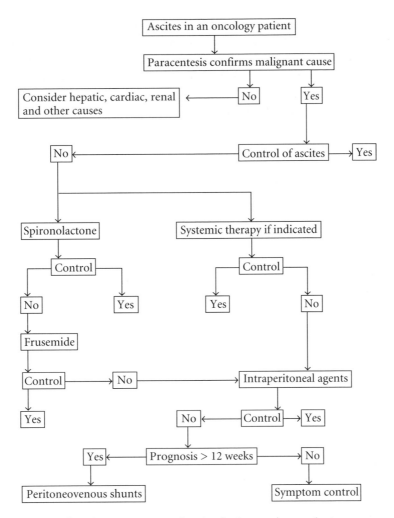

Fig. 7.3 Management of ascites in the oncology patient.

sodium and water retention. The diagnosis should be considered in patients with hepatic dysfunction with rising serum creatinine who do not have sepsis, shock, recent fluid losses (vomiting, diarrhea, excessive diuresis, or paracentesis), renal disease, or who are on nephrotoxic drugs.

Investigations are aimed at excluding other causes of renal insufficiency and include serum and urinary electrolytes, creatinine clearance, blood cultures, urinalysis, and urinary tract ultrasound (to exclude obstruction or renal parenchymal disease). The usual findings are serum creatinine >200 µmol/l, creatinine clearance <40 ml/min, hyponatremia, oliguria, absence of urinary casts and proteinuria, and low urinary sodium.

Management involves withdrawal of nephrotoxic drugs including non-steroidal anti-inflammatory drugs and aminoglycosides, treatment of any sepsis, and fluid, sodium, potassium and protein restriction. The outcome is poor with a two-month survival rate of 10 percent, and the only effective therapy is orthotopic liver transplantation.

7.6 Hepatic encephalopathy

Hepatic encephalopathy is a reversible state of altered cognitive function or level of consciousness in patients with impaired liver function or portosystemic shunts. There is a failure of hepatic clearance of nitrogenous compounds including ammonia derived from the gut or elsewhere. There is new evidence suggesting that the gamma-aminobutyric acid (GABA) receptor complex also contributes to neuronal impairment. Table 7.2 gives the main precipitants of encephalopathy in hepatic impairment.

Clinical features include altered level of consciousness (ranging from drowsiness to coma), flapping tremor, slow and slurred speech, constructional apraxia, and altered reflexes. Investigations are aimed at excluding other causes of altered level of consciousness and include chemistries, serum ammonia, blood sugar, vitamin B_{12}, complete blood count, coagulation studies, arterial blood gases and perhaps computed axial tomography (CT) scan of brain.

The main features in the treatment of hepatic encephalopathy are outlined in Fig. 7.4. The involvement of the GABA receptor has led to use of the benzodiazepine anatagonist flumazenil, but responses tend to be both brief and incomplete.

Table 7.2 Precipitants of encephalopathy in hepatic impairment

Cause	Examples
Electrolyte imbalance	Uremia, diuretics, dehydration, vomiting, diarrhea
Gastrointestinal	Constipation, excess dietary protein, bleeding
Infections	Spontaneous bacterial peritonitis, urinary tract, respiratory
Drugs	Benzodiazepines, alcohol excess, opiates

- Monitor volume status and vital signs
- Identify precipitant and correct if possible (e.g. gastrointestinal bleed)
- Monitor and correct electrolyte, calorie, and fluid balance
- Discontinue nephrotoxic and sedative drugs
- Stop dietary protein
- Empty colon with lactulose 50 ml every 2 hours
- Neomycin 1 g orally q 6 hourly for 1 week
- Gradually increase dietary protein with recovery

Fig. 7.4 Treatment of hepatic encephalopathy.

Table 7.3 Causes of fulminant hepatic failure in oncology patients

Cause	Examples
Tumors	Widespread infiltration by primary or metastatic tumors, rapid growth (angiosarcoma)
Vascular disorder	Budd–Chiari syndrome, veno-occlusive disease
Infections	Viral (Hepatitis A, B and others), tuberculous
Others	Paracetamol, idiosyncratic drug reactions, toxins, metabolic disorders

7.7 **Fulminant hepatic failure**

Fulminant hepatic failure is either rapid development of hepatic dysfunction leading to coagulopathy and/or encephalopathy with no prior liver disease or liver disease leading to coagulopathy and/or encephalopathy soon after the onset of jaundice. Table 7.3 gives the main causes of fulminant hepatic failure in oncology patients.

Many cases of fulminant hepatic failure are drug or toxin-related, necessitating a careful history on use of medications (including over the counter ones), vitamins, complementary and alternative medicines. Investigation should include toxicology screen, hepatitis and other viral serology, and imaging with ultrasound scan, CT or magnetic resonance imaging (MRI). Complications of fulminant hepatic failure include hypoglycemia, sepsis, hemorrhage, hypotension, respiratory and renal failure.

Treatment is principally supportive in an intensive care setting, with liver transplant-ation as the only option for irreversible cases. Supportive measures include prophylaxis against upper gastrointestinal hemorrhage with proton pump inhibitors, treatment of any coagulopathy, reversal of hypoglycemia and hypoxia, and treatment of any sepsis. If specific therapy is available, then it should be given, for example, acetylcysteine in paracetamol poisoning, chemotherapy (if indicated) for primary or metastatic malig-nancy. The survival rate for fulminant hepatic failure is under 50 percent, but increases to 60–70 percent after liver transplantation.

7.8 **Painful liver capsule**

Stretching of the fibrous capsule surrounding the liver parenchyma is associated with visceral pain. It may occur with any disease state that causes rapid enlargement or increased pressure within the liver. Metastatic infiltration or replacement of normal liver parenchyma with primary or metastatic tumor is a common cause. Clinically, there is right upper quadrant pain that may radiate to the back, epigastrium, or shoulder tip. Nausea, vomiting, and other autonomic symptoms may also occur. Management involves adequate analgesia (often requiring opiates), anti-emetics and corticosteroids (e.g. prednisolone 40 mg orally daily). Depending upon the type of tumor and patient performance status, chemotherapy and palliative hepatic irradiation may be considered.

7.9 **Hepatic bleeding**

Primary benign or malignant liver tumors may cause spontaneous bleeding, while this is less frequent with metastatic lesions. In South East Asia ruptured hepatocellular carcinoma is a common cause of fatal hemoperitoneum. Metastatic lesions tend to maintain the vascular characteristics of their primary tumor, so some metastases have a greater propensity for hemorrhage into the host organ than others. Intraparenchymal hematomas at sites of tumors may become subcapsular by detaching and elevating the liver capsule and this may tear causing either a localized collection or free intraperitoneal hemorrhage.

Clinical suspicion is important in diagnosing localized hematomata prior to rupture. Symptoms range from right upper quadrant pain, nausea, vomiting and a drop in hemoglobin and hematocrit to frank peritonism and hypotension. Ultrasound or preferably CT scanning should be performed immediately once the diagnosis is considered.

Conservative management may be used unless the patient is hemodynamically unstable following adequate resuscitation. This approach will involve fluid and blood product replacement, analgesia, careful monitoring (in a High Dependency or Intensive Care Unit if necessary), observation by a surgical team, and repeat scanning to check for resolution. Vigilance is necessary as delayed rupture can occur after several weeks.

For patients who require intervention, hepatic angiography and transcatheter embolization may be considered (see section on embolization below). The complications of this approach are hepatic abscess, sepsis and gallbladder ischemia.

Surgery is indicated for hemodynamic instability, ongoing blood loss, and expanding hematomata on observation. After aggressive resuscitation, laparotomy is performed and the hematoma evacuated. Diathermy, topical hemostatic agents, suturing, packing, vascular ligation or resection may be used dependent on the operative findings. Post-operative complications include rebleeding, disseminated intravascular coagulation, cardiopulmonary problems and sepsis.

7.10 **Budd–Chiari syndrome**

Budd–Chiari syndrome is caused by decreased hepatic venous outflow, classically due to obstruction by acute thrombus formation at the junction of the inferior vena cava and hepatic veins. However, flow may be reduced at any site between the right atrium and small hepatic venous radicles. Table 7.4 gives the main causes of Budd–Chiari syndrome in oncology patients.

In fulminant Budd–Chiari syndrome, features are severe pain, jaundice, ascites, hepatomegaly, rapidly deteriorating liver function, and progression to encephalopathy and liver failure. In acute cases, there are several weeks of tender hepatomegaly, pain, and ascites. Features vary dependent upon the site of obstruction and proportion of normally functioning liver. Chronic Budd–Chiari syndrome is less common in oncologic practice, and includes hepatomegaly, cirrhosis with venous collateralization, and chronic ascites.

Table 7.4 Causes of Budd–Chiari syndrome in oncology patients

Cause	Examples
Tumors	Adrenal, renal cell, lung, hepatocellular, leukemia, rhabdomyosarcoma, leiomyosarcoma
Hypercoagulable state	Advanced malignancies especially pancreatic, coagulation factor mutations, myeloproliferative diseases
Infections	Hepatic abscess, pelvic sepsis, tuberculosis, aspergillosis
Others	Idiopathic, hypotension, post-hepatobiliary surgery

Investigations reveal altered liver function tests with a pattern of acute liver damage, and is diagnosed by doppler ultrasound scan. Typical features include absence of hepatic venous waveform, non-visualization of contiguous venous flow from hepatic veins into inferior vena cava, and maybe intrahepatic collateral vessels.

Management depends upon the underlying cause and rapidity of progress. Liver transplantation is advised for fulminant liver failure and deterioration after shunting procedures. Transjugular intrahepatic portosystemic shunts have been successfully used in patients with severe disease who would not survive until transplantation. For acute cases, thrombolytic agents with or without resection of tumor and abscess drainage is performed. Balloon angioplasty may be used in localized disease. In chronic Budd–Chiari syndrome, surgical shunting is used. Lifelong anticoagulation is necessary after initial therapy because of the high risk of recurrent thrombosis.

7.11 **Portal hypertension and portal vein thrombosis**

The differential diagnosis of upper GI bleeding in the cancer patient must include portal hypertension and esophago-gastric varices. Variceal bleeding is a medical emergency.

Portal hypertension occurs when the portal venous pressure (usually 6–10 mmHg) exceeds 12 mmHg. This results in the development of a portosystemic collateral circulation with portosystemic shunting and altered intrahepatic circulation. Table 7.5 gives the main causes of portal hypertension in oncology patients. Variceal bleeding is the presenting symptom in approximately 5 percent of cases of hepatocellular carcinoma.

Complications include splenomegaly and hypersplenism; bleeding from portosystemic varices in the gallbladder bed, esophagus, stomach, duodenum, jejunum, ileum, colon, and anorectal region; ascites; coagulopathy; hepatic encephalopathy; hepatorenal syndrome and liver failure. Venous congestion of the stomach and gut may lead to non-variceal bleeding, especially in the presence of infection and aspirin or NSAID ingestion. The usual presentation of portal hypertension is variceal bleeding leading to hematemesis and/or melena.

A common cause of portal hypertension in oncology practice is portal vein thrombosis. Table 7. 6 gives the main causes of portal vein thrombosis in oncology patients.

Table 7.5 Causes of portal hypertension in oncology patients

Type	Examples
Pre-hepatic	Budd–Chiari syndrome, right heart failure, constrictive pericarditis due to tumor infiltration or irradiation
Hepatic	Alcoholic or post-hepatitic cirrhosis
Post-hepatic	Portal vein thrombosis, splenic vein thrombosis, extrinsic compression by tumors

Table 7.6 Causes of portal vein thrombosis in oncology patients

Cause	Examples
Tumors	Bladder cancer
Hypercoagulable state	Advanced malignancies especially pancreatic, coagulation factor mutations, myeloproliferative diseases
Infections	Abdomino-pelvic sepsis, fungal infections
Iatrogenic	Splenectomy, hepatic surgery including OLT, chemoembolization, alcohol injection, TIPS
Others	Cirrhosis, pancreatitis

Investigations include endoscopy and radiologic imaging. Doppler ultrasound reveals abnormalities of flow, portal vein thrombus, collateralization, and splenomegaly. If ultrasound scan is diffficult, CT scanning or MRI with angiography should be used. Diagnostic endoscopy is usually combined with either variceal sclerotherapy or band ligation.

Figure 7.5 outlines the treatment of variceal bleeding. Balloon tube tamponade is used if endoscopy is delayed or visualization difficult. This allows esophageal and gastric aspiration whilst compressing the esophageal varices. Complications include ulceration, perforation and aspiration pneumonitis. In sclerotherapy, a sclerosing agent is injected into the varix and/or adjacent submucosa, and this controls bleeding in 75–90 percent of cases. Complications include fever, chest pain, dysphagia, ulceration, stricture, and esophageal perforation and there is an in-hospital mortality rate of 20 percent for an episode of variceal bleeding. Sclerotherapy has been largely replaced with rubber band ligation, where 1–3 bands ligate an aspirated varix causing thrombosis. Controlled trials show equivalent control of acute bleeding and rate of variceal eradication, with the advantages of lower morbidity and fewer repeated sessions for eradication than sclerotherapy.

Further management involves repeated endoscopy and sclerotherapy/ligation. Oral beta-blockers may reduce portal pressure, but are not used during acute bleeds. Indications for surgery in selected candidates are bleeding from varices anatomically not amenable to endoscopic therapy, or rebleeding despite endoscopic manouveres. Surgical shunting (portocaval or splenorenal) has a low operative mortality and good survival, but carries the risk of encephalopathy.

ACUTE

- Monitor volume status and vital signs
- Resuscitate and correct coagulopathy—colloids, packed red cells, fresh frozen plasma, vitamin K, platelets
- Reduce splanchnic blood flow—IV infusional octreotide, IV vasopressin, transdermal or IV glyceryl trinitrate
- Balloon tube tamponade if necessary
- Emergency endoscopy—confirm varices present, define bleeding site
- Treat varix—sclerotherapy or band ligation

ELECTIVE

- Endoscopy programme with sclerotherapy/ligation
- Oral beta-blockers
- Surgery if necessary

Fig. 7.5 Treatment of variceal bleeding.

Gastric varices cause 10–30 percent of variceal bleeds. Isolated gastric varices can occur and may be due to splenic vein thrombosis secondary to malignancy. This is an important diagnosis as it can be cured by splenectomy with gastric devascularization. Other procedures used for gastric varices include endoscopic administration of "superglue," and insertion of transjugular intrahepatic porto-systemic shunts.

7.12 **Hepatic veno-occlusive disease**

The syndrome of veno-occlusive disease, usually seen following stem cell or bone marrow transplantation, has the clinical features of weight gain, ascites, edema, tender hepatomegaly, and jaundice. It usually occurs early, at 1–3 weeks after the conditioning regimen, and is common, affecting 50–70 percent of patients following allogeneic bone marrow transplantation. It appears to be caused by a combination of factors, including high dose combination chemotherapy, total body irradiation, pre-existent liver dysfunction and drugs, especially cyclosporin. The differential diagnosis includes acute hepatic graft-versus-host disease, sepsis with cholestasis, viral or fungal hepatitis, total parenteral nutrition-induced liver injury and congestive heart failure.

Investigations reveal increased bilirubin, alkaline phosphatase, and then transaminases. The doppler ultrasound or CT scan changes of ascites, hepatomegaly, and diminished hepatic venous blood flow are not specific, but can exclude other diagnoses. Liver biopsy features are centrilobular sinusoidal congestion, hepatocyte necrosis, and sinusoidal and central venous fibrosis.

Outcome depends upon the severity of the veno-occlusive disease. Mild and moderate (requiring diuretics) cases recover, whereas severe veno-occlusive disease results in encephalopathy, hepatorenal syndrome and multi-organ failure with death usually between 4 and 8 weeks later. Therapy is supportive, with careful fluid balance and judicious use of diuretics. Ursodiol, a naturally occurring bile salt, has been used as a hepatic protectant against veno-occlusive disease with partially encouraging results. Recombinant human tissue plasminogen activator, glutamine and vitamin E have all been tried in established veno-occlusive disease but with uncertain efficacy. Defibrotide is a molecule with thrombolytic, anti-ischemic and anti-inflammatory actions and is very promising. Randomized controlled trials are ongoing in both prevention and therapy of veno-occlusive disease.

7.13 Radiation hepatitis

Radiation hepatitis (also known as radiation-induced liver disease) is characterized clinically by ascites, weight gain, fatigue, and right upper quadrant pain. Less commonly, jaundice occurring 1–2 months after completion of radiotherapy is seen. Laboratory tests reveal marked elevations of alkaline phosphatase, moderate transaminase rises and no, or minimal, increases in bilirubin. Histologic features are sinusoidal congestion and fibrosis with adventitial and sub-endothelial central vein fibrosis.

The radiation tolerance of the liver, expressed as total dose, is 30–35 Gy to whole liver alone, 20 Gy to the liver during whole abdominal irradiation, 15–20 Gy after partial hepatectomy or when delivered concurrently or sequentially with chemotherapy, and 70 Gy to a limited area only. These tolerances assume single daily fractions of 1.5–2.0 Gy five times per week in adult patients. Immature livers in children are very sensitive to radiation damage, and require lower total doses and fraction sizes of 1.2–1.8 Gy. Combined use of vincristine, dactinomycin, and doxorubicin have been associated with severe radiation hepatitis at lower than expected radiation doses. Advances in radiotherapy techniques with three-dimensional treatment planning permit delivery of high radiation doses to liver tumors with sparing of normal liver.

Most patients recover within 3 months, but chronic fibrotic disease or progressive liver failure may occur, and the overall mortality rate is estimated at 10–20 percent. There is no established therapy, and treatment is supportive in nature, and is similar to that of veno-occlusive disease and drug-induced hepatic fibrosis. This includes avoidance of alcohol and other potentially hepatotoxic drugs, and diuretics, steroids and anticoagulants have all been tried.

7.14 Hepatic acute graft-versus-host disease

Graft-versus-host disease occurs in up to 70 percent of patients undergoing allogeneic bone marrow transplantation despite immunosuppressants, and up to 20 percent die from it. Acute graft-versus-host disease usually occurs by day 14–20 post-bone marrow transplantation, concurrent with engraftment of donor stem cells. Hepatic graft-versus-host disease usually occurs in association with cutaneous and/or intestinal manifestations. The differential diagnosis of hepatic graft-versus-host disease includes Budd–Chiari syndrome, infectious hepatitis, other sepsis, drug toxicity and veno-occlusive disease. If the diagnosis is in question, a liver biopsy should be performed. Characteristic histo-logic features include biliary duct epithelial atypia and apoptotic loss, periportal lymphocytic infiltrate, and cholestasis. There are progressive increases in bilirubin and alkaline phosphatase followed by transaminases. Treatment involves alteration of the immunosuppressant regimen with inclusion of prednisolone. However, results are poor with over two-thirds of cases failing to resolve fully, and over half progressing to chronic hepatic graft-versus-host disease with cholestatic changes and features resembling primary biliary cirrhosis.

7.15 Hepatic surgery

Resection of liver metastases provides the only hope for cure for patients with metastases confined to the liver with colorectal and functioning neuroendocrine tumors. For hepa-tectomy for colorectal metastases, the 5-year survival is 25–35 percent and operative mortality 1–2 percent in specialist units. Post-operative problems include bile leaks, bleeding, hypoglycemia, liver failure, biliary obstruction, acute renal failure, cardio-pulmonary problems, and sepsis.

Orthotopic liver transplantation for malignant disease is indicated in few tumors. These currently include hepatocellular carcinoma (restricted to those with <3 sites, 5 cm maximal diameter, and no vascular, nodal or extra-hepatic involvement) and slow-growing neuroendocrine tumors such as carcinoids. Likely complications and relationship to time from surgery are in Table 7.7.

7.16 Hepatic artery embolization

This interventional radiologic procedure is used to control bleeding, pain, hormone secretion, and tumor size. Any accessible tumor can be embolized but it is most effective when used for metastatic neuroendocrine tumors. Percutaneous selective angio-graphy is used to identify the feeding vessels. A shower of small particles embolizes the

Table 7.7 Complications of liver transplantation

Week 1	Week 2–4	Week 5 onwards	Late
Hyperacute rejection	Acute rejection	Acute rejection	Chronic rejection
Ischemic injury	Preservation injury	Infectious hepatitis including Cytomegalovirus	Tumor recurrence
Biliary obstruction	Bile leaks	Biliary strictures and calculi	Lymphoproliferative disease
Drug toxicity	Drug toxicity	Drug toxicity	Drug toxicity
Sepsis	Sepsis		Bone loss
Hepatic artery Thrombosis	Pleural effusion		

smaller peripheral vessels (reducing collateral vessel formation) then the main feeding vessels are embolized. Agents include iodized oil, Gelfoam, polyvinylchloride, and coils, and concurrent intra-arterial chemotherapy may be used.

As all embolized tumors undergo selective aseptic necrosis, the post-embolization syndrome (characterized by right upper quadrant pain, nausea, pyrexia, leucocytosis and deranged liver function tests) is ubiquitous to a greater or lesser extent. Symptomatic treatment in the early stages with analgesia and anti-emetics is sufficient. Prolonged symptoms for >5 days should be investigated to exclude rarer complications. These include abscesses which can be drained percutaneously or at laparotomy, bleeding requiring laparotomy, gallbladder ischemia requiring cholecystectomy, pancreatic pseudocyst requiring drainage for non-resolution, sepsis, hepatic artery aneurysm, carcinoid crisis, and embolization of unrelated arteries by release of the material elsewhere in the circulation.

7.17 **Acalculous cholecystitis**

Acute acalculous cholecystitis is acute gallbladder inflammation in the absence of gallstones, and accounts for up to 10 percent of all cases of cholecystitis. It occurs in ill, hospitalized patients and is associated with prolonged fasting, immobility, and hemodynamic instability. Other predisposing features are bone marrow transplantation, trauma, burns, salmonella, cytomegalovirus (CMV) in immunocompromised patients, and systemic vasculitis. Clinical features are right upper quadrant pain and tenderness on palpation or sonography. The investigation of choice is an ultrasound scan, which reveals a thickened gallbladder wall and often adjacent fluid collections. Complications include septicemia, gangrene of the wall, and perforation. Management involves initial resuscitation and antibiotics to cover gram-negative gut or bilary flora and anaerobes. Definitive options include percutaneous cholecystotomy under ultrasound scan control; endoscopic placement of a nasobiliary catheter for drainage and lavage; and either laparoscopic or open cholecystectomy.

7.18 **Hepatic abscess**

Pyogenic hepatic abscesses present with high fever, rigors, anorexia, malaise, and right upper quadrant pain which may radiate to the epigastrium, back, or shoulder tip. Investigations reveal non-specific changes of leucocytosis, anemia, raised acute phase reactants, decreased albumin, mildly elevated transaminases, and alkaline phosphatase (but rarely bilirubin). Blood cultures must be done and are positive in half of cases. Ultrasound scan or CT will show multiple small lesions in one or both lobes, which may coalesce to form one large mass. Predisposing causes are ascending cholangitis (usually E. coli or anaerobes), pancreatitis or perihepatic sepsis, cholelithiasis, immunosuppression, chronic liver disease, septicemia and portal pyemia in diverticulitis and following bowel or biliary tract surgery. Figure 7.6 outlines the treatment plan for hepatic abscesses.

- Antibiotics guided by presumptive then cultured organisms
- Needle aspiration under ultrasound scan guidance
- Placement of fine-bore catheters under ultrasound scan guidance
- Continue antibiotics for 4–6 weeks
- Surgery is indicated for ongoing sepsis despite conservative measures, deteriorating patient status, or increasing abscess size
- Open drainage
- Open placement of wide-bore drains

Fig. 7.6 Treatment of hepatic abscesses.

7.19 Ascending cholangitis

Ascending bacterial cholangitis must be recognized and treated promptly, as otherwise there is a high mortality rate due to early septicemia. The most common cause is an impacted stone in the common bile duct, and other causes include neoplastic obstruction, biliary strictures, parasitic infections, and congenital biliary anomalies. Biliary obstruction is not sufficient on its own for cholangitis, as it only occurs in 15 percent of cases of malignant obstruction. The biliary tree must already contain bacteria prior to the onset of obstruction. The usual cultured species are coliforms, Klebsiella, Pseudomonas, Proteus, enterococci, bacteroides, and clostridia.

Symptoms include Charcot's triad of pain, jaundice and fever (70 percent of cases). Signs include fever (95 percent), right upper quadrant tenderness (90 percent), jaundice (80 percent), peritonism (15 percent), and altered mental state (15 percent). Laboratory findings are leucocytosis (80 percent), elevated alkaline phosphatase (90 percent) and bilirubin (80 percent), and positive blood cultures (80 percent), often growing multiple organisms such as *E. coli*, Klebsiella, enterococci, Pseudomonas, Proteus, and Bacteroides. The best imaging modalities are the gold standard of endoscopic retrograde cholangio-pancreatography (ERCP), with useful alternatives being magnetic resonance cholangio-pancreatography and percutaneous transhepatic cholangiography.

Management involves immediate blood cultures followed by broad spectrum antibiotics effective against the likely organisms (third generation cephalosporin as single agent, or triple therapy with a penicillin, aminoglycoside and metronidazole in severe cases). If clinical improvement does not occur within 12 hours, then emergency decompression of the common bile duct at ERCP with sphincterotomy, stenting, and calculus removal as appropriate. If necessary, definitive surgical therapy may be performed electively.

7.20 Sclerosing cholangitis

Sclerosing cholangitis is a spectrum of hepatobiliary disorders characterized by diffuse extra- and intrahepatic biliary inflammation and fibrosis resulting in stricturing. This

Table 7.8 Causes of sclerosing cholangitis in oncology patients

Cause	Examples
Tumors	Cholangiocarcinoma, hepatocellular carcinoma, lymphoma, metastatic carcinoma
Immunological	Transplant rejection, graft-versus-host disease, immunodeficiencies
Toxic	Fluorodeoxyuridine
Obstructive	Choledocholithiasis, anastomotic stricture, fungal infection
Others	Primary sclerosing cholangitis, chronic inflammatory bowel disease, collagen vascular disease

process may lead ultimately to biliary cirrhosis and liver failure. Table 7.8 gives the main causes of sclerosing cholangitis in oncology patients.

A finding of a cholestatic pattern of liver function tests should be followed by cholangiography endoscopically or by MRI. The beaded appearance of diffuse stricturing with segmental dilatation is diagnostic. Cholangiocarcinoma may produce dense biliary fibrosis and be difficult to distinguish from primary or other secondary causes of sclerosing cholangitis.

Management is initially supportive and symptomatic, aiming at relief of pruritus, correction of nutritional deficiencies and treatment of episodes of bacterial cholangitis. Endoscopic or percutaneous dilatation of dominant strictures with sphincterotomy and removal of calculi is useful when large ducts are principally involved, but extensive small duct destruction may eventually result in biliary cirrhosis. Hepatic arterial infusion of fluorodeoxyuridine produces sclerosing cholangitis via direct toxic biliary damage and secondary ischemic damage from vasculitis. Although resolution can occur on discontinuation of fluorodeoxyuridine therapy, palliation with percutaneous transhepatic biliary drainage may be necessary. Transplantation is the treatment of choice for end-stage liver disease from sclerosing cholangitis but does not have a role in the presence of incurable malignant disease.

7.21 Acute pancreatitis

There is a spectrum of disease, ranging from a mild and self-limited process of edematous interstitial pancreatitis to a fulminant course involving a necrotizing process involving the pancreas and surrounding tissues with multiple organ impairment or failure. The pathogenesis of acute pancreatitis is unclear, but appears to involve activation of proteolytic enzymes within pancreatic cells, initiating a localized inflammatory process which may become systemic. Table 7.9 gives the main causes of acute pancreatitis in oncology patients.

The hallmark of acute pancreatitis is abdominal pain. This is sited in the epigastrium and radiates to the back, but may become more generalized in the upper and then also the lower abdomen. Pain tends to be severe and associated with nausea and vomiting, and may mimic a perforated viscus or myocardial infarction. The diagnosis should

Table 7.9 Causes of acute pancreatitis in oncology patients

Cause	Examples
Tumors	Pancreatic ductal obstruction by primary or metastatic pancreatic tumors
Iatrogenic	Post-operative, endoscopic retrograde cholangiopancreatography, sphincterotomy, other biliary instrumentation, embolization of hepatic tumors
Infection	Adenovirus, Coxsackie virus, CMV, Epstein–Barr virus, varicella, candida, aspergillosis, tuberculosis
Medication	Angiotensin converting enzyme inhibitors, frusemide, metronidazole, octreotide, thiazides
Antineoplastic agents	Single agent or combination regimens containing azathioprine, bleomycin, cisplatin, cyclophosphamide, cytarabine, fluorouracil, ifosfamide, interferon, methotrexate, mitomycin C, estrogens, pentamidine, steroids, vinca alkaloids
Others	Gallstones, alcohol, hypercalcemia, hyperlipidemia

Mild cases

• Fluid resuscitation

• Analgesia, preferably with patient controlled devices

• Fasting followed by gradual refeeding

Severe cases

• As above, with care in an Intensive Care Unit and aggressive fluid resuscitation with colloids

• Supplemental oxygen or intubation and ventilation depending upon degree of hypoxia

• Inotropic support

• Dialysis for renal impairment

• Treatment of infected necrosis/abscesses by radiological or surgical drainage

• Correction of metabolic disturbances such as hyperglycemia and hypocalcemia

• Nutritional support with total parenteral nutrition

Fig. 7.7 Treatment of acute pancreatitis.

always be considered as a possible cause of abdominal pain in oncology patients. The diagnosis is based on clinical features and raised serum or urine amylase or lipase. Scoring systems are used to predict the severity of the attack, as early admission of severe cases to high dependency or intensive care units is important. Abdominal CT is used to confirm the diagnosis, and assess for complications and the severity of inflammation. Local complications include pancreatic and peripancreatic necrosis, pseudocyst and abscess formation. Systemic complications include septicemia, hypotension, renal and respiratory failure. Figure 7.7 outlines the treatment of acute pancreatitis. The overall mortality is 10–20 percent, but this depends upon severity, with mortality <5 percent in mild cases and 20–30 percent in severe cases, especially in the presence of infected necrosis.

7.22 Pancreatic resection

Immediate post-operative complications include hyperglycemia, bleeding, hepatic and/or renal failure, sepsis, mesenteric thrombosis, anastomotic leaks, cardiovascular problems, pulmonary embolism, and pneumonia. Later, pancreatic exocrine insufficiency must be treated with careful diet and pancreatic enzyme replacement, and insulin-dependent diabetes mellitus may be difficult to control, with hypoglycemia a frequent problem.

Suggested reading

Alison, D.M., Modln, I.M., and Jenkins, W.J. (1977) Treatment of carcinoid liver metastases by hepatic artery embolisation. *Lancet*, 2, 1323–5.

Badalamenti, S., Graziani, G., Salerno, F., and Pontcelli, C. (1993) Hepatorenal syndrome: new perspectives in pathogenesis and treatment. *Arch Int Med*, 153, 1957–67.

Barie, P.S. and Fischer, E. (1995) Acute acalculous cholecystitis. *J Am Coll Surg*, 180(2), 232–44.

Baron, T.H. (2001) Expandable metal stents for the treatment of cancerous obstruction of the gastrointestinal tract. *N Engl J Med*, 344(22), 1681–7.

Bearman, S.I. (2000) Veno-occlusive disease of the liver. *Curr Opin Oncol*, 12(2), 103–9.

Beckingham, I.J. and Bornman, P.C. (2001) Acute pancreatitis. *Br Med J*, 332, 595–8.

Beckingham, I.J. and Ryder, S.D. (2001) Investigation of liver and biliary disease. *Br Med J*, 322, 33–6.

D'Amico, G., Pagliaro, L., and Bosch, J. (1995) The treatment of portal hypertension: a meta-analytic review. *Hepatology*, 22(1), 332–54.

Fong, Y. (1999) Surgical therapy of hepatic colorectal metastasis. *CA Cancer J Clin*, 49(4), 231–55.

Gimson, A.E., Ramage, J.K., Panos, M.Z., Hayllar, K., Harrison, P.M., Williams, R., and Westaby, D. (1993) Randomised trial of variceal banding ligation versus injection sclerotherapy for bleeding oesophageal varices. *Lancet*, 342, 391–4.

Greenway, B., Johnston, P.J., and Williams, R. (1982) Control of malignant ascites with spironolactone. *Br J Surg*, 69, 441–2.

Hanau, L.H. and Steigbigel, N.H. (2000) Acute (ascending) cholangitis. *Infect Dis Clin North Am*, 14(3), 521–46.

Kim, W.R., Ludwig, J., and Lindor, K.D. (2000) Variant forms of cholestatic diseases involving small bile ducts in adults. *Am J Gastroenterol*, 95(5), 1130–8.

King, P.D. and Perry, M.C. (2001) Hepatotoxicity of chemotherapy. *Oncologist*, 6, 162–76.

Lawrence, T.S., Robertson, J.M., Anscher, M.S., Jirtle, R.L., Ensminger, W.D., and Fajardo, L.F. (1995) Hepatic toxicity resulting from cancer treatment. *Int J Radiat Oncol Biol Phys*, 31(5), 1237–48.

Lee, W.M. (1996) Management of acute liver failure. *Semin Liver Dis*, 16(4), 369–78.

McDonald, G.B., Shulman, H.M., Wolford, J.L., and Spencer, G.D. (1987) Liver disease after human marrow transplantation. *Semin Liver Dis*, 7(3), 210–29.

Mas, A., Salmeron, J.M., and Rodes, J. (1994) Diagnosis and therapy of hepatic encephalopathy. *Adv Exp Med Biol*, **368**,119–23.

Souter, R.G., Wells, C., Tarin, D., and Kettlewell, M.G. (1985) Surgical and pathologic complications associated with peritoneovenous shunts in management of malignant ascites. *Cancer*, **55**, 1973–8.

Starzl, T.E., Demetris, A.J., and Van Thiel, D. (1989) Liver transplantation. *N Engl J Med*, **321**(16), 1092–9.

Terkivatan, T., de Wilt, J.H., de Man, R.A., van Rijn, R.R., Tilanus, H.W., and Ijzermans, J.N. (2001) Treatment of ruptured hepatocellular adenoma. *Br J Surg*, **88**(2),207–9.

Tilanus, H.W. (1995) Budd–Chiari syndrome. *Br J Surg*, **82**(8), 1023–30.

Chapter 8

Bone Emergencies

Ruth Eakin

8.1 Introduction

Cancer patients are at risk of severe and distressing bone pain, with or without associated pathologic fractures. Given the relatively high percentage of cancers which metastasize to bone, this type of clinical presentation is not uncommon. In the emergency setting, clinical examination and plain X-rays are often all that are required to diagnose the majority of problems quickly. The importance of appropriate management cannot be underestimated if good palliative care is to be part of modern medicine.

8.2 Bone cancer

Cancer affecting the bone may be from a primary or secondary malignancy. The vast majority (99 percent) are metastases from distant primary sites, but 1 percent of bone cancer arises in the bone itself.

8.2.1 Primary bone tumors

Primary bone tumors are rare, accounting for less than 0.5 percent of all cancers. The most common is osteosarcoma (or osteogenic sarcoma), followed by chondrosarcoma and Ewing's sarcoma (Table 8.1). There is an increased incidence of osteosarcoma associated with bilateral retinoblastomas, and this has been linked to the presence of specific deletions in the Retinoblastoma (Rb) gene arrangement. The Rb gene product is recognized to play an important part in regulating the cell cycle. Likewise, mutation of the p53 gene have found to be associated with a number of different cancers. In the Li Fraumeni syndrome, there is an association with malignancies such as breast cancer, gliomas, and hematologic malignancies in first-degree relatives of children and adolescents presenting with osteosarcoma.

A detailed account of the management of these tumors is beyond the scope of this text. However, it is important to note that the outlook for these often young patients has significantly improved over the past two decades. Long-term survival has risen from less than 20 percent in the 1960s to around 60 percent in the 1990s, with average survival at 3 years in 2001 in excess of 50 percent. Reasons for this include better diagnostic imaging, more effective systemic chemotherapy, improvements in radiation therapy techniques, advances in surgical techniques, but most importantly an increasing move

Table 8.1 Primary bone cancer—classification

Osteosarcoma	High grade
	Periosteal
	Post-radiation
	Paget's osteosarcoma
Chondrosarcoma	
Round cell tumors	Ewing's sarcoma
	Askin tumor
	Primitive neuroectodermal tumor (PNET)
Giant cell tumor	
Malignant fibrous histiocytoma	
Non-Hodgkin's lymphoma of bone	
Other	Fibrosarcoma
	Liposarcoma
	Hemangiosarcoma

towards combined modality assessment and treatment. Less aggressive surgery has been possible with the combination of pre- or post-operative radiotherapy and neo-adjuvant or adjuvant chemotherapy. It is by continuing the entry of these patients into clinical trials that further progress will be made.

8.2.2 **Bone metastases**

Solid tumors commonly metastasize to lung, liver, and bone. The axial skeleton is often affected in adults (ribs, vertebrae, pelvis, and skull), with primary tumors originating from breast cancer, prostate cancer, lung cancer, Hodgkin's disease, thyroid carcinoma, and renal cell carcinoma (Table 8.2). The femur and humerus are also commonly involved. In contrast, primary tumors such as leukemia and neuroblastoma in pediatric patients, more frequently metastasize to the long bones.

Patterns of metastases are poorly understood, but are nonetheless recognized to be unique in several ways. It is more common for tumor cells to metastasize to bone than to any other organ, more so than can be explained by expected blood flow patterns alone. The vertebral-venous plexus is thought to play a significant role, in that blood returning to the heart via the vena cava can be easily diverted through this system by changes in intra-abdominal pressure, unlike blood returning through the hepatic or pulmonary systems. These anatomical features alongside other factors such as bone physiology (see Section 8.3) are felt to represent major reasons for predilection to bone. However much is still unknown in this area. In addition, the symptoms and difficulties caused by bony metastatic deposits are variable, and include pain, fracture, hypercalcemia, bone marrow impairment, and/or painful nerve pathway disruption such as spinal cord compression. The survival of these patients is also variable, and in breast and prostate cancer especially, may be many years. The appropriate and timely

Table 8.2 Secondary bone cancer—incidence of primary sites

	Median incidence (%)
Breast	73
Prostate	68
Thyroid	42
Kidney	35
Lung	36
Rectum	11
Esophagus	6

management of bone metastases is, therefore, extremely important if optimum palliation is to be achieved.

8.3 Pathophysiology of bone metastases

8.3.1 Normal physiology of bone

Bone is made up mostly of a collagenous matrix which is 95 percent type I collagen fibers. The principal crystalline salts of calcium and phosphate are deposited in this matrix, along with magnesium, sodium, potassium, and carbonate ions. These salts form hydroxyapatite crystals and this is where almost all calcium is stored.

There are two main types of bone, but both have great tensile and compressional strength. The collagen fibers extend primarily along the lines of tension, while the mineral salts provide resistance to compression. Compact bone is the main component of long bones and provides the skeleton with a solid structure, whereas cancellous bone is much less dense, although also strong, and provides a housing for bone marrow and other metabolic processes.

There is a constant turnover of collagen and mineral salts, with osteoblasts synthesizing collagen, and osteoclasts tunneling into bone causing erosion and resorption. Osteocytes are thought to play an important role in the movement of minerals. The precise mechanism of remodeling is not well-understood, and the regulation of bone turnover even less well-defined. However, osteoblasts have been shown to be involved in synthesis of collagen, while osteoclasts are intricately linked with the resorption process. The achievement of a normal balance between osteoclastic activity and osteoblastic activity seems to be related to environmental factors, as well as growth factors found within the matrix. Their specific roles in the normal process also differ depending on the type of bone studied. Stimulators of bone resorption include cytokines such as interleukin-1, granulocyte colony-stimulating factor, and tumor necrosis factor, and hormones such as parathyroid hormone (PTH) may enhance the presence of these products.

8.3.2 Pathophysiology of bone

Precise mechanisms and reasons for preferential tumor spread to bone, how, and why, have all eluded scientists for decades. Nonetheless, there is increasing knowledge about some of the issues, and many products and factors have been isolated from individual types of malignant cells, which have been found to influence metabolic activity in bone. For example, an osteoblastic stimulating factor has been isolated from prostate cancer cells, and human melanoma cells have been shown to produce a macrophage stimulating factor, which causes them to release tumor necrosis factor and interleukin-1. Several breast cancer cell lines have been found to secrete transforming growth factor α, transforming growth factor β, epithelial growth factor, parathyroid-related protein, prostaglandins, and procathepsin D, all related to bone destruction.

Tumor metastases appear to be either osteoblastic, or more commonly osteolytic. Osteoblastic metastases occur in prostate cancer, breast cancer, renal cell carcinoma, thyroid carcinoma, and Hodgkin's disease. It would seem that in osteoblastic metastases, the imbalance is shifted towards excess bone formation, whereas in osteolytic metastases, bone is destroyed to a greater extent than it is laid down. Whichever occurs, the bone involved is often weakened, and the patient is at risk of complications. The distribution of solitary or multiple metastatic deposits in any individual is not predictable, although the anatomy of blood supply to the vertebrae or long bones is thought to play a pivotal role. The clinical picture will naturally depend on the site, size and extent of metastases, and deserves careful and thorough evaluation in each individual, so that management can be tailored appropriately.

8.4 Presentation of bone emergencies

8.4.1 Fractures and impending fractures

Bone pain is the most common presenting feature of either pathologic fracture, or of impending pathologic fracture, but it is not absolutely essential for the diagnosis. For many patients, the presentation of a pathologic fracture may be the first sign of metastatic disease, and it may not signal the only site of spread. Around 50 percent will be due to metastasis from breast cancer (Table 8.3), and the commonest site for pathologic fracture is the femur (Table 8.4), although almost any tumor can be responsible for disease at a variety of sites.

Life expectancy of these patients has gradually improved with increasing progress in the combined modality therapy of different tumors, and must be taken into account. Whether fractures are displaced, non-displaced, impending in weight-bearing bones or in non-weight-bearing bones are all important factors when management decisions are being made. These tumor-related factors, along with patient-related factors, such as performance status and previous mobility, need to be assessed and collated. For example, operative intervention for fractures in non-weight-bearing bones may be considered worthwhile when survival is expected to be at least 3 months, whereas for fractures

Table 8.3 Tumors causing pathologic fractures

Primary tumor	No. of patients	No. of fractures
Breast	101	116
Lung	21	22
Prostate	21	22
Kidney	7	7
Rectum	6	6
Bladder	3	3
Stomach	3	3
Melanoma	2	2
Uterus	2	2
Thyroid	1	1
Colon	1	1
Esophagus	1	1
Bile Duct	1	1
Cervix	1	1
Penis	1	1
Lymphoma	4	5
Leukemia	6	6
Myeloma	24	34
Not known	4	4
Total	211	239

in weight-bearing bones it should be considered even with a life expectancy of as little as 1 month. Pain relief may be as important an objective as stability or mobility, and in fact surgical intervention is desirable for most pathologic fractures.

Impending fractures need to be identified and managed as early as possible, in order to reduce pain, disability, and obvious consequences of proceeding to fracture. If they involve the hip or proximal femur, then urgent assessment and preventative action should be taken. Indications for active intervention are not always clear-cut, but certain criteria and a scoring system have been proposed, based on the site of impending fracture, clinical and radiologic findings, and the size of the abnormality (Table 8.5). Given the overlap of clinical outcomes between the groups, it can only be considered as a guide, but nonetheless, it can give some useful additional information about the likelihood of fracture, or not.

8.4.2 **Spinal cord compression**

It is estimated that up to one in every five patients who have vertebral metastases, will develop spinal cord compression at some time during their illness. Moreover, it is

Table 8.4 Sites of pathologic fractures

Site	Subsite	Number
Pelvis		2
Femur	Transcervical	57
	Intertrochanteric	25
	Subtrochanteric	26
	Shaft	40
	Distal	10
Humerus	Proximal	19
	Shaft	47
	Distal	3
Tibia	Proximal	2
	Shaft	1
Radius	Shaft	2
Ulna	Shaft	1
Clavicle		3
Mandible		1
Total		239

Table 8.5 Mirel's criteria and scoring system for impending fractures

Variable	Points			Score	No. of patients	Fracture rate (%)
	1	2	3			
Site	Upper extremity	Lower extremity	Peri-trochanteric	0–6	11	0
				7	19	5
Pain	Mild	Moderate	Severe	8	12	33
X-ray	Blastic	Mixed	Lytic	9	7	57
Size	0–33%	34–67%	68–100%	10–12	18	100

second only to brain metastases as a neurologic complication of cancer. The most common types of tumor responsible for spinal cord compression are lung, breast, "unknown primary," lymphoma, myeloma, sarcoma, prostate, kidney, gastrointestinal, and thyroid tumors. Spinal cord compression occurs by direct pressure from an enlarging mass within the vertebra, vertebral fracture and retropulsion of fragments into the canal, epidural metastases behind intact vertebrae, and rarely by intradural metastases. It should be emphasized that cord compression is usually a late manifestation of spinal metastasis. Although these patients have an incurable disease, many can live for some considerable time with their cancer, and so the importance of early active intervention cannot be over-stated, given the difference in quality of life on which good management depends. The restoration of function, prevention of deterioration, and relief of pain, must be given a high priority.

In a variable proportion of patients, spinal cord compression is the presenting scenario to specialist hospital services. As neurologic status at initiation of treatment is the single most important determination of outcome, it is vital that there are no delays in the appropriate management pathway. Back pain is often the first symptom of spinal metastasis and usually predates spinal cord compression. Ninety percent of patients with spinal cord compression have back pain. In patients with a known history of cancer, the development of back pain should be regarded as sinister, warranting immediate referral and investigation. Pain may be due to infiltration or mechanical effects. It may be localized to the back or in a root distribution. Mechanical events may have an effect, but the cardinal feature is that the pain is progressive with time, and eventually interferes with sleep. Motor symptoms generally predate sensory symptoms as spinal cord compression is usually anterior. Unexplained reduced mobility in a cancer patient should raise the suspicion of neurologic involvement. Sensory symptoms usually ascend. As a result, prediction of level of spinal involvement from sensory examination is unreliable until late in the clinical course at which time there may already be loss of bladder and bowel control.

Clinical examination varies depending on the site of compression. The most commonly involved site is the thoracic spine (70 percent), and is classically associated with lower limb weakness and exaggerated deep reflexes, upgoing plantars, and sometimes a sensory level. Tone varies depending on the acuteness of onset. Below L1 where the spinal cord ends, a lower motor neuron cauda equina syndrome may occur. Once suspected, the patient should be immobilized to protect from further neurologic injury. If there is any question of bladder involvement, a urinary catheter should be inserted to protect bladder function. Dexamethasone 8 mg given intravenously may help to stabilize or improve neurologic function temporarily while investigations are instituted. The extent of spinal cord involvement needs to be determined. It is important to be aware that metastases often occur at multiple sites along the spine.

Magnetic resonance imaging (MRI) should be obtained (Fig. 8.1) of the whole spine. Radiographs should be obtained of any areas where there is pathologic fracture. If spinal cord compression is the presenting symptom then a rapid confirmation of the histologic diagnosis should be sought. If a primary site is identified and is accessible, then this should be biopsied. However this may not be possible. In osteolytic lesions a percutaneous vertebral biopsy usually by the transpedicular route with a 3 mm needle such as a Craig needle may give enough tissue to allow histologic diagnosis in >90 percent of cases where the tumor is confined to the vertebral body. If the tumor has significantly spread into the surrounding soft tissues, a CT guided Trucut needle biopsy can be used. In emergency cases sufficient information may be obtained by using a smear technique rather than waiting for routine histologic preparation to differentiate between metastatic tumor, lymphoma, myeloma, and infection.

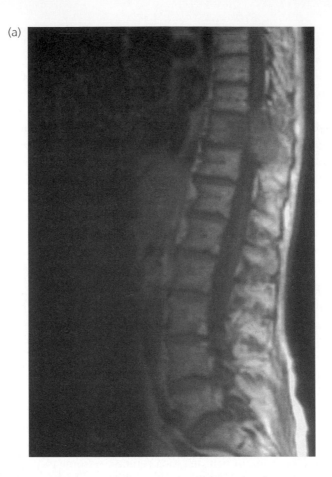

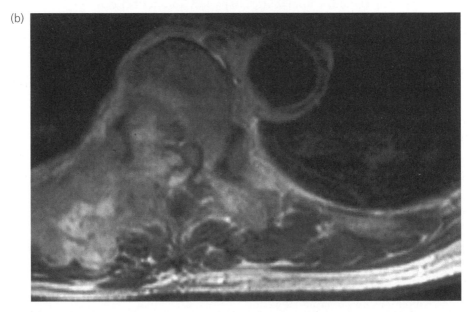

Fig. 8.1 MRI scan showing spinal cord compression—(a) saggital view, (b) MRI scan showing spinal cord compression—axial view.

Once the site, extent of spinal cord compression and the histology of the tumor are known, treatment can be rationalized. Patients who are still ambulatory at presentation and treatment, have a fairly good chance of remaining so. Once function has gone, it is most unlikely to be restored. Despite the obvious need for early diagnosis, up to 80 percent of patients still present too late. The key to successful management is a high index of suspicion leading to early referral and investigation.

8.5 Management of bone emergencies

8.5.1 Assessment and general supportive measures

History taking, careful clinical examination, pain relief, and stabilization of the anatomical region concerned, are all part of the immediate management of a pathologic fracture, impending pathologic fracture, or compression of the spinal cord. Immobilization will help control pain and bleeding, and the patient may need to be admitted if there are associated neurologic deficits, fractures through lesions presenting for the first time, or significant structural fractures requiring immediate operative intervention. Plain X-rays will be done in the emergency setting, and other urgent investigations depending on the situation. These are difficult and frightening times for patients and their relatives, and due consideration for the associated apprehension of all concerned, should not be overlooked at this time.

8.5.2 Management of bone pain *(Algorithms 8.1, 8.2)*

Pharmacologic methods of treating pain (see Chapter 9) need to be used in the immediate setting. Opiate analgesia is almost always required because of the intensity of pain associated with a pathologic fracture, but where appropriate, the analgesic ladder should be followed. Neuropathic pain occurs as a result of a different physiologic mechanism, and is not thought to be particularly opioid responsive. Corticosteroids and non-steroidal anti-inflammatories may also be used, particularly when nerve compression is an obvious problem. Many of these patients have several forms of pain, and additional types of medication such as anti-depressants and anti-convulsants may also be useful. As part of the multidisciplinary team involved in managing these situations, palliative medicine physicians and anesthesiologists often have an invaluable role to play.

Definitive treatment is most often orthopedic, and will involve stabilizing the fracture or impending fracture, either by internal or external fixation. Whether it is done at all, and what procedure is performed, needs to be decided by the orthopedic surgeon, as part of the multidisciplinary team, and must be tailored to each individual case. Orthopedic intervention should be considered in all situations where there is instability, a risk of fracture or where a fracture has occurred, whatever the stage of the illness, and (usually) however poor the prognosis. It is by far the most effective way to establish durable pain relief.

As an alternative, or more often as an adjunct, palliative radiotherapy has an important role to play. It can relieve bone pain, help to prevent pathologic fractures or vertebral

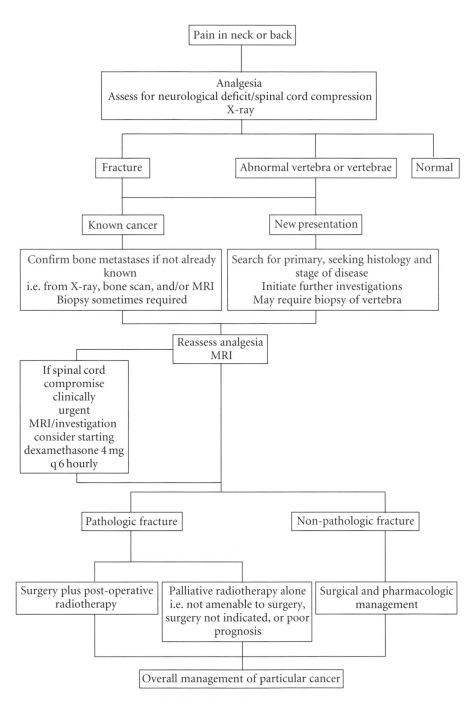

Algorithm 8.1 Spinal symptoms.

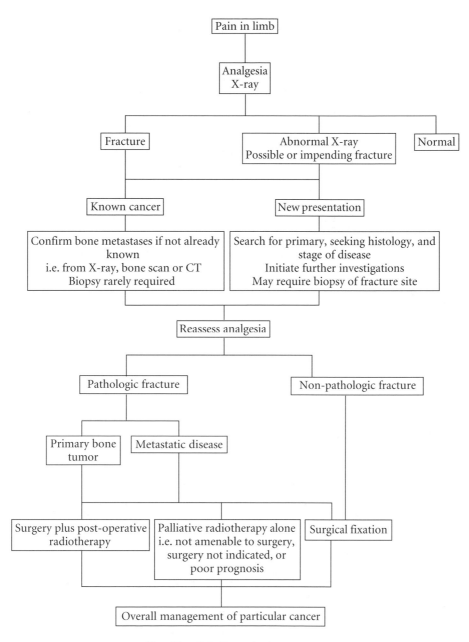

Algorithm 8.2 Non-spinal symptoms.

collapse, and promote healing of fractures, preferably after orthopedic fixation. Dose and fractionation regimes are discussed later in this chapter. Radiation treatment is highly effective, with overall symptomatic response rates in excess of 80 percent. In addition, it is non-invasive, and depending on the site being treated, often delivered without any side effects. Commonly it is given using external beam therapy, but radioactive isotopes such as strontium or sumarium can also be used, although not in the emergency setting. These isotopes are given by intravenous injection, commonly where there are multiple and symptomatic bony metastases. Minimal radioprotection precautions are required for a short period of time afterwards, as the half-life of sumarium is only 46 hours. This property also allows for repeated injections if clinically indicated. Isolation is not required, but avoidance of mingling with the public, or holding children closely, for a few days, will always be discussed before treatment, as part of the standard protocol. Bone marrow suppression is a possible side effect, easily avoidable by ensuring adequate bone marrow function prior to treatment.

Other methods of controlling pain include the use of intravenous or oral bisphosphonates, and other strategies such as physiotherapy and occupational therapy, all have their part to play. An important issue is that many professionals must be able to work as a team in order to bring the necessary wide expertise together in a timely and appropriate fashion, for each individual patient.

8.5.3 Orthopedic intervention

Surgical management involves reducing displaced fractures, stabilization and may or may not include excision of the defective bone. If tumor is excised, then the remaining deficit can be filled with methylmethacrylate cement prior to fixation. In some situations, it may be appropriate to attempt to 'downstage' the tumor prior to surgery, as this might allow the removal of a smaller volume of tissue. In less fit patients, a closed reduction may be the appropriate option, with either internal or external fixation. The general condition of the patient, their co-morbidity, the size and site of the lesion, and the type of tumor with its associated responsiveness to systemic or other local therapies, are all important factors in the decision-making process. Plates and screws tend to concentrate the load at the end of the device, and are best suited to metaphyseal lesions, where intramedullary devices would be difficult to insert. They are better for diaphyseal lesions, and tend to spread the load throughout the affected bone. Endoprostheses fixed with cement give good stability, thus good pain relief, and often good return of function. Issues pertinent to managing individual fractures and impending fractures are discussed later.

8.5.4 Radiation therapy

Radiation therapy is a highly effective modality for treating painful bony metastases. Where a fracture has occurred, surgical intervention should always be considered in the first instance, unless it involves regions not amenable to orthopedic intervention such as ribs, scapula, or pelvis. In these cases, radiotherapy can provide pain relief in up to 80 percent of patients, while promoting bone healing. For long bone fractures, rigid immobilization with internal fixation should be performed prior to irradiation, in order to give the lesion the best chance of healing. In addition, radiotherapy is likely to impede local tumor progression which is thought to reduce the risk of failure of the fixation device.

The dose of radiation which should be given, is controversial. Thirty Gy in ten 300 cGy fractions over a two-week period was considered to be standard since the early part of the twentieth century, when fractionation was revealed as a way of achieving maximum tumor cell kill while allowing normal tissue regeneration. However, the desire to reduce the number of fractions in the palliative setting, in order to reduce inconvenience for patients, and overall cost, led to many studies worldwide. As a result of these, there is probably more uncertainty than ever, as to which fractionation regime is optimum. Nonetheless, where there are painful bony metastases and no fracture or impending fracture, it is entirely appropriate to treat with a single fraction of 800 cGy. Several recent surveys have reported current practice in Europe, USA, and Canada. Longer fractionation regimes are still most commonly used in the United States, quite commonly used in Europe, with Canadian oncologists using the shorter one-week regimes.

Another recent study tried to break down the reasons for oncologists' reluctance to use single fractions, despite evidence to support it. Factors such as prognosis, performance status, site of lesion (e.g. weight bearing or not), type of cancer, fracture or no fracture, and the presence or absence of neurologic signs, all seemed to be taken into consideration. Currently, single fractions are given to poor performance status patients, with uncomplicated bone metastases and a poor prognosis. Otherwise, fractionated courses are preferred, especially for weight-bearing regions, where there are neurologic complications, and where there are pathologic fractures, or impending fractures.

As well as local field (LF) irradiation, hemibody or wide field irradiation can be used. As an alternative, or as complementary to external beam radiotherapy, systemic radioisotopes can be used. Hemibody irradiation is considerably more toxic than LF, and requires intensive pre-medication plus intravenous hydration, because of gastrointestinal toxicity. Neither hemibody nor radioisotopes are normally used in the emergency setting, and will, therefore, not be discussed in detail.

8.5.5 Management of pathologic fractures

Lower extremity long bone fractures

Weight-bearing requirements are clearly significant when considering the clinical impact of fractures of the femur, or neck of femur. Replacement arthroplasty is the operation of choice, and the prosthetic device used should aim to allow immediate full weight-bearing, for the anticipated duration of the patient's life. There is a fairly high failure rate for internal fixation devices due to the stresses and strains of this part of the skeleton, and healing can be slow. Prostheses can be inserted as a total hip replacement, with or without an acetabular reconstruction, depending on the extent and position of disease involvement. In certain situations, such as where there are several lesions in close proximity or the tumor is known to be relatively radio-resistant, a long-stemmed endoprosthesis may be required to reinforce the bulk of the long bone, especially where prognosis is uncertain, and disease progression likely.

There is much more controversy over the management of inter-trochanteric fractures, for which there are good arguments for using an open reduction and internal fixation with a compression device. Even with this approach, there is some uncertainty as to whether the cement should be injected before or after the compression screw is inserted, that is, whether it is better to embed the screw into bone or cement. Long or short intramedullary hip screws can also be used, but have some disadvantages as well as advantages. In particular, fractures have been reported to occur at the tip of the short hip screws, and although few reports have been published on the use of long hip screws, they seem to have the advantage of strengthening the entire bone. If there is extensive involvement, then prosthetic replacement should be the procedure of choice, despite the risks of disrupting gait and recurrent dislocation.

Fractures of the sub-trochanteric region need to be treated with intramedullary devices, where interlocking nails, proximally and distally, help to secure the necessary degree of fixation (Fig. 8.2a). Fractures of the shaft or diaphysis, require conventional, closed, intramedullary stabilization (Fig. 8.2b), and in some cases, where the lesion is large, replacement of bone can be achieved with methylmethacrylate filling. For fractures

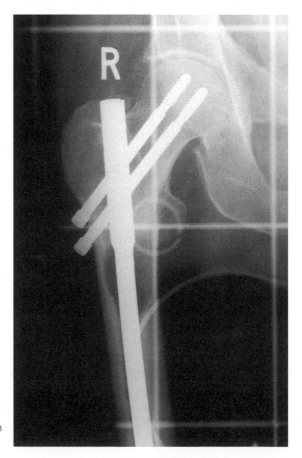

Fig. 8.2a Patient with sub-trochanteric lytic lesion from renal cell carcinoma, showing intramedullary fixation with interlocking nails.

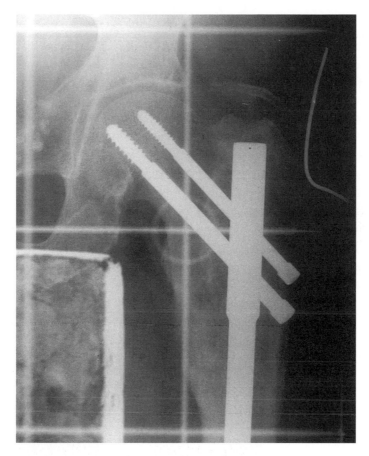

Fig. 8.2b Patient with prostate carcinoma and fixation of typical expanding sclerotic lesion of the upper femur.

of the distal femur, again internal fixation is normally used, except where there is significant bone destruction, in which case replacement arthroplasty may be necessary.

In most of these circumstances, post-operative radiotherapy is to be recommended, and can be given by simple parallel opposed fields. Fractionated dose regimens are generally preferable, that is, treating daily over 1–2 weeks.

Upper extremity long bone fractures

The aim of treatment here is to ensure stability of the shoulder joint and thereby achieve pain relief. Rotator cuff damage is not possible to repair. Because of the smaller size of the humerus, internal intramedullary devices are used with extreme caution, and open bone grafting is often required. Replacement arthroplasty may be necessary if stabilization is not possible otherwise, however the vast majority can usually be dealt with satisfactorily by intramedullary nailing (Fig. 8.3a). Fractures around the metaphyses generally require plate and screw fixation. Post-operative radiotherapy giving 20–30 Gy over 1–2 weeks is usually recommended, and should be commenced around 4–6 weeks post-operatively, whenever the wound has healed satisfactorily (Fig. 8.3b).

Pelvic fractures

Acetabular fractures, in general, require total hip replacement arthroplasty. Because of the often extensive metastatic involvement around the acetabulum and femur, this major operation is not often recommended, given the potential morbidity and mortality in often frail patients. Where it is offered, the procedure will depend on the class of fracture:

Class I   The lateral cortices and superior and medial walls are intact. In this situation, there is sufficient surrounding intact bone to attempt a total hip arthroplasty.

Class II   The medial wall is involved, therefore reconstruction must aim to transfer weight bearing away from the medial wall on to the intact acetabular rim.

Class III   All the above locations are deficient. This scenario is the most challenging, and requires an accurate transfer of the weight-bearing structures to be aligned at

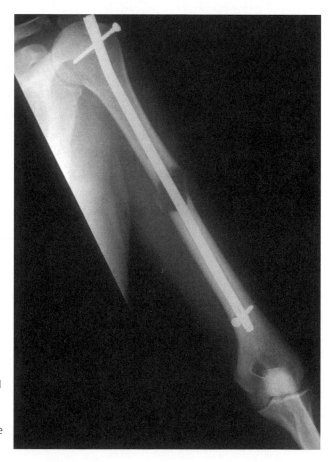

Fig. 8.3a Patient with renal cell carcinoma, showing intramedullary fixation of a minimally displaced fracture of the left humerus.

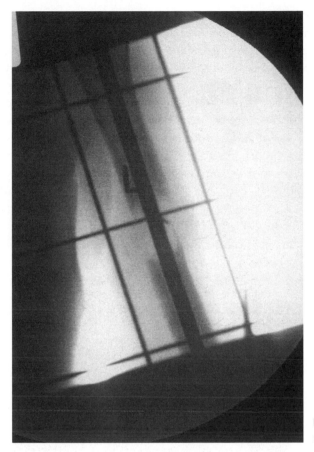

Fig. 8.3b Simulator film of radiation treatment portal.

15 degrees medial to the vertical, in other words along the direct line across the pelvis from femur to vertebrae. Several groups of pins are placed to produce a lattice-type structure from a prosthetic cup and acetabulum. Blood loss during this operation can be a significant issue, and embolization may be needed as part of this technique.

Class IV   In this group, there is a solitary metastasis which if resected, may result in long-term survival. This includes patients with a previous hypernephroma, or occasionally thyroid carcinoma.

Spinal fractures

Ideally all pathologic vertebral fractures should be assessed jointly by an oncologist and spinal surgeon soon after diagnosis. The primary goals of therapy in fractures of the vertebrae, are to ensure stability of the spine and local tumor control, hence obtaining pain relief and maintenance of neurologic function for the patient.

Patients with spinal collapse can present with two clinical problems—pain or neurologic involvement. If there is pain without neurologic involvement it is important to assess whether the pain is due mostly to tumor expansion/infiltration or whether it is mechanical in nature. The first category will respond to local tumor control by non-surgical means such as radiation therapy, chemotherapy, or hormone manipulation, and is best managed by an oncologist. These represent the majority of patients with pathologic spinal fracture.

A smaller number of patients develop major mechanical pain. Such pain is much better understood and treated by a spinal surgeon. X-rays may give a strong clue to the likely mechanical behavior of an involved vertebra. Biomechanically the spine can be considered to be made up of two columns, an anterior weight-bearing column (vertebral body), and a posterior column (lamina/facets/pedicles), which largely resists tension and checks abnormal movement. If the anterior column (vertebral body) is largely destroyed, the vertebra becomes susceptible to deformity under axial load. If, in addition, the posterior column is affected the spine also becomes capable of abnormal movement under rotation and shear (Fig. 8.4). Hence instability is not a black and white situation but a spectrum from mild to severe depending on the degree of involvement of the vertebral body. This could be thought of as a stage in which there is a varying

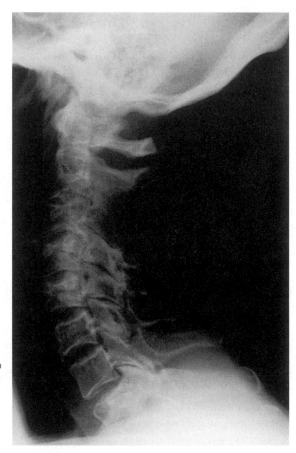

Fig. 8.4 Patient with rectal carcinoma who was found to have extensive destruction of the spinous processes and posterior elements of C2 and C3, with retained spinal alignment.

degree of risk of impending neurologic upset. Although several different methods of classifying individual vertebral involvement have been suggested in an effort to predict mechanical behavior and aid surgical planning, none have been validated clinically. In some instances the degree of loss of bone integrity is so obvious that instability can almost be assumed (Fig. 8.5a). In situations of doubt, mechanical insufficiency can be judged by a trial of appropriate immobilization either by bedrest or a suitable orthosis. If pain is improved dramatically the diagnosis is confirmed and surgical stabilization may be indicated if there are no confounding variables (Fig. 8.5b,c,d). It is a relatively uncommon indication for surgery.

More commonly spinal surgery is offered to the patient with a pathologic fracture associated with spinal cord compression where there is spinal cord impingement by retropulsed fragments. This is usually a late manifestation of spinal metastatic disease. Other indications for spinal surgery where there are spinal metastases, include progressive neurologic defects by a radio-resistant tumor or recurrent tumor after maximum radiotherapy irrespective of whether or not the vertebra has collapsed.

For the treating surgeon it is not always easy to decide whether an operative strategy is appropriate in an individual patient due to other variables. The basic premise is that all patients in whom there is a reasonable chance of preserving or restoring mobility and continence, and who will live long enough to enjoy the benefits of successful surgery, should be considered. The three most important factors known to be predictive of outcome are the *histology* of the tumor, and the *degree* and *rapidity* of progression of the neurologic upset. Patients with lung tumors rarely live longer than three months

(a)

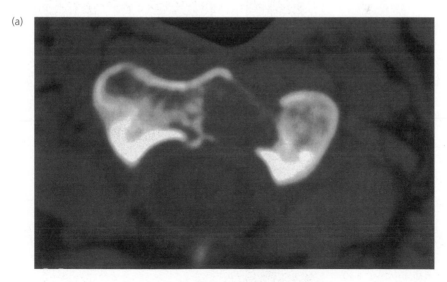

Fig. 8.5a MRI scan through cervical vertebra of a patient with breast cancer, showing metastatic infiltration of the lateral process, with complete destruction of the posterior cortex and significant thinning of the anterior cortex.

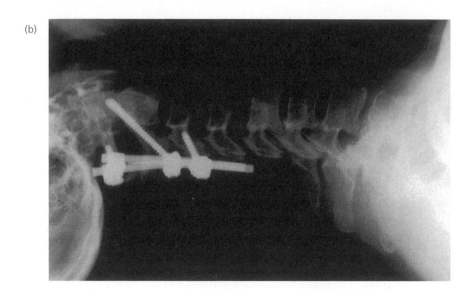

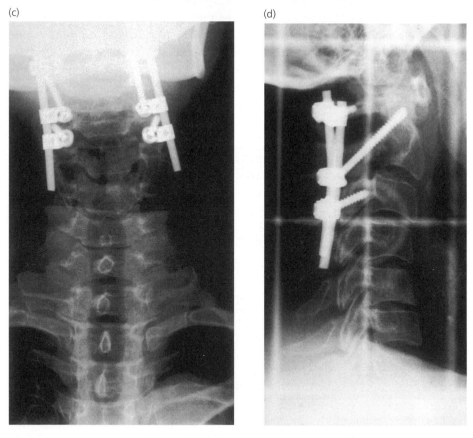

Fig. 8.5b–d (b) Lateral view of surgical fixation. (c) Anterior view of surgical fixation. (d) Simulator film of radiation treatment portal.

following the onset of spinal cord compression and it is debatable whether they should be considered routinely for surgery. Patients who are unable to move their lower limbs against gravity (grade III power) pre-operatively, especially if the neurologic deficit came on rapidly, have a poor neurologic outcome irrespective of treatment. If the disease process is spread over several levels very occasionally it may not be possible to produce a stable biomechanical fix to the spine, or the patient's general medical condition may suggest that they will not live long enough to derive benefit from the surgery. Tokuhashi *et al.* produced a scoring system in an effort to predict outcome of surgery based on the Karnofsky performance status, number of extraspinal metastases, number of metastases in the vertebral body, number of metastases to major internal organs, primary site, and extent of paresis. If the patients scored less than five they did not survive longer than 3 months. Those who scored more than nine lived longer than 12 months. The scoring system has not been widely adopted and independent validation is very limited. It is not suitable for use in emergency cases when it is often not possible to gather all the necessary information quickly. Although there are now many surgical series in the literature confirming the favourable results of surgery for late metastatic spinal disease with cord compression, further work is needed to allow more accurate prediction of surgical outcome in emergency cases.

The surgical approach is dictated by a number of factors. The goals of surgery are to decompress or stabilize or both. Biomechanically stable fixation methods for virtually all regions of the spine for both anterior and posterior aspects have been available for approximately 10 years. Where possible a single approach to the spine is employed to limit morbidity. Debate still exists whether this should be performed from an anterior or posterior approach. As the compression is anterior to the cord in 85 percent of cases decompression must be directed to this area irrespective of the surgical approach used. An anterior approach gives a better direct approach to decompression. The disadvantage of an anterior approach is its potential for increased morbidity if the thoracic cavity has to be opened and the special expertise required to instrument the anterior thoraco-lumbar spine. The posterior approach usually allows a postero-lateral decompression to be fashioned. A posterior decompression in the thoracic region is only indicated in the rare instance that there is involvement purely posterior to the cord or there is tumor restricted to a doughnut-shaped ring of tumor around the cord requiring decompression. A posterior approach allows for long segments of the spine to be fixed which is particularly useful when disease is multilevel. If the tumor is below the level of the conus a purely posterior approach can usually achieve stabilization and decompression adequately.

Palliative radiotherapy should be given post-operatively, or can be used as a single modality of treatment, and is normally delivered to the thoracic or lumbar spine using a direct posterior field (Fig. 8.6). The cervical spine needs to be treated by lateral opposing fields. As the lumbar vertebrae are significantly deeper than thoracic vertebrae, an anterior and posterior parallel-opposed field arrangement is sometimes used, or else the single posterior field is prescribed to depth. Prophylactic anti-emetics are recommended when

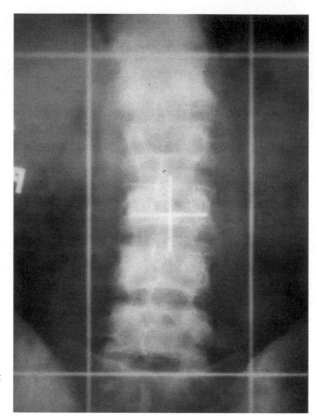

Fig. 8.6 Radiation treatment portal for direct posterior field.

a significant amount of small bowel is likely to be included in the treatment volume. A single fraction of palliative radiotherapy is generally considered to be adequate and effective where the primary objective of treatment is pain relief in patients who have a poor prognosis, or those who have poor performance status. Side effects are uncommon, but can include marginally increased pain over a few days, temporarily, before the desired symptomatic improvement. Otherwise, a fractionated course of radiotherapy, of 20–30 Gy over 2–3 weeks, should be considered. The importance of early recognition, (i.e. within 24 hours of presentation), joint oncology/surgical spine team assessment followed by prompt investigation and management, cannot be overemphasized.

8.5.6 Impending pathologic fractures and prevention

Recognized indications for prophylactic intervention of impending long bone fractures, can be summarized as follows:

1. Cortical bone destruction of 50 percent or more (Fig. 8.7)
2. A lesion of 2.5 cm or more in the proximal femur

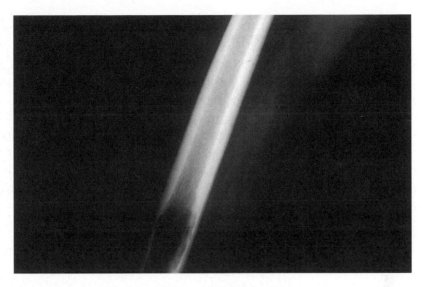

Fig. 8.7 Impending pathologic fracture of the femur in a patient with renal cell carcinoma.

3. Pathologic avulsion fracture of the lesser trochanter

4. Persisting pain despite irradiation.

It is also important to recognize that pain will only be present in less than half of these patients, and is often a sign of a fracture having occurred. As soon as an impending or possible fracture is suspected, simple measures such as avoiding weight bearing, or providing ambulatory aids should be instituted, until full evaluation with plain X-rays has taken place and an assessment of risk of fracture, performed. Before and after any intervention, physiotherapy input should be initiated, as rehabilitation is an extremely important part of the overall management strategy.

Once the decision has been made to physically intervene, every effort must be made to avoid fracture during the operation, and dissection to surrounding soft tissue needs to be kept to a minimum in order to preserve periosteal blood supply. Cement will be required where there is significant tissue deficit, and debulking of tumor should be attempted prior to post-operative irradiation. Otherwise, surgical and radiotherapy techniques do not differ dramatically from those described above for pathologic fracture.

8.5.7 Other bone emergencies

Hypercalcemia

Symptoms of hypercalcemia include nausea, vomiting, abdominal pain, polydipsia, polyuria, malaise, weight loss, and constipation. It is a medical emergency and is covered in more detail in Chapter 3. Suffice to say that it affects about 70 percent of all cancer patients at some stage of their illness, and is often, but not always, associated with bone metastases. Active management including rehydration and intravenous bisphosphonates can rapidly alleviate symptoms. For those with proven bone metastases, other palliative measures should be considered, as appropriate.

Infection

Bone infection or abscesses occur in the immunocompromised patient with cancer who may have had chemotherapy as part of their treatment regime. Neutropenic sepsis is very common, and the possibility of an abscess should always be considered when the patient is being assessed. Needle aspiration can be performed for diagnosis and as part of management and broad-spectrum antibiotics commenced. Joints can also become infected and surgical drainage with irrigation may be required. Occasionally, aggressive surgical intervention is unavoidable, but again, prompt recognition and appropriate management should keep this to a minimum.

Pediatric bone emergencies

Children with cancer are at risk of tumor or treatment-related bone complications. Most can be diagnosed by plain radiology and treated without delay. However, as with adults, some difficulties can occur. There is a different spectrum of tumors in children, and fractures tend to occur in those who have had previous surgery for primary bone tumors, most commonly osteosarcoma. Certain chemotherapy drugs, such as methotrexate, and steroids may also contribute to insufficiency fractures related to treatment-induced osteopenia. A detailed account is beyond the scope of this text, and pediatric oncology literature should be consulted.

8.5 **Summary and conclusions**

Community and hospital physicians should have a low threshold for suspecting a pathologic fracture or an impending fracture in any patient who is known to have cancer. It can of course be the presenting scenario. In any case, investigations should be initiated without delay, so that a decision can be made whether admission is necessary or not in the first instance. In the case of possible spinal cord compression, the urgency is even greater if significant morbidity is to be avoided. Increasingly, it is essential to conduct a multidisciplinary team approach to management in order to effect the optimum response for each individual emergency situation. All aspects of the patient's care must be dealt with in totality.

Suggested reading

Amling, M., Takeda, S., and Karsenty, G. (2000) A neuro (endo)crine regulation of bone remodelling. *Bioessays*, **22**(11), 970–5.

Ben-Josef, E., Shamsa, F., Williams, A.O., and Porter, A.T. (1998) Radiotherapeutic management of osseous metastases: a survey of current patterns of care. *Int J Radiat Oncol Biol Phys*, **40**(4), 915–21.

Chow, E., Danjoux, C., Wong, R., *et al.* (2000) Palliation of bone metastases: a survey of patterns of practice among Canadian radiation oncologists. *Radiother Oncol*, **56**(3), 305–14.

Galasko, C.S.B. (1995) *Oxford textbook of oncology* (ed. M. Peckham, H.M. Pinedo, and U. Veronesi), pp. 2286–95, Oxford University Press.

Galasko, C.S.B. (1981) The anatomy and pathways of skeletal metastases. In *Bone metastasis* (ed. L. Weiss and A.H. Gilbert), pp. 49–63, GK Hall, Boston.

Harrington, K.D. (1997) Orthopedic surgical management of skeletal complications of malignancy. *Cancer*, **80**(Suppl 8), 1614–27.

Lievens, Y., Kesteloot, K., Rijnders, A., *et al.* (2000) Differences in palliative radiotherapy for bone metastases within Western European countries. *Radiother Oncol*, **56**(3), 297–303.

Manglani, H.H., Marco, R.A.W., Picciolo, A., and Healy, J.H. (2000) Orthopedic emergencies in cancer patients. *Seminars in Oncology*, **27**(3), 299–310.

Nielsen, O.S., Bentzen, S.M., Sandberg, E., Gadeberg, C.C., and Timotyh, A.R. (1998) Randomized trial of single dose versus fractionated palliative radiotherapy of bone metastases. *Radiother Oncol*, **47**(3), 233–40.

Roebuck, D.J. (1999) Skeletal complications in pediatric oncology patients. *Scientific Exhibit*, **19**(4), 873–85.

Roos, D.E. (2000) Continuing reluctance to use single fractions of radiotherapy for metastatic bone pain: an Australian and New Zealand Practice survey and literature review. *Radiother Oncol*, **56**(3), 315–22.

Tokuhashi, Y., Matsuzaki, H., Toriyama, S., Kawano, H., and Ohsaka, S. (1990) Scoring system for the preoperative evaluation of metastatic spine tumor prognosis. *Spine*, **15**(11), 1110–3.

Tomita, K., Kawahara, N., Kobayashi, T., Yoshida, A., Murakami, H., and Akamaru, T. (2001) Surgical strategy for spinal metastases. *Spine*, **26**(3), 298–306.

Chapter 9

Acute Pain Emergencies

Sheila Kelly and Bernadette Corcoran

9.1 Introduction/definition

Pain is something we feel. It can be described as an unpleasant sensory and emotional experience associated with actual or potential damage, or described in terms of such damage.

Pain recognition, assessment, and management have been shown to be challenging. Pain measurement is necessarily subjective. There are no objective measures of pain as in blood tests, or X-rays. Observation of physical signs and change in behavioral patterns may provide some information.

Research has found pain to be a common symptom among patients with cancer. Research has also shown that oncologists tend to focus on the physical domain and use information from assessment more for treatment decisions than to address the impact the pain has on the patient's life. This approach fails to recognize that pain is a dynamic construct made up of interweaving layers of physical, social, emotional, and existential distress. Saunders first recognized this and used the term "total pain" to emphasize the interlinking between physical pain and the patient's suffering. Suffering can be defined as the state of severe distress associated with events which threaten the intactness of the person.

Assessment and management, therefore, are more effective when approached from a holistic stance which addresses physical, emotional, social, and spiritual factors. Because of the variety of skills needed, the patient's pain may be best addressed by appropriate members of a multi-professional team.

9.2 Pain prevalence

Patients (and relatives) commonly express a fear of developing severe intractable pain when a diagnosis of cancer is made. The reported prevalence varies from study to study, depending on the setting (hospital, cancer hospital or hospice) and stage of disease. Pain tends to increase as disease progresses. There is a wide variation in prevalence figures depending on tumor type. Prevalence figures range from 33 percent of patients in a cancer hospital, where one-third of patients in active therapy had pain versus two-thirds of patients with advanced disease, to 84 percent of patients in the hospice setting.

Although two-thirds of cancer patients experience severe pain, one-third does not. In a Danish study, by Banning and colleagues, the majority of patients attending a cancer pain clinic had at least two causes of pain.

9.3 Neuroanatomy and neurophysiology

Nerve fibers are classified on the basis of the fiber diameter. A, B, and C nerve fibers with alpha, beta, delta, and gamma subcategories are identified. Of these A-beta, A-delta, and C are sensory fibers and play a role in pain perception. Their nerve endings are known as nociceptors.

A-delta nociceptors respond to pinching and squeezing and result in the fast sharp pain of injury.

C fibers ("polymodal nociceptors") respond to noxious mechanical thermal or chemical stimuli. They are also stimulated by pain producing substances such as acetycholine, bradykinin, histamine, and capsaicin. These C fibers respond to produce a slow throbbing diffuse pain.

A-delta and C fibers synapse in the dorsal horn neurons, which may modulate or inhibit the transmission of the painful stimulus to the thalamus and cortex. This theory was first described by Melzach and Wall in 1965 and is known as the Gate Control Theory. This theory has been modified in light of more recent understanding of the dorsal horn neuronal activity. Descending inhibitory neural pathways to the dorsal horn also modulate incoming nociceptive stimuli.

A variety of neurotransmitters have been recognized and play a role in pain perception.

1. Excitatory amino acid receptors have been identified in the dorsal horn. In the context of pain modulation attention has focused on the N-methyl D-asparate (NMDA) receptor.

2. Serotonin and noradrenaline are involved in the descending inhibitory pathways.

3. Opioid peptides are found in the brain and throughout the spinal cord. These endogenous opioid peptides, endorphins, dynorphins, and enkephalins have morphine-like properties, and have specificity for the opioid receptor sites. At least three types of opioid receptor subtypes, mu, kappa, and delta subserve opioid analgesia.

The interplay of the nerve stimulation, neurotransmitters, the dorsal horn inter-neurone activity and influence of the descending inhibitory pathway together modulate pain perception.

9.4 Classification and pathophysiology of pain

Pain can be classified into different types. Understanding the difference in these pain types may indicate the pathophysiology and guide treatment options.

Common approaches include:

1. Acute and chronic pain based on different symptoms, expressions and behavior (Table 9.1).

2. Nociceptive and neuropathic pain based on whether the pain results from noxious stimuli being detected by nociceptive nerve endings or pain resulting from a pathologic change in the nervous system (Table 9.2).

3. Constant and episodic or incident pain based on temporal nature of the pain. This can be either nociceptive, neuropathic or a combination of both.

Table 9.1 Acute and chronic pain based on different symptoms, expressions and behavior

	Acute	**Chronic**	
Time course	Transient	Persistent	
Meaning to patient	Positive: Draws attention to injury or illness	Negative: Serves no useful purpose	Positive: As patient obtains secondary gain
Accompanying features	Fight or flight: Pupillary dilatation Increased sweating Tachypnea Tachycardia Shunting of blood from viscera to muscles	Vegetative: Sleep disturbance Anorexia Decreased libido No pleasure in life Constipation Somatic pre-occupation Personality change Lethargy	

Reproduced with permission of Radcliffe Medical Press.

Table 9.2 Nociceptive pain/neuropathic pain

Category	Characteristics	Examples	Response to opioids
Nociceptive			
Somatic pain	Dull, aching, throbbing, or gnawing Well localized	Bone pain Incisional pain Myofascial, musculofascial, and musculoskeletal pain	Excellent
Visceral pain	Originates from injury to sympathetically innervated organs Caused by infiltration, compression, distention, or stretching of thoracic/abdominal viscera Poorly localized, deep, dragging, squeezing, or pressure-like When acute, may be colicky and associated with autonomic symptoms (nausea, vomiting, sweating, tachycardia) Often referred to cutaneous sites remote from the lesion (e.g. shoulder pain of hepatic origin)	Bowel obstruction Stretching of liver capsule	Good

Table 9.2 (continued)

Category	Characteristics	Examples	Response to opioids
Neuropathic pain	Results from injury to peripheral and/or central nervous system, by tumor compression or infiltration or damage from surgical, radiation, or chemotherapy Superficial burning, stinging, sometimes with superimposed lancinating, electric shock-like pain Often associated with sensory changes There may also be associated muscle atrophy, autonomic changes, and trophic changes in the skin	Brachial/lumbosacral plexopathies Post-herpetic neuralgia Vincristine or cisplatin neuropathy Diabetic neuropathy	Poor

Reproduced with permission of Radcliffe Medical Press.

Chronic pain is not merely an extension of acute pain. It is understood that in chronic pain there is central nervous system modification induced by the chronic afferent neuronal activity. Repeated C fiber stimulation leads to increased neuronal responses in the dorsal horn leading to increased and prolonged pain. This is called "wind-up" and is thought to be mediated via the excitatory amino acid NMDA receptor.

Some neuropathic pains are sympathetically maintained. This is recognized where there are accompanying signs of autonomic dsyfunction such as sweating and temperature changes.

9.5 Pain management approach

9.5.1 Pain assessment

Successful pain management relies on an accurate assessment which should be holistic, that is, inclusive of the impact of the pain on the psychosocial and spiritual well-being of the patient. Because of the many variables in pain it is essential to have a standard approach to assessment. This includes:

- Taking an accurate pain history
- Using an assessment tool
- Standard clinical examination
- Appropriate laboratory and radiologic investigation.

Pain assessment tools help in understanding the patient's pain and facilitate monitoring of the effects of analgesics and other interventions. These include questionnaires, categorical scales, visual analogue scales (VAS), body charts and pictorial scales for children; the more complex are used for research only.

Most patients can grade their pain out of ten, where 0 = no pain and 10 = worst pain ever or use a simple VAS.

Least Possible Pain 0 → 10 Worst Possible Pain

Physical examination should aim to identify causes of pain, for example, tenderness from bone metastases; evidence of bowel obstruction; neurologic dysfunction as a pointer to neuropathic pain or patterns suggestive of cancer pain syndromes.

Investigation may be necessary to confirm areas of suspected disease.

Altered skin sensation associated with neuropathic pain:

1. Numb area of skin
2. *Dysesthesia* An unpleasant abnormal sensation spontaneous or evoked
3. *Hyperesthesia* An increased sensitivity to stimulation
4. *Allodynia* Pain caused by stimuli which does not normally evoke pain
5. *Hyperalgesia* Increased response to a stimulus that is normally painful
6. *Hyperpathia* Explosive and often prolonged painful response to a stimulus.

9.5.2 **Principles of pain management**

This aim of optimal pain management is to maximize quality of life and independence.

To achieve this aim attend to the following principles:

1. Identify the type or classification of the pain:
    (a) *Nociceptive* Somatic or visceral pain. This is usually opioid sensitive. Use the WHO Analgesic Ladder.
    (b) *Neuropathic pain* This may be poorly opioid responsive. Adjuvant analgesic drugs may help. Optimal pain management may be difficult.
    (c) *Acute/episodic pain* Frequently has mixed pathophysiology. May need advice from a Specialist Palliative Care Team.

2. Accurately diagnose the cause of each pain and correct the cause if possible.

3. Communicate to the patient the likely cause of the pain and with the patient set realistic goals of pain relief.

4. Use regular analgesia in doses titrated to the individual's pain threshold, and in the most appropriate route of administration.

5. Manage the patient at the lowest effective dose of the most appropriate drug.

6. Communicate clearly with patient regarding medication changes, likely side effects and benefits.

7. Pain levels change frequently, therefore review regularly, especially after change in dose or choice of medication.

8. Remember to attend to the multidimensional aspects of "total pain." The "meaning" of pain varies with each patient, and each culture and this may need to be explored.

9. Provide support for family and carers of patients with pain.

9.5.3 Pain management options

Effective pain management may be achieved by any one of the following modalities. Frequently a combination is necessary.

- **Retard tumor progression**
  Palliative chemotherapy
  Radiotherapy
  Hormonal therapy

- **Palliative surgery**
  Orthopedic procedure to stabilize a fracture, or decompress the spinal cord will relieve pain. Defunctioning colostomy in bowel obstruction may relieve visceral pain.

- **Analgesics**
  Non-opioids
  Opioids

- **Adjuvant analgesic drugs**

- **Transcutaneous electrical nerve stimulation** (TENS)

- **Physiotherapy**

- **Nerve blocks**
  Local nerve block
  Spinal analgesia
  Sympathetic ganglion block

- **Acupuncture**

- **Complementary medicine**

- **Relaxation therapy**

- **Alterations in life style**

9.5.4 Analgesic pain management

Before addressing management of acute pain or cancer pain syndromes it is necessary to have an understanding of available analgesics, their pharmacokinetics, how to make the appropriate analgesic option/combinations, and how to minimize or treat side effects.

The World Health Organization *3 Step Analgesic Ladder* effectively combines analgesic agents to achieve optimum pain control using a stepwise approach (Fig. 9.1). This 3-step ladder is based on pain severity rather than on pain etiology. It works on the premise that patients with advanced disease will have constant pain. Using this treatment strategy up to 88 percent of patients obtain satisfactory pain relief.

1. *By the mouth* The oral route is the preferred route for analgesia. This includes morphine.

2. *By the clock* Constant pain requires regular analgesics. Analgesics should be given prophylactically rather than on a "PRN" rescue pattern.

3. *By the ladder* If a drug fails to relieve pain move up the ladder. It is not helpful to move laterally in the same efficacy group.

Step 1—Non-opioid analgesics

Because of the risk factors associated with aspirin, paracetamol is usually the drug of choice. It has no anti-inflammatory action but acts by inhibition of prostaglandin mediated pathways in the spinal cord.

Step 2—Opioids for mild/moderate pain

This group includes tramadol, dextropropoxyphene, and codeine. The latter two are available in combination with paracetamol.

Tramadol is a synthetic centrally acting analgesic which has both opioid and non-opioid properties. The latter are related to stimulation of neuronal serotonin release and inhibition of presynaptic re-uptake of noradrenaline and serotonin. Parenterally it is 1/10 as potent as morphine.

Step 3—Opioids for moderate to severe pain

These drugs were previously known as 'strong opioids.' Morphine oral formulation and diamorphine parenteral formulation remain the first line drugs of choice in the UK.

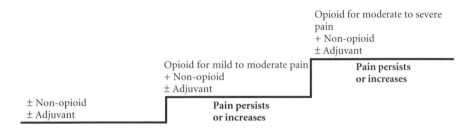

Fig. 9.1 World Health Organisation analgesic ladder.

The short duration of action of pethidine (1–2 hours) and potentially toxic metabolites make it unsuitable for the treatment of chronic pain. Alternative opioids include fentanyl, hydromorphone, oxycodone, and methadone. The alternative strong opioids may be useful where dose titration is limited by side effects of morphine/diamorphine. (see opioid switching)

9.6 Opioids

9.6.1 Morphine: preparations (Tables 9.3, 9.4)

Tho WHO/EAPC guidelines recommend morphine as the opiate of first choice for cancer pain management. There is no ceiling dose on morphine; the correct dose for each patient is the dosage that relieves the patient's pain without intolerable side effects. On oral administration it is readily absorbed in the upper small bowel and metabolized mainly in the liver to Morphine-3-Glucuronide (M3G) and Morphine-6-Glucuronide (M6G). Morphine-6-Glucuronide is an active metabolite and is more potent than morphine. Morphine and its glucuronides are excreted renally and may accumulate in patients with impaired renal function.

Commencing a patient on morphine

Guidelines on the use of morphine in cancer pain were published by the European Association for Palliative Care in 1996, these guidelines were recently reviewed together with the indications for the use of alternative opioid by Hanks *et al.*

A normal release morphine preparation given orally four hourly facilitates rapid pain management. The starting dose for severe pain is usually 10 mg four hourly in robust patients (reduce to 2.5–5 mg four hourly in the frail or elderly). Pain occurring between the four-hourly doses of morphine is called "breakthrough pain." When this occurs a "rescue" normal release dose equivalent to the four-hourly dose is given. The scheduled four-hourly dose continues even if the rescue dose has been administered.

Dose titration

After 24 hours, the total morphine given (four hourly plus breakthrough) is calculated, one-sixth of this is then given four hourly as the new regimen. This continues until pain is

Table 9.3 Morphine: preparations

Oral	Normal release (dose titration and breakthrough pain) Modified release (maintenance treatment)
Rectal	Normal release Modified release
Parenteral/spinal	Poor solubility, diamorphine is used in the UK due to its greater solubility

Table 9.4 Relative potency ratios for oral administration of morphine when changing routes of administration

	Ratio to oral morphine
Rectal morphine	1 : 1
Subcutaneous morphine	1 : 2
Intravenous morphine	1 : 3
Subcutaneous diamorphine	1 : 3

stable. When pain control has been achieved, the total dose of morphine taken over the 24 hours is calculated. This total dose is then given as a modified released preparation, either as a 12- or 24-hourly formulation. It may be impractical in a community setting to commence a patient on four-hourly normal release morphine and patients outside the hospital and hospice setting are frequently commenced on modified release preparations.

Normal release preparations should always be available for "breakthrough pain," given as one-sixth of the 24-hour dose, as pain levels in cancer patients frequently change.

9.6.2 Diamorphine

This is the preferred preparation for parenteral use in the UK. It is highly soluble in small volumes.

Management of morphine side effects

- *Constipation*   A laxative should always be prescribed with opioids.
- *Nausea and vomiting*   This occurs in about 30 percent of patients first starting on opioids, but is self-limiting. Appropriate anti-emetics such as metoclopramide 10 mg q 6 hourly or haloperidol 1.5–3 mg at night should be prescribed.
- *Dry mouth*   Artificial saliva preparations are recommended.
- *Undue sedation*   This commonly occurs when commencing morphine or when the dose has been increased. It is self-limiting within 2–3 days on the same dose. Excessive sedation indicates early toxicity.
- *Less frequent side effects*   Itching, sweating, and occasional hypotension.

Addiction/dependence

When using opioids for the management of pain, addiction is not a problem. There may be a degree of physical dependence which on withdrawal presents as agitation, restlessness, mild confusion and signs of sympathetic overdrive. This is avoided by ensuring that reduction of opioids is gradual rather than precipitous.

Tolerance

The mechanism for tolerance is not well understood. Clinical practice confirms that tolerance is rare. It is more likely to do so with repeated intravenous use of opioids.

Signs of morphine toxicity

- Persistent drowsiness
- Pinpoint pupils
- Persistent nausea and vomiting
- Myoclonic jerks/seizures
- Respiratory depression

Opioid—switching/rotation

While there is no ceiling dose in using opioids, in effect dose escalation may be limited by side effects, possibly due to the accumulation of toxic metabolites in frail, dehydrated patients. For patients with side effects despite inadequate analgesia, there are three main approaches:

1. Opioid dose reduction—to reduce side effects, with use of adjuvants to improve analgesia.
2. Switching to an alternative opioid—may allow titration to adequate analgesia without the same disabling effects.
3. Switching route of opioid delivery—much smaller drug doses can be given by the spinal (intrathecal) route (local anesthetic can also be given).

To date there are no Randomized Controlled Trials(RCTs) to establish if switching between opioids is effective and there are no agreed indications of the optimal frequency of switching. This is a developing practice in countries where effective alternatives to morphine are available. Specialist advice may be necessary.

Alternative opioids increasingly used include:

- Fentanyl
- Methadone
- Hydromorphone
- Oxycodone

9.6.3 Fentanyl: preparations

- Transdermal patch (maintenance treatment)
- Oral transmucosal (breakthrough pain)
- Parenteral/spinal

Fentanyl is a semi-synthetic opioid and an established intravenous anesthetic and analgesic drug. It is a highly selective mu agonist and is about 80 times as potent as parenteral morphine. Orally, it rapidly undergoes extensive first pass metabolism. As it has less effect on gastrointestinal transit time it causes less constipation. Metabolism occurs in the liver and the metabolites are inactive, therefore, it causes less toxicity than morphine in the presence of renal impairment.

Transdermal fentanyl

The transdermal fentanyl patch is a newer pain control option for patients with stable pain. Fentanyl patches are available in four sizes: 25, 50, 75, and 100 µg. The amount of drug delivered is proportional to the patch size: a 25 patch delivers 25 µg of fentanyl per hour. Following application of the first patch the plasma levels rise reaching analgesic level by 8–16 hours, steady state is reached before the next dose at 72 hours. The patch should be replaced every 3 days. On removal a depot remains in the skin for approximately 24 hours. Transdermal fentanyl is not suitable for patients with acute pain in whom rapid dose titration is required, and may also present a problem when rapid reduction in opioid levels is desired.

Indications for transdermal fentanyl patch

Patients with opioid responsive *stable* pain

(1) who are severely constipated on other opioids;

(2) who are unable to take oral medication;

(3) who have poor compliance with oral medication;

(4) who have unacceptable side effects with other opioids (see opioid switching).

Key points when converting between morphine and a transdermal fentanyl patch

The choice of the appropriate patch strength should be guided by the relationship between oral morphine dose and patch size (Table 9.5).

1. If converting from four-hourly oral morphine, continue to give regular doses for 12 hours.

2. If converting from 12-hourly morphine preparations, apply the fentanyl patch at the same time as giving the final 12-hourly dose.

Table 9.5 Relationship between oral morphine and patch size

4-hourly oral morphine (mg)	24-hourly oral morphine (mg)	Fentanyl patch size (µg/hour)	24-hourly s.c. diamorphine (mg)
5–20	30–130	25	10–40
25–35	140–220	50	50–70
40–50	230–310	75	80–100
55–65	320–400	100	110–130

Systemic analgesia concentrations are generally reached within 12 hours.

3. If converting from a syringe driver, maintain the syringe driver for about 12 hours after applying the first patch.

4. In patients for whom pain was not controlled while on the fentanyl patch, when converting to diamorphine calculate the equivalent dose of diamorphine and increase the dose by 30 percent. It is important to review the patient frequently during this opioid changeover time period.

Oral transmucosal fentanyl citrate (OTFC)

The oral mucosa is highly vascularized and permeable and presents a large surface area for absorption, in addition transmucosal drug delivery avoids first pass metabolism. Oral transmucosal fentanyl citrate, therefore, has a rapid onset of action.

The OTFC consists of a fentanyl impregnated sweetened and hardened lozenge on a plastic handle. The lozenge dissolves in contact with the buccal mucosa and a portion of the drug is absorbed across the oral mucosa. The remaining drug is swallowed and absorbed in the stomach and intestine. The OTFC is available in six dosage strengths (200, 400, 600, 800, 1200, and 1600 µg fentanyl-base per unit).

The rapid absorption and time-to-peak plasma concentration are associated with onset of pain relief in 5–10 min. The successful dose of OTFC cannot be predicted and is not directly related to the daily dose of regular opioid being received for background pain, the dose has to be titrated to the individual patient's pain intensity.

Indications for OTFC   Patients who have acute episodic opioid responsive pain.

- Hanks and colleagues in 2001 completed a UK multi-center study showing that OTFC is an effective and well-tolerated treatment for breakthrough pain.

9.6.4 **Methadone: preparations (Table 9.6)**

Methadone is a synthetic opioid which is rapidly absorbed after oral administration. Its plasma half-life is long, averaging approximately 24 hours but there is considerable inter-individual variability in its pharmacokinetics. It has both mu and delta receptor effects and the recent literature describes its NMDA blocking effects.

Indications for Methadone (Specialist only)

- Patients who have unacceptable side effects with other opioids (see opioid switching)
- Patients with neuropathic pain (NMDA blocking effect).

Specialist advice should be sought before commencing methadone because of its complex pharmacokinetics and its inter-individual variability. There are difficulties determining an

Table 9.6 Methadone: preparations

Oral	low and high concentration
Parenteral	

equi-analgesic dose of methadone when changing from another opioid. It should be used with caution in the elderly because of its long half-life and potential for accumulation.

9.6.5 Hydromorphone: preparations

Table 9.7

Oral	Normal release (dose titration and breakthrough pain)
	Modified release (maintenance treatment)
Parenteral/spinal	Available in some countries (UK-named-patient basis only)

Hydromorphone is pharmacologically similar to morphine with a similar efficacy and adverse effect profile, but 5–6 times more potent. Its potential advantages are potency, thus small volumes when used parenterally, (where available) and possibly less accumulation of active metabolites in renal failure. A conversion ratio of morphine: hydromorphone of 7.5 : 1 is recommended.

Indications for hydromorphone

• Patients who have unacceptable side effects with other opioids (see opioid switching)

• Renal impairment (unproven).

9.6.6 Oxycodone: preparations (Table 9.8)

Oxycodone is a semi-synthetic opioid which has been available in a rectal preparation for many years. It is twice as potent as morphine. It is postulated that the analgesic effects of oxycodone are primarily mediated by the kappa opioid receptor while having a weak affinity for the mu receptor. A morphine : oxycodone of ratio 2 : 1 is recommended.

Indications for oxycodone

• Patients who have unacceptable side effects with other opioids (see opioid switching).

Adjuvant analgesics

The following groups are frequently used.

• Non-steroidal anti-inflammatory drugs (NSAIDs)

• Tricyclic antidepressant drugs

• Anticonvulsant drugs

• Corticosteroids

• NDMA receptor antagonists (e.g. Ketamine)

• Bisphosphonates

Table 9.8 Oxycodone: preparations

Oral	Normal release (dose titration and breakthrough)
	Modified release
Rectal	Limited availability
Parenteral	Variable in some countries (not UK)

These adjuvant analgesics are drugs which are not analgesic in their own right but can produce analgesia in certain situations. They are particularly useful for neuropathic pain which may be "opioid poorly responsive."

Non-steroidal anti-inflammatory drugs (NSAIDs)

The mechanism of action is through inhibition of the enzyme cyclo-oxygenase (Cox) involved in prostaglandin synthesis. Two forms of Cox enzyme exist: Cox-1 is present in all normal tissue; Cox-2 is normally undetectable in tissues but is induced in the presence of inflammation. It is postulated that the anti-inflammatory and analgesic effects of NSAIDs are related to inhibition of Cox-2 and that selective Cox-2 inhibitors reduce the renal and gastric toxicity of NSAIDs.

Despite their recognition as adjuvant analgesics the literature has no definite information on the efficacy of NSAIDs as adjuvants with opioids, therefore the choice of NSAID and the duration of treatment must be individualized. NSAIDs are available in oral, rectal and parenteral formulations. Diclofenac and ketorolac may be delivered by subcutaneous route via a syringe driver.

Ketorolac is a potent NSAID but has a high risk of gastrointestinal side effects; it has been advocated as an opiate-sparing analgesic. It may be appropriate to set up a ketorolac subcutaneous infusion by syringe driver as a temporary measure to gain control in acute pain. Patients prescribed NSAIDs should be monitored for adverse effects.

They are indicated for painful bony metastases, inflammatory pain, pleuritic chest pain, and musculoskeletal pain, for example, rheumatoid and osteoarthritis.

Antidepressants

There is evidence that tricyclic antidepressant drugs are analgesic in a variety of chronic pain syndromes but their usefulness is unclear in cancer pain; there is also less evidence to support the use of other antidepressants such as Selective Serotonin Re-uptake Inhibitors. Amitriptyline has been established as the antidepressant drug of choice in this category. The mechanism of action probably involves inhibition of re-uptake of noradrenaline and serotonin in the spinal cord. Anticholinergic side effects can inhibit increase in dose or continuing use. If no response has been achieved on titration to maximum tolerated dose, or following 3 weeks of treatment the drug ought to be discontinued.

Anticonvulsants

Anticonvulsants are used in the management of both chronic non-malignant and cancer-related neuropathic pain, carbamazepine, sodium valporate, and clonazepam are among those most frequently used. A number of newer anticonvulsant drugs have been promoted for the management of neuropathic pain, gabapentin is licensed for this use. Its precise mechanism of action as an analgesic is unknown. The commencement dose is titrated against response. Optimal pain response may be achieved in days or weeks. If no response is achieved gabapentin is discontinued.

N-methyl D-aspartate (NMDA) receptor antagonists

Ketamine, an anesthetic agent, has analgesic properties at sub-anesthetic doses. It also has sedative properties without causing respiratory depression.

Ketamine analgesia seems to be mediated through inhibition of the NMDA receptor in the dorsal horn, however, ketamine may also have an opioid receptor property. A synergistic effect between ketamine and opioids has been observed in cancer pain patients who have lost an analgesic response to high doses of morphine.

It can be used either as a continuous subcutaneous infusion by syringe driver or by the oral route. Ketamine S isomer has a lower side effect profile than the racemic mixture. Psychomimetic side effects may limit dose escalation. It is considered for neuropathic and other difficult pain management problems. When used, it is best commenced by palliative care/pain specialists.

Bisphosphonates

These drugs inhibit osteoclast activity and bone resorption. They are used to treat hypercalcemia and have a role in bone pain of malignancy. They are adsorbed onto bone surface and bind to hydroxyapatite, thus they may have a prolonged action. There is evidence from RCTs that they reduce pain (and morbid events) in metastases in multiple myeloma and breast cancer. Palliative Care Clinical Guidelines suggest their use in bone metastases from any malignancy where conventional treatment is unsuccessful or inappropriate. They are discussed elsewhere in this text (see Chapter 3).

9.6.7 Nerve blocks: spinal anesthetic

Approximately 10 percent of patients with difficult pain who do not respond to opioids and/or adjuvant analgesics may benefit from a nerve block or spinal analgesia.

When it is possible to locate neuropathic pain to a single nerve distribution or dermatome it is frequently possible to block that particular nerve using local anesthetic with or without steroids. This gives pain relief for weeks to months. However, depending on the patient's debility and degree of symptoms, neuro-ablation may be performed using phenol or cryotherapy. Common nerve blocks include:

(1) intercostal nerve block for chest wall pain,
(2) brachial plexus and/or stellate ganglion block for sympathetically maintained arm pain,
(3) lumbar sympathectomy for tenesmus or pelvic visceral pain.

Spinal analgesia includes both the epidural and intrathecal route. There is evidence to suggest that catheters via the epidural route may be more prone to complications than intrathecal catheters. It is important to select carefully who will best benefit from this method of pain management.

Indications for spinal analgesia

(1) Unacceptable side effects with other opioids despite opioid switching and other measures,

(2) severe pelvic/lower limb pain,

(3) acute control of pain in limb fractures.

Both epidural and intrathecal catheters deliver opioids, local anesthetics and other adjuvant drugs for neuropathic pain. Diamorphine (UK) is the usual opioid formulation and the conversion ratio calculated is 100 mg diamorphine subcutaneous = 10 mg epidurally = 1 mg intrathecally. Bupivacaine is the usual choice of local anesthetic. The dosage, strength and volume are titrated to optimize pain management and minimize power loss. Clonidine, ketamine, and fentanyl have also been used as spinal analgesics.

9.7 **Cancer pain syndromes**

Recognized cancer pain syndromes have been described. These help to identify the site and causation of the pain and may direct appropriate investigation, oncologic and pain management. Assessment should include consideration of the role of preexisting painful disorders such as arthritis and osteoporosis in the causation of the patient's pain.

The following are some of the more common syndromes.

9.7.1 **Treatment-related syndromes**

1. *Mucositis*   This is a painful condition of the mouth and pharynx caused by mucosal injury and inflammation, due to local radiation and some forms of chemotherapy. It may also affect the colorectal mucosa. Morphine analgesia may be necessary along with treatment of secondary infection.

2. *Steroid pseudo-rheumatism*   This is due to relatively rapid reduction of steroid dose and presents as a diffuse myalgia and arthralgia with associated muscle and joint tenderness. It is managed by reinstating the previous steroid dose and reducing more slowly.

3. *Chemotherapy-related polyneuropathy*   This is associated with a number of chemotherapeutic agents, in particular the vinca alkaloids. Management can be problematic. Opioids and adjuvants for neuropathic pain are used.

4. *Post-surgical pain syndromes*   These include post-mastectomy pain, post-thoracotomy pain and post-radical neck dissection pain. This is a mixed group and includes pain caused by nerve damage at the time of surgery and pain due to recurrent disease. Opioid, neuropathic adjuvant analgesia, and specific nerve blocks are indicated.

5. *Radiation neuropathy, plexopathy, and myelopathy*   This damage to nervous tissue occurs some years after radiotherapy and occurs less commonly than post-chemotherapy damage. Disease recurrence has to be excluded. These syndromes can cause challenging acute neuropathic pain which require a multimodal analgesic approach.

9.7.2 **Disease-related syndromes**

Bone pain is the most common cancer related pain, occurring in 60–84 percent of patients with solid tumors, followed in frequency by visceral pain and finally nerve infiltration pain. Pattern recognition allows early identification and intervention.

1. *Base of skull metastases* There are a number of syndromes relating to the specific areas of skull involvement and all share the features of pain (head and neck), cranial nerve dysfunction and difficulty with plain X-ray localization. Identification involves careful neurologic examination and MRI examination.

2. *Vertebral metastases* Metastases occur most frequently to the thoracic spine, followed by the lumbar and finally the cervical spine. Of note, (a) the atlanto-axial syndrome (destruction of the atlas or fracture of the odontoid process) with severe pain in occiput and neck, worsened particularly by neck flexion, (b) C7-T1 syndrome with referral of pain to the interscapular area and (c) T12/L1 syndrome, with referral of pain to the sacro-iliac joint and iliac crest.

3. *Spinal cord compression/cauda equina compression* This may be due to bony collapse or epidural extension of tumor and less commonly paraspinal tumor extension and hematogenous spread. Features include local bone pain, uni- or bilateral nerve root pain and neurologic dysfunction.

4. *Plexopathy* Infiltration of the brachial and lumbar plexuses give rise to pain with sensory and motor dysfunction. Brachial plexopathy is associated with lower cervical nerve root sensory and motor dysfunction. The patient may have a Horner's syndrome and lymphoedema. There is aching pain in the shoulder, upper back and paraspinal region with dysesthesia in the hand. In lumbosacral plexopathy the upper and/ or lower roots are involved with back, pelvic and thigh or leg pain and muscle weakness. With malignant psoas syndrome there is pain on hip extension with painful limitation of mobilization due to psoas muscle infiltration. Benign causes such as surgical trauma and radiation damage may sometimes be responsible.

Visceral pain

Visceral pain is poorly localized. Sensory nerves are present in the capsule of solid organ and the muscle coats of hollow organs and are stimulated by distension, inflammation, ischemia, and malignant infiltration.

Debility-related pain

This is a very diverse group and includes such conditions as myofascial pain and muscle cramp which are best managed by physical therapy and non-analgesic methods.

Management of cancer pain syndromes

See Table 9.2. Many patients have neuropathic and mixed nociceptive/neuropathic pain which are often opioid poorly-responsive and require tailored approaches to management. To avoid the problems of very high opioid dose, the use of adjuvant medication, such as anticonvulsants/corticosteroids for neuropathic pain and cortico-steroids/NSAIDs for visceral capsular pain may be helpful. There is a role for NMDA antagonists such as ketamine. Anesthetic procedures such as nerve blocks and spinal drug administration need to be considered.

In some cases, the difficulty lies in the episodic nature of the pain. For these patients, strategies include the use of adjuvant medication, alternative opioids and alternative routes, for example, the spinal route as well as non-pharmacologic approaches such as TENS and relaxation.

Referral to a Palliative Medical Consultant and the pain clinic may be helpful for these acute complex pain issues.

9.7.3 Breakthrough pain/incident pain

Pain which occurs against a background of stable pain relief is known as breakthrough pain. If there is a precipitant such as movement, micturition or passing flatus, this is known as incident pain.

Cancer-related pain frequently is constant, nociceptive in nature and is opioid sensit-ive. It therefore may not present management challenges to clinicians. The converse is true when cancer pain is episodic/acute incident pain. Patients frequently present to general practitioners, hospitals, or hospices as an emergency for crisis management. A recent study by Swanwick and colleagues, on the prevalence of episodic pain in cancer in 245 consecutive admissions to four hospices in Yorkshire, established that 232 patients (93 percent) had at least one experience of episodic pain during the 24 hours preceding admission. This pain frequently is a mixed nociceptive and neuropathic pain, and can be associated with significant patient debility.

Causes of acute-on-chronic pain or incident pain

- Fracture
- Hemorrhage
- Infarction or thrombosis
- Obstructed viscus
- Perforated viscus
- Nerve compression or inflammation
- Infection within tumor or surgical wound

Management of acute incident pain

The management of these events will depend on appropriate assessment and will need to be individualized for each patient.

Pathologic fractures may need to be stabilized temporarily, for example, with close fit-ting slings for upper arm fractures, and splints for femoral fractures while awaiting more definitive treatment such as orthopedic fixation and radiotherapy. Femoral nerve block may provide good temporary relief. Spinal or psoas compartment infusion may be used to manage pain if surgery is inappropriate in the terminal stage.

Hemorrhage into a tumor may cause an additional change in the quality of the pain if it causes nerve compression, corticosteroids may be useful for pain management.

Hemorrhage into hepatic secondaries may cause rapidly increasing right upper quadrant pain presenting like an acute abdomen. The opioid dose will require temporary rapid escalation with dose reduction as the hematoma resolves. Corticosteroids/NSAIDs may help.

Colicky pain of gastrointestinal obstruction may be palliated by antispasmodic anticholinergics in addition to opioids, if surgery is not feasible.

Infection should be considered if there is a rapid increase in pain in ulcerated tumor masses with associated swelling, induration and edema of surrounding tissues. Empirical antibiotics may provide dramatic benefit in 3–4 days.

Depending on the severity of the acute pain, and the patient's general condition, spinal analgesia may be the option of choice to gain rapid pain control. This, together with anxiolytics to contain the patient's emotional distress, allows the team to carry out appropriate investigations, to review the pathophysiology, and plan other treatment options if indicated and available (Figs. 9.2 and 9.3).

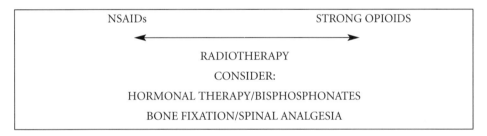

Fig. 9.2 Summary of management of skeletal pain.

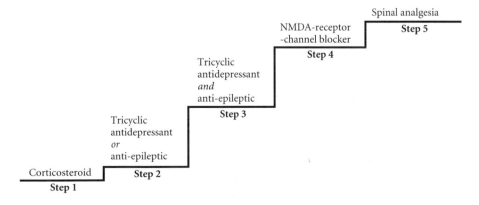

Fig. 9.3 Summary of management of neuropathic pain.

Suggested reading

Banning, A., Sjogren, P., and Henrisken, H. (1991) Pain causes in 200 patients referred to a multidisciplinary cancer pain clinic, *Pain*, 45(1), 45–8.

Casell, E. (1991) *The nature of suffering and the goal of medicine*, Oxford University Press, Oxford.

Davis, M. and Walsh, D. (2000) Cancer pain syndromes. *Eur J Palliat Care*, 7(6), 206–9.

Hanks, G. (2001) Oral transmucosal fentanyl citrate for the management of breakthrough pain. *Eur J Palliat Care*, 8(1), 6–9.

Hanks, G.W., de Conno, F., Cherny, N., Hanna, M., Kalso, E., McQuay, H.J., *et al.* (2001) Morphine and alternative opioids in cancer pain: the EAPC recommendations. *Br J Cancer*, 84(5), 587–93.

International Association for the Study of Pain Task Force on Taxonomy (1994) *Classification of chronic pain* (2nd edn) ISAP Press, Seattle.

Ripamonti, C., Groff, L., Brunelli, C., Polastri, D., and de Conno (1998) Switching from morphine to oral methadone in treating cancer pain: what is the equi-analgesic dose ratio? *J Clin Oncol*, 16, 3216–21.

Simpson, K.H. and Russon, L. (2000) The use of intrathecal drug delivery systems in pain management. Continuing medical education bulletin. *Palliat Med*, 2(1), 17–20.

Swanwick, M., Haworth, M., and Lennard, R.F. (2001) The prevalence of episodic pain in cancer: a survey of hospice patients on admission. *Palliat Med*, 15, 9–18.

Twycross, R.G. (2001) *Symptom management in advanced cancer* (3rd edn) Radcliffe Medical Press.

Waller, A. and Caroline, N.L. (1996) *Palliative care in cancer*. Butterworth-Heinemann.

Chapter 10

Psychiatric Emergencies

Chris B. Kelly and Roy J. McClelland

10.1 Disease-related psychiatric problems

10.1.1 Personal crises and adjustment

For the majority of patients a diagnosis of cancer is both a major psychologic event as well as a physical one. About one-third will experience some form of adjustment difficulty. As many as 80 percent of breast cancer patients report significant distress during initial treatment. Additional illness-related stresses are treatment with radiotherapy, chemotherapy, and diagnosis of recurrence of the illness. Patient concerns are often multiple and particularly in situations where the illness has progressed, issues other than the cancer or symptom control may come to the fore. Heaven and Maguire reported commonest concerns among hospice patients to be loss of independence and issues surrounding the family. Concerns surrounding life expectancy and death are inevitably raised and issues of an existential nature are common and no less a basis for acute suffering than any of the physical aspects of the disease process or its management. A strong relationship has been found between the number and severity of unresolved concerns and the later development of anxiety or depressive disorder.

Anticipating, recognizing and acknowledging patient concerns is likely to play a significant part in ameliorating distress and may prevent the development of more serious psychologic reactions. It is often nursing staff and junior medical staff who encounter patients at moments of existential crises. Such encounters are more likely in the terminal phases. Staff often feel ill equipped to respond to such situations as the focus of their training is mostly on physical care and disease management. Added to this is the tendency within modern culture, reflected in medical practice, that a diagnosis of a terminal illness signals the end of meaningful life. Such attitudes are counter to modern palliative care. A most important tenant within cancer care is that the patient is living with cancer. A key principle for any member of the clinical team encountering someone at crisis points is never to abandon the patient. At such moments clinicians can best serve their patient by simply being present. In their study of brain tumor patients Adelbratt and Strang noted the gratitude of patients for the opportunity to talk about questions of death and that they had few previous opportunities. Byock identified a series of goals the achievement of which can give meaning for people at the end of life (Table 10.1).

Table 10.1 Developmental landmarks and tasks for the end of life

---

Sense of Completion with Affairs
Transfer of fiscal, legal and formal social responsibilities

Sense of Completion in Relationships
Closure of multiple social relationships (employment, commerce, organisational, congregational).
Components include: expressions of regret, expressions of forgiveness, acceptance of gratitude
  and appreciation
Leave-taking; the saying of goodbye

Sense of Meaning About One's Individual Life
Life review
The telling of "one's stories"
Transmission of knowledge and wisdom

Experienced Love of Self
Self-acknowledgement
Self-forgiveness

Experienced Love of Others
Acceptance of worthiness

Sense of Completion in Relationships with Family and Friends
Reconciliation, fullness of communication and closure in each of one's important relationships.
Component tasks include: expressions of regret, expressions of forgiveness and acceptance,
  expressions of gratitude and appreciation, acceptance of gratitude and appreciation, expressions
  of affection
Leave-taking; the saying of goodbye

Acceptance of the Finality of Life—of One's Existence as an Individual
Acknowledgement of the totality of personal loss represented by one's dying and experience of
  personal pain of existential loss
Expression of the depth of personal tragedy that dying represents
Decathexis (emotional withdrawal) from worldly affairs and cathexis (emotional connection) with an
  enduring construct
Acceptance of dependency

Sense of a New Self (Personhood) Beyond Personal Loss
Sense of meaning about life in general
Achieving a sense of awe
Recognition of a transcendent realm
Developing/achieving a sense of comfort with chaos

Surrender to the Transcendent, to the Unknown—"Letting Go"

Reduction in distress and improvements in adjustment and mood can also be facilitated
through the use of group therapy.

How well a person adjusts to the cluster of stresses associated with a diagnosis of
cancer is dependent on many different factors usually unrelated to the illness process
itself. Rodrigue *et al.* identified the following important predictors of adjustment
difficulties: poor coping styles (acceptance/resignation or avoidance), low social support,
and family disturbance. Depending on the balance of strengths and vulnerabilities within

the person and in their situation a person may fail to cope with the illness and associated stresses. The commonest psychologic reactions among patients with serious difficulty in adjusting are anxiety and depressive disorders which are reported in up to one-third of cancer patients.

10.2 Anxiety disorders and post-traumatic disorder

10.2.1 Anxiety disorders

Presentation/description

Two clinical states predominate, in general anxiety disorder symptoms are generalized and persistent but not restricted to any particular circumstance. The dominant symptoms are variable but include complaints of persistent nervousness and fear, trembling, muscular tensions, sweating, dizziness, palpitations, and epigastric discomfort.

The second state is panic disorder which is characterized by recurrent attacks of severe anxiety (panic). As with general anxiety disorder the dominant symptoms include palpitations, chest pain, choking, dizziness, and feelings of unreality. There is often a secondary fear of dying, and losing control.

Anxiety states can be of sudden onset as a reaction to severe external stress in previously stable personalities with low trait anxiety. This can be considered a normal reaction to stress. Other individuals with high trait anxiety (described by relatives as worriers or nervous) may be more prone to the development of an anxiety state, and may have suffered from this in the past.

Prevalence

As with other disorders there is wide variation in reported prevalence of anxiety states in cancer patients. One study by Aass *et al.* reported 13 percent of a large cohort of patients, with cancer attending hospital, suffered from an anxiety disorder. Patient selection, stage of illness and difference in rating instruments account for the wide differences.

Emergency presentation

The most likely emergency presentation of an anxiety state is in the form of panic disorder. The patient is acutely distressed, fearing death with marked somatic symptoms which they may link with their cancer diagnosis.

Anxiety symptoms, including panic, can occur secondarily in other disorders. Care should be taken to check for features of depressive disorder which can present with prominent anxiety particularly in the elderly. Alcohol and benzodiazepine withdrawal can present with severe anxiety symptoms or even frank psychosis. Finally, the effects of other drug treatments should be considered. Anti-emetics, in particular, can induce akathesia or restlessness, similar to a severe anxiety state.

Emergency management

In the first instance supportive reassurance that the patient will not die and that they are suffering from a common disorder is important (Fig. 10.1). During a severe panic

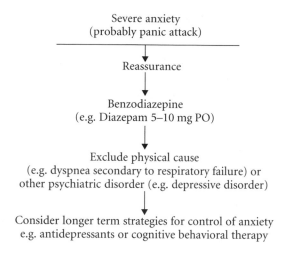

Fig. 10.1 Management of acute anxiety attack.

attack pharmacologic treatment is often necessary. A benzodiazepine, such as diazepam at a dose of 5–10 mg orally, is indicated. This is rapidly absorbed because of high lipid solubility. The benzodiazepines remain the most effective drugs for the short-term relief of anxiety. Benzodiazepines can be used for up to several weeks. Although longer term use may be indicated problems of tolerance and dependence mean this would not be routine for the majority of patients. Care should be taken in reducing benzodiazepine dosage after prolonged use (months) as this can induce withdrawal symptoms unless carried out slowly (weeks to months).

Once the acute attack has subsided other options for long-term control of anxiety states can be implemented. Selective Serotonin Re-uptake Inhibitors (SSRI's) have been shown to be effective in the treatment of panic disorder also. These agents may need to be prescribed in a higher dosage than used in depressive disorder. Some patients with severe anxiety notice a transient worsening of their symptoms when an antidepressant is prescribed; in this group starting at a lower dose often prevents this problem.

Tricyclic antidepressants are also effective in resolving panic disorder and general anxiety disorder. Cognitive therapy can be useful in the treatment of anxiety disorders. The cognitive theory of panic predicts that panic disorder patients are more likely to interpret bodily sensations in a catastrophic fashion and that this leads to anxiety. If the patient learns the early symptoms of an attack and assign them to an appropriate cause, the attacks can be prevented.

Pain which may exacerbate anxiety should be treated actively. Anxiety secondary to the dyspnea of respiratory failure in patients with terminal cancer can respond well to opioid drugs.

10.2.2 **Post-traumatic stress disorder**

Presentation/description

The diagnosis of Post-Traumatic Stress Disorder (PTSD) refers to the emergence of severe and disabling anxiety reactions in the wake of severe traumatic experiences. According to criterion A in DSM-IV a qualifying trauma is defined as one which involves 'actual or threatened death or serious injury' and which invokes 'feelings of horror and intense fear' in those exposed to it. DSM-IV* specifies additional criteria that must be met before a diagnosis can be made. According to criterion B, symptoms must include persistent re-experiencing of the trauma such as flashbacks and nightmares. Criterion C states that the individual engages in efforts to avoid reminders of the trauma. This can assume many forms such as attempting to suppress thoughts about the trauma. Criterion D states that the individual must experience symptoms of increased arousal and irritability such as difficulty falling or staying asleep, hyper-vigilance, exaggerated startled response, and concentration difficulties. These symptoms must not have been present prior to the trauma. For diagnostic purposes an individual must display a minimum of one re-experiencing symptom, three avoidance symptoms, and two symptoms of hyper-arousal, present for at least one month and of sufficient intensity to have impaired the individual's ability to function.

Prevalence

While cancer differs from many other known PTSD stressors in not being a discrete, short-lived event, it is by no means unique; other causes include war trauma with active combat exposure and repeated abuse in childhood. Estimates of the prevalence of PTSD among adult survivors of cancer varies from 1.9 to 14 percent. In one study by Tjemsland *et al.* the rates of PTSD were similar—6 weeks and 12 months post-surgery. Risk factors for PTSD include the intensity of emotional distress, early onset of depression, and lack of emotional support. Individuals with poor pre-morbid health (physical and mental) have been found to be at greater risk of developing PTSD.

Management

The management of patients with PTSD requires the use of both pharmacotherapy and cognitive-behavioral therapy (CBT). Serotonin re-uptake inhibitors can reduce hyper-arousal symptoms and co-morbid depression. Cognitive-behavioral therapy has proven especially effective in PTSD.

10.2.3 **Depressive disorder**

Presentation/description

Depressive disorder is characterized by low mood or loss of interest as cardinal symptoms. Associated symptoms include fatigue, sleep, and appetite disturbance, although

---

* DSM-IV Classification of mental disorder reflects a consensus of current knowledge and is widely accepted throughout the western world.

these symptoms can be difficult to interpret in patients with advanced cancer or severe pain. Cognitive symptoms include low self-esteem, pessimism, guilt, and tearfulness. Suicidal ideas and plans are core symptoms of depressive disorder and should always be enquired about when assessing mood state. Anxiety symptoms may be prominent, particularly in elderly patients with depression. A distinction may be drawn between sustained depressed mood with several of the above symptoms for several weeks and symptoms present for brief or fluctuating periods, which are usually a psychologic adjustment or secondary to other physical causes.

Prevalence

The reported prevalence of depression varies widely with a range between 0 and 49 percent. The variation probably reflects different instruments used for detection which have included rating scales, clinical interviews, and standardized diagnostic schedules. Other sources of variation include type of cancer, stage of illness, and treatments being undertaken. A meta-analysis of such studies by Vant Spyker and colleagues suggests levels of depression are higher in cancer patients than in the general population. It is possible that adjustment disorders with depressive symptoms may account for a considerable proportion of the excess.

Emergency presentation

Depressive disorder should rarely present as an emergency, unless the developing symptoms have not been reported or been misinterpreted. Adjustment disorder may occur more rapidly, often with some precipitant.

The most common emergency presentation of depressive disorder is with suicidal ideation (see below). Other possible emergency presentations include self-neglect and poor nutrition, though the significance of these may be difficult to interpret in patients with advanced cancer. Factors associated with suicidal ideation are severity of depression and older age. It is unclear if prospective screening would prevent emergency presentation.

Emergency management

The majority of presentations with depressive disorder will respond to either pharmacotherapy with an antidepressant or psychologic treatments such as CBT. All currently available antidepressants act to increase brain synaptic concentrations of amines such as noradrenaline or serotonin. For most patients there is no difference in outcome between classes. Side effects represent the major practical pharmacologic difference between antidepressant groups. Older tricyclic antidepressants affect multiple chemical systems giving a wide range of side effects, for example, anticholinergic, antihistaminergic (sedation). Newer agents with more specific chemical actions tend to have less extensive side effects, appropriate to the brain chemical systems on which they act. An example being the side effects of nausea and headache which occur commonly with SSRI's. The reduced range of side effects may make the newer agents (such as SSRI's) preferable for first line treatment. The SSRI's are also less likely to be prescribed at sub-therapeutic dosages. Examples of different antidepressant classes are given in Fig. 10.2.

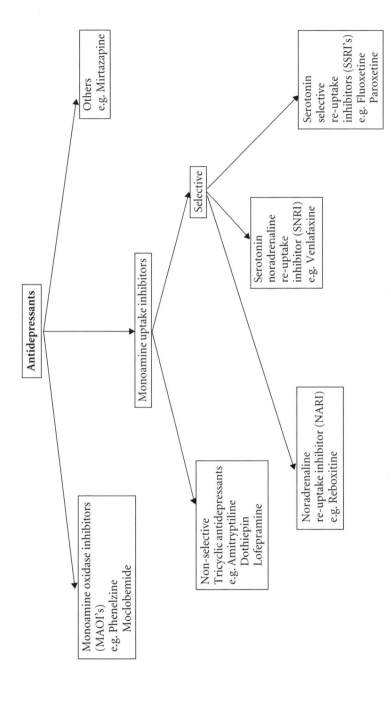

Fig. 10.2 Classes of antidepressants.

The presence of pronounced suicidal ideation in the setting of a depressive disorder may necessitate psychiatric admission or "one to one" observation depending on the situation of the patient. Although rarely used, electro-convulsive therapy may be indicated in severe cases with high suicide risk or in depressive psychosis.

Depressive illness may be precipitated by other medications that should be discontinued. In such cases antidepressant treatment may still need to be commenced. Another cause of secondary depression is severe and persistent pain, treatment of which may alleviate the need for antidepressants.

10.2.4 Suicidality

Presentation/description

It is important to remember that suicidal ideation, to some degree, is not uncommon in the population at large. The severity ranges from infrequent feelings that life is not worth living to concrete suicidal plans or attempts at self-harm. Individuals inexperienced in the assessment of suicidal risk may be alarmed and overact to off-hand comments, alternatively the listener who is uncomfortable may fail to probe adequately.

The assessment of suicide risk should occur in an uninterrupted setting and in an unhurried manner. It is generally best to begin with non-directive, open questions. It is important to ask about the severity and frequency of suicidal thoughts. For many patients such thoughts are likely to be transitory and associated with low risk of suicide. It is important to ask if the patient has made a definite plan. Other important information includes history of psychiatric disorder or suicide attempts, recent stressors, hopelessness, and availability of social supports. A review of the patient's mental state should be carried out to detect any current psychiatric disorder precipitating suicidal thoughts. Any worsening of pain or physical health which may be contributing should not be overlooked.

The main risk factors for suicide in cancer patients are psychiatric disorder, substance abuse, advanced disease, previous suicide attempts, and severe pain.

Prevalence

There are little available data on the frequency of suicidal ideation in large samples of cancer patients. Information for selected groups such as those with pain (17 percent with suicidal ideation), breast cancer (2 percent) and terminal disease (2.3 percent) are reported from small studies.

Emergency presentation

It is likely that suicidal ideation will present in one of three ways. Either the patient will disclose that he has had such thoughts, request assistance from a physician in completing suicide or will attempt self-harm.

Emergency management

Thorough assessment is the cornerstone of management (Fig. 10.3). While a distinction can be made between suicidal patients with low intent and those at high risk, all such

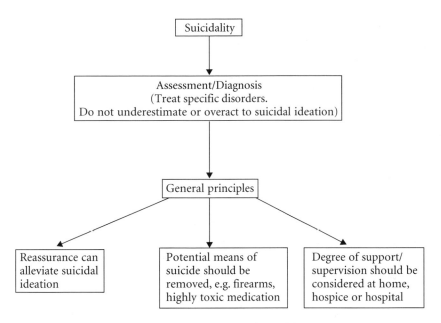

Fig. 10.3 Management of suicidality.

patients should have the option of clarifying their problems with the possibility of establishing realistic and specific goals. Patients may have difficulties related to the diagnosis of cancer or in other areas of their lives.

Specific disorders require detection and prompt treatment. The presence of a depressive disorder is usually an indication to commence an antidepressant agent. Likewise detection of delirium, alcoholism, etc. should trigger emergency management of these separate disorders (see other sections). While treatment of these conditions may take days or even weeks to be fully effective, a clear explanation of their likely benefits can have important therapeutic effects in alleviating suicidal ideation.

Potential means of suicide should be removed in any patients with suicidal ideation. Enquiries should be made about access to firearms and medications that are least toxic, in overdose, should be dispensed. If potentially more toxic drugs are prescribed, the quantities should be reviewed. Due to its disinhibiting effects, alcohol should be avoided.

A family member may be involved to support the patient and help with treatment planning. For actively suicidal patients the possibility of a psychiatric hospital admission should be considered, though this may be less appropriate for a terminally ill patient with cancer. Other options include "one to one" supervision in a hospital ward.

Requests for physician-assisted suicide are not uncommon. While they should trigger a thorough assessment as noted above, they are unlikely to trigger an emergency response. Management of such requests varies between cultures and countries.

10.2.5 **Alcohol problems**

Presentation/description

Alcohol is only one of many drugs of abuse, however there are two reasons why it may be more likely to present in patients with a cancer diagnosis. Firstly alcohol is the preferred drug of abuse in most countries—approximately 5 percent of the United States population is alcoholic. Secondly alcohol misuse is associated with the development of a variety of cancers, particularly those of the head and neck.

The diagnostic terminology for alcohol-related disorders can be confusing to non-specialists. Problems related to alcohol can be most easily divided into harmful use and dependence. Harmful use is indicated by damage to health that can be physical (e.g. falls, cirrhosis) or mental (episodes of depressive disorder secondary to heavy consumption of alcohol). Dependence is characterized by a cluster of behavioral, cognitive, and physiologic phenomena that develop after heavy repeated use of alcohol. These include a strong desire to take alcohol, difficulties in controlling its use, persisting in its use despite harmful consequences, a higher priority given to alcohol than other obligations, increased tolerance and sometimes physical withdrawal.

Prevalence

Reported rates for alcohol abuse/dependence vary from 1 to 12 percent for a variety of patient groups with cancer. The prevalence varies from one site-specific neoplasm to another with the highest rate found in the head and neck cancer population.

Emergency presentation

There are several routes by which alcohol problems may come to light in the oncology setting. Patients may spontaneously divulge the extent of their alcohol intake and associated problems. In those where alcohol may be related to the neoplastic disease, the diagnosis of cancer may be a watershed encouraging them to confront and deal with alcohol problems. All medical histories should enquire about specific quantities of alcohol intake. Where alcohol intake is high or problems suspected enquiries about possible medical, legal, or social problems secondary to alcohol can be made to help confirm the diagnosis. Past problems with stopping alcohol should be investigated. Patients may present repeatedly at the clinic smelling of alcohol or routine blood tests may show unexplained macrocytosis or altered liver function tests. The latter findings should raise suspicion but are not diagnostic.

The above are unlikely to present as emergencies. The most serious alcohol-related emergency is the presentation of a patient in withdrawal or delirium tremens (DT's). Mild forms of withdrawal are characterized by tremulousness, sweating, tachycardia, nausea, and vomiting. This can progress to full DT's which in addition presents with restlessness, disorientation, illusions, and terrifying hallucinations which are most often visual but can be auditory or tactile. Delirium tremens commence 24–72 hours after cessation of alcohol and usually subside within 4 days. Patients with cancer at greatest risk are those who are suddenly debilitated by physical complications of the neoplasm or who are admitted to an oncology unit for treatment where the supply of alcohol is terminated and they are either not questioned about alcohol use or deny it. Individuals in DT's are at risk from physical complications such as dehydration, shock, and epileptic seizures. Untreated there is a considerable mortality. In addition the development of agitation with psychotic symptoms can result in fearful patients attempting to flee from their environment with risk of self-injury.

Patients with alcohol abuse/dependence may also have poorer coping strategies and react to the difficulties of diagnosis and treatment of cancer with suicidal ideation.

Emergency management

The most serious emergency presentation specific to alcohol dependence is the patient in withdrawal or DT's (Fig. 10.4). Many presentations are preventable given a full medical history and high index of suspicion.

Milder forms of withdrawal can be managed at home with adequate support and monitoring. DT's require a medical admission. The keystones to management are adequate hydration and the use of benzodiazepines. A variety of benzodiazepines can be used, choice often depending on individual experience. One option is chlordiazepoxide starting at 100–150 mg per day orally and reducing as symptoms subside. Lower doses may be required in the elderly, physically debilitated and can be used in milder forms of

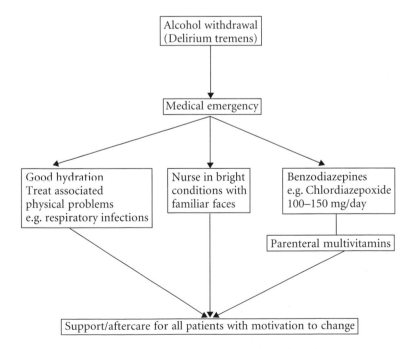

Fig. 10.4 Management of alcohol withdrawal.

withdrawal. Alcohol dependence is associated with several neuropsychiatric complications, particularly affecting memory (especially the Wernicke–Korsakoff syndrome). Parenteral multivitamin preparations may be required, especially if there is evidence of sustained disorientation, ataxia, acute neuropathy, opthalmoplegia, or marked short-term memory difficulties.

Safe cessation of alcohol use is important but encouraging individuals to maintain abstinence is also critical to prevent recurrence. A range of clinical and voluntary services is available to aid after-care and local options should be offered to all motivated patients.

10.2.6 Neuropsychiatric sequelae

Prevalence

Organic mental disorders are the second most common group of psychiatric problems occurring in cancer patients, found in up to 20 percent of inpatients and in over 75 percent of terminally ill cancer patients. Neuropsychiatric problems can arise from the direct effects of the cancer on the nervous system (primary CNS cancers, secondary metastatic spread), from non-metastatic effects (metabolic, endocrine, paraneoplastic) or through the side effects of treatment (see below).

Paraneoplastic neurologic complications of cancer include encephalopathies which may involve the cerebral cortex. Dementia is a prominent feature. In one variant, *limbic encephalopthy*, pathologic changes occur in the limbic grey matter leading either to acute memory loss, confusion and hallucinations, or a more gradual dementia. The most common cause is small cell lung cancer. While the underlying mechanism remains elusive, the prevailing view is that the pathogenesis involves an immune response to tumor antigens cross-reacting with nerve cells.

Non-metastatic effects of cancer

The two most common neuropsychiatric responses of the higher nervous system to non-metastatic effects of cancer are forms of delirium (acute confusional state) and dementia. The former is an acute response and, depending on causation, reversible while the latter is seen as a more chronic and often progressive response particularly in the terminal stages of cancer. Hormonal effects arising from some cancers or their treatment can produce specific neuropsychiatric effects. Best recognized are the effects of corticosteroid hormones on mood (depression and elation) and thyroxine on anxiety.

Delirium

Presentation/description   Delirium, or acute confusional state, is characterized by impairment of consciousness and global cognitive impairment of acute onset. Other key features include disorientation and disturbance of the sleep–wake cycle. Psychomotor behavior may be altered. Patients may be hypoactive or hyperactive, the latter can be agitated and even physically combative.

Perception can be altered with patients experiencing illusions (misinterpretations of external stimuli, for example, believing patterns in the bed sheets are insects) or hallucinations (perceptions in the absence of stimuli). Frank paranoid ideas or delusions may occur. The syndrome is frequently worse at night, and periods of relative lucidity can occur.

Delirium is caused by a widespread disturbance of cerebral metabolism. It is a common feature of physical illness or drug intoxication particularly in the elderly. In contrast to dementia it begins suddenly and is of relatively short duration (hours to weeks).

Prevalence   Delirium has been under-recognized and under-researched in general medical patients with cancer. Obviously the prevalence will vary with the stage and type of cancer, being more common with advanced disease. Studies in patients with advanced cancer suggest that 40–50 percent may have delirium at time of admission to a palliative care unit. Over 80 percent of patients with terminal cancer develop delirium, in the days and weeks before death.

Emergency presentation   Delirium can indicate the development or worsening of a wide variety of physical disorders. For this reason it is a medical emergency for which a cause should be sought. Even in advanced cancer delirium is potentially reversible in up to 50 percent of patients. Common causes of delirium, with good prognosis, in these patients include dehydration and opioid toxicity. Behavioral manifestations including wandering, agitation, perceptual abnormalities, and paranoid ideation may also present as emergencies.

Emergency management (Fig. 10.5)   Treatment of any physical cause underlying the delirium should be started promptly.

General principles include nursing in bright conditions with familiar staff members. If wandering is problematic "one to one" nursing management may have to be implemented for the patient's safety.

The most effective supportive treatment is haloperidol. Patients with advanced cancer may not tolerate high doses and 0.5 mg twice daily should be used at initiation. This dose may need to be increased. Parenteral doses are approximately twice as potent as oral doses. Benzodiazepines may worsen or precipitate delirium.

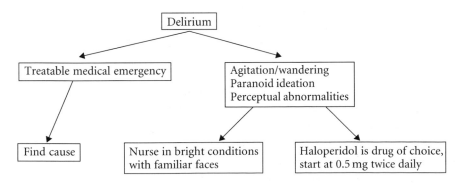

Fig. 10.5 Management of delirium.

Psychoses

Presentation/description   The term psychosis refers to a group of mental disorders characterized by the potential for loss of contact with reality. The latter presents typically with hallucinations or delusions. Mental disorders which fall into this category include schizophrenia, mania, and psychotic depression. However, it is well recognized that under extreme stress (such as the diagnosis and treatment of cancer) some individuals may develop transient psychotic disorders (in the absence of signs of organic cerebral disturbance) often characterized by persecutory beliefs involving the staff treating the patient. These episodes are usually brief and prognosis is generally felt to be good. Although delirium is a psychotic disorder, its frequent presentation in patients with advanced cancer, organic precipitants and different management mean it is best considered separately.

Finally treatments used against cancer are recognized to precipitate psychotic symptoms in some patients. The management of such iatrogenic crises will be considered in this section, although further details of causative agents will be considered later.

Prevalence   It is important to remember that both psychiatric disorders and cancer are common in the general population. Even after excluding suicide, patients with psychiatric illness have higher than expected mortality rates, cancer being one of the illnesses over-represented. It is therefore not unlikely that a proportion of patients with psychotic disorders may develop cancer. In addition, patients susceptible to stress may suddenly develop transient psychotic disorders of short duration. In one large multi-center study by Grassi and colleagues at least 4 percent of patients (excluding those with delirium) referred from oncology units to psychiatric liaison services suffered from psychotic disorders.

Emergency presentation   Psychotic disorders present most typically with hallucinations or delusions. Delusions may be persecutory, referential (believing others talk about or refer to the patient) or occasionally of a grandiose nature where the individual feels they have special powers or abilities. Hallucinations are usually auditory. Visual hallucinations occur rarely in a number of psychotic disorders, but characteristically occur in delirium and illnesses with an organic basis. For patients with a known past diagnosis, recurrences often have the same cardinal features. The behavioral presentation is dictated by the mental symptoms but may range from the suspicious individual who is increasingly withdrawn, to frank aggressive outbursts or the patient trying to leave hospital.

Emergency management   In medically ill patients, especially those with advanced cancer it is important not to confuse delirium with psychoses of non-organic origin (Fig. 10.6). The concern here is less with psychiatric management but that an active physical disorder is missed.

If a patient has suffered a previous psychotic illness, it is prudent to obtain information from psychiatric services involved. Many community psychiatric services have management plans *in situ* for such relapses, based on knowledge of the patient and any relevant risks. Such plans may have to be altered in response to current cancer care.

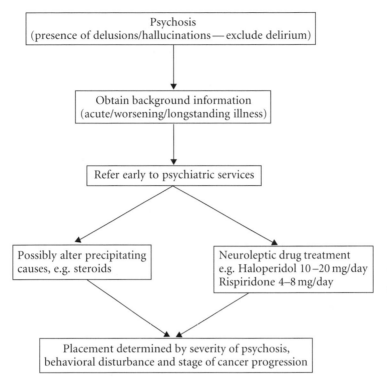

Fig. 10.6 Management of psychosis.

Individuals undergoing treatment for cancer who develop a new psychotic episode, should be referred to psychiatric services either via a liaison psychiatry service for patients attending hospital or through community services. The issue of psychiatric hospitalization depends on the severity of psychosis, level of behavioral disturbance and support available. Transient psychotic disorders often settle within a few days.

Acute psychosis usually requires pharmacologic treatment. Consideration should be given to altering anticancer treatment possibly associated with the onset of the psychotic symptoms. For patients with prior episodes, treatment may be guided by previous dosage and response, bearing in mind changes in physiologic status occurring with cancer and associated drug treatment. A selection of neuroleptic drugs is available. Older neuroleptic agents such as haloperidol can be given at a starting dose of 5–10 mg orally, with a maintenance dose of 5–20 mg per day. For the emergency control of disturbed behavior haloperidol can be given at 5–10 mg by the intramuscular route. Haloperidol may induce Parkinsonian or dystonic (this may range from clenching of jaw muscles or protrusion of the tongue to an oculogyric crisis) symptoms which are best treated with an anticholinergic agent (e.g. procyclidine 5–10 mg twice daily). Newer neuroleptic drugs are less likely to give rise to such extrapyramidal side effects. One such agent is rispiridone which has a three day dose escalation schedule with usual maintenance between 4 and 8 mg per day.

Metastatic and primary cerebral tumors

The great majority of cerebral tumors, whether primary or secondary, produce mental symptoms at some stage in their course. Depending on the rate of progression two syndromes predominate, the acute confusional state (delirium) and dementia. While tumors commonly present with symptoms of raised intracranial pressure, seizures or focal neurologic signs, in some the earliest manifestation may be mental symptoms. Carcinoma of the lung is the most frequent metastatic cancer of the nervous system though other tumors which commonly metastize to the brain include breast, alimentary tract, prostate, and pancreatic cancers. Not infrequently such metastases may give rise to symptoms before the primary lesion.

Dementia due to cerebral malignancy

Presentation/description   Cognitive impairment is the commonest psychiatric finding with tumor involvement of the cerebral cortex. At its earliest stages this may simply consist of reduced concentration, mental fatigue, and forgetfulness. As the disease progresses the more characteristic features of dementia, progressive intellectual decline, severe memory impairment, and personality change, manifest themselves. While many of the symptoms and signs are a reflection of raised intra-cranial pressure, tumors in specific cortical areas can produce variations in the general dementia pattern. Tumors, particularly slower growing tumors, in the frontal lobe and temporal lobe may produce changes in personality which are more prominent than any subtle impairment in memory or intellect. Characteristic personality changes include irritability, loss of social judgement, disinhibition, apathy, or euphoria.

Cognitive decline will generally be a reflection of progress of the intracerebral neoplasm. While this may be due to local effects, including infiltration, a rise in intracranial pressure is common and often treatable. Acute behavioral disturbance will usually respond to a major tranquillizer such as haloperidol often in small doses (0.5 mg twice daily).

10.3 Treatment related neuropsychiatric problems

10.3.1 Chemotherapeutic drugs

While most anticancer drugs do not readily cross the blood–brain barrier, with greater innovation and aggressive use of chemotherapy there is increasing recognition of the neurotoxic side effects of this form of therapy. From a psychiatric perspective confusion and even frank delirium have been found secondary to many of the chemotherapy drugs (Table 10.2). There is also growing evidence of milder cognitive impairments including memory impairment and intellectual impairment in patients being treated with these agents. Psychiatric impairments are often accompanied by other evidence of neurotoxicity including peripheral neuropathy, seizures, ototoxicity, and autonomic changes.

10.3.2 Immunologic agents

Subtle cognitive effects have been found in patients treated with cytokines including interferon alpha and interleukin-2. Disorders of mood have also been found, particularly

Table 10.2 Chemotherapeutic agents which can cause delirium

L-Asparaginase	Interleukin
Bleomycin	Ifosfamide
Carmustine (BCNU)	Methotrexate
Cisplatin	Prednisone
Cytosine arabinoside (Ara-C)	Procarbazine
Fludarabine	Vinblastine
Fluorouracil	Vincristine
Interferon	

depression. Cognitive impairment, particularly memory impairment, can arise in patients treated with bone marrow transplantation and have been attributed to the neurotoxic effects of both chemotherapy and radiation.

10.3.3 **Corticosteroids**

These drugs have long been known to cause a wide range of neuropsychiatric problems. The frequency of steroid-induced psychiatric disorder increases with the dosage of medication ranging from 4 percent of those taking 40–80 mg prednisone (or equivalent) to 18 percent of those taking more than 80 mg. The psychiatric complications include cognitive impairment, delirium, sleep disturbance, and affective disturbance, which can run the full spectrum between mania and depression. While treatment of the cancer should take priority, staff should have a low threshold for suspecting behavioral or psychologic change including changes reported by a relative as this may herald the onset of psychoses.

As part of the screening for side effects of anticancer treatments questions related to cognitive impairment including memory impairment and disturbances of mood should be considered.

Suggested reading

Aass, N., Fossa, S.D., Dahl, A.A., and Moe, J.J. (1997) Prevalence of anxiety and depression in cancer patients seen at the Norwegian Radium Hospital, *Eur J Cancer*, **33**, 1597–604.

Akechi, T., Okanura, H., Kugaya, A., Nakano, T., Nakanishi, T., Akizuki, N., *et al.* (2000) Suicidal ideation in cancer patients with major depression, *Jpn J Clin Oncol*, **30**, 221–24.

Adelbratt, S. and Strang, P. (2000) Death anxiety in brain tumor patients and their spouses, *Palliat Med*, **14**, 499–507.

Baile, W.F. (1996) Neuropsychiatric disorders in cancer patients, *Curr Opin Oncol*, **8**, 182–7.

Boston, Collaborative Drug Surveillance Program (1972) Acute adverse reactions to prednisone in relation to dosage, *Clin Pharmacol Ther*, **13**, 694–98.

Butler, R., Rizzi, L.P., and Handwerger, B.A. (1996) Brief report: the assessment of PTSD in pediatric cancer patients and survivors, *J Pediatr Psychol*, **21**, 499–504.

Byock, I.R. (1996) The nature of suffering and the nature of opportunity at the end of life, *Clin Geriatr Med*, **12**, 237–52.

Doherty, M., Garstin, I., McClelland, R.J., Rowlands, B.J., and Collins, B.J. (1991) A steroid stupor in a surgical ward, *Br J Psychiatry*, **158**, 125–27.

Edelman, S., Bell, D.R. and Kidman, A.D. (1999) A group cognitive behaviour therapy programme with metastatic breast cancer patients, *Psycho-Oncology*, **8**, 295–305.

Freedman, S.A., Brandes, D., Peri, T., and Shalev, A. (1999) Predictors of chronic post-traumatic stress disorder, *Br J Psychiatry*, **174**, 353–9.

Goldberg, R.J. and Cullen, S.C. (1985) Factors important to psychosocial adjustment to cancer: a review of the evidence, *Soc Sci Med*, **20**, 803–7.

Grassi, L., Gritti, P., Rigatelli, M., and Gala, C. for the Italian Consultation-Liaison Group (2000) Psychosocial problems secondary to cancer: an Italian multicentre survey of consultation-liaison psychiatry in oncology, *Eur J Cancer*, **36**, 579–85.

Green, B.L., Rowland, J.H., Krupnick, J.L., Epstein, S.A., Stockton, P., Stern, N.M., *et al.* (1998) Prevalence of post-traumatic stress disorder in women with breast cancer, *Psychosomatics* **39**, 102–11.

Haverkate, I., Onwuteaka-Philipsen, D., Van der Heide, A., Kostense, P.J., Van der Wal, G., and Van der Mass, P.J. (2000) Refused and granted requests for euthanasia and assisted suicide in the Netherlands: interview study with structured questionnaire, *Br Med J*, **321**, 865–86.

Heaven, C.M. and Maguire, P. (1998) The relationship between patients' concerns and psychological distress in a hospice setting, *Psycho-Oncology*, **7**, 502–7.

Hecaen, H. and Ajuriaguerra, J. de (1956) Troubles Mentaux au cours des Tumeurs Intracraniennes, Masson Paris, 218–31.

Hinton, J. (1994) Can home care maintain an acceptable quality of life for patients with terminal cancer and their relatives? *Palliat Med*, **8**, 183–96.

Lawlor, P.G., Gagnon, B., Mancini, I.L., Pereira, J.L., Hanson, J., Suanez-Almazor, M.E., *et al.* (2000) Occurrence, causes and outcome of delirium in patients with advanced cancer, *Arch Int Med*, **160**, 786–94.

Lishman, W.A. (1998) Organic psychiatry. *The psychologic consequences of cerebral disorder*, Oxford Blackwell Science.

Lundberg, J.C. and Passik, S.D. (1997) Alcohol and cancer a review for psycho-oncologists, *Psycho-Oncology*, **6**, 253–66.

Perry, S., Difede, J., Musngi, G., Frances, A.J., and Jacobsberg, L. (1992) Predictors of post-traumatic stress disorder after burn injury, *Am J Psychiatry*, **149**, 931–35.

Rodrigue, J.R., Behen, J.M., and Tumlin, T. (1994) Multidimensional determinants of psychological adjustment to cancer, *Psycho-Oncology*, **3**, 205–14.

Roth, A.J. and Breitbart, W. (1996) Psychiatric emergencies in terminally ill cancer patients, *Pain Palliat Care*, **10**, 235–59.

Sellick, S.M. and Crooks, D.L. (1999) Depression and cancer: an appraisal of the literature for prevalence, detection and practice guideline development for psychological interventions, *Psycho-Oncology*, **8**, 315–33.

Slaughter, J.R., Iain, A., Holmes, S., Reid, J.C., Bobo, W., and Sherrod, N.B. (2000) Panic disorder in hospitalised cancer patients, *Psycho-Oncology*, **9**, 253–8.

Spiegel, D., Morrow, G.R., Classen, C., Raubertas, R., Stott, P.B., Mudaliar, N., *et al.* (1999) Group psychotherapy for recently diagnosed breast cancer patients: a multicenter feasibility study, *Psycho-Oncology*, **8**, 482–93.

Tjemsland, L., Søriede, J.A., and Malt, U.F. (1998) Post-traumatic distress symptoms in operable breast cancer III: status one year after surgery, *Breast Cancer Res Treat*, **47**, 141–51.

Vant Spyker, A., Trijsburg, R.W., and Duivenvoorden, H.J. (1997) Psychological sequelae of cancer diagnosis: a meta-analytic review of 58 studies after 1980, *Psychosom Med*, **59**, 280–93.

Chapter 11

Pediatric Emergencies

Kenneth J. Cohen and Lee J. Helman

All of the oncologic emergencies detailed in this textbook can be seen in the pediatric setting. Often, establishing a diagnosis can be complicated by the age of the patient, the inability of the patient to articulate specific concerns, and the subtle presentation of many of these diagnoses in the pediatric patient. In addition, there are a number of diagnoses unique to the pediatric cancer patient that pose specific risks for oncologic emergencies. This chapter attempts to highlight the breadth of emergencies seen in the pediatric setting with particular emphasis on complications related to tumors predominantly seen in children. For the convenience of the reader, when possible this chapter follows the outline of the book as a whole.

11.1 Cardiovascular and pulmonary emergencies

Cardiovascular complications are frequently seen in the pediatric oncology patient. Certain complications predominate including: superior vena cava and tracheal obstruction, pleural and pericardial effusions, cardiac tamponade, deep vein thromboses, and anthracycline associated cardiotoxicity.

11.1.1 Superior vena cava syndrome

Superior vena cava syndrome (SVCS) refers to obstruction or compression of the superior vena cava. Tracheal compression may coexist (superior mediastinal syndrome (SMS)). Pediatric patients are at particular risk for both syndromes due to the relatively thin wall of the superior vena cava coupled with the small intraluminal diameters of both this vessel and the adjacent trachea and bronchi. This region is susceptible to external compression due to the many adjacent lymph nodes sandwiching the vena cava and the adjacent thymus, which is prominent in the pediatric patient. Signs include: swelling, plethora, and cyanosis of the face, neck, and upper extremities; suffusion and edema of the conjunctivae; distended neck and chest wall veins; diaphoresis; wheezing and stridor; and pulsus paradoxus. Symptoms include: respiratory findings of cough, hoarseness, dyspnea, orthopnea, and chest pain; central nervous system (CNS) findings of headache, visual impairment, lethargy, and irritability and anxiety in the young patient. Hematologic malignancies predominate with non-Hodgkin's lymphoma (NHL), acute lymphoblastic leukemia (ALL) and Hodgkin's disease (HD) all implicated. Thoracic neuroblastoma, particularly common in infants, may present with vascular and/or tracheal compression. Germ cell tumors and sarcomas complete the list of common pediatric tumors. Diagnosis can be challenging because of the risks of anesthesia or conscious sedation, particularly in the youngest of patients. The least invasive method should be utilized in attempting to establish a diagnosis. Strategies include: a complete blood count with evaluation of the peripheral smear often coupled with a bone marrow aspirate or biopsy; thoracentesis, which may be therapeutic as well as diagnostic; biopsy of a superficial node; or evaluation of tumor markers including β-HCG and alpha-fetoprotein. Once a diagnosis is established, specific therapy is initiated and may include the use of steroids, chemotherapy or regional radiation therapy. Increasingly, SVCS is seen in patients following the initiation of therapy due to the presence of indwelling central venous catheters. Treatment centers on the use of thrombolytic therapy.

11.1.2 Pleural and pericardial effusions

Pleural and pericardial effusions may be seen with a variety of tumors including lymphomas and metastatic solid tumors. For patients at presentation, thoracentesis or pericardiocentesis may be diagnostic as well as therapeutic. Prompt initiation of therapy following diagnosis will often eliminate further symptomatic effusions. In contrast, for patients with recurrent disease causing effusions, reaccumulation of fluid following therapeutic taps may be common. In that setting, sclerosing therapy may be indicated.

Cardiac tamponade is an extremely rare symptom in the pediatric oncology patient. A variety of tumors have been implicated including the leukemias and lymphomas and sarcomas and rare tumors, including desmoplastic small round cell tumor. In addition, extension of Wilms' tumor to right-sided heart structures can result in compromised output. Management is complex and has included utilization of chemotherapeutics or cardiopulmonary bypass with tumor thrombus removal.

11.1.3 Deep venous thrombosis

Deep-vein thromboses (DVT) are increasingly seen in the pediatric setting. Similar risk factors exist in adults, including prolonged periods of immobility (e.g. osteosarcoma patients' post limb-salvage), the presence of indwelling catheters, the apparent increased risk of thrombus in oncology patients due to generation of procoagulants in certain tumors, genetic susceptibility to clotting (e.g. Factor V Leiden deficiency), and the frequent use of chemotherapeutic agents associated with thrombosis (e.g. L-asparaginase). Pulmonary embolism as a complication of DVT is relatively rare in pediatrics. Detection of a DVT can be problematic, particularly in the young patient where irritability and failure to ambulate may present. Similar to SVCS due to indwelling catheters, treatment revolves around the use of anticoagulant therapy.

11.1.4 Anthracycline cardiotoxicity

Anthracycline cardiotoxicity is a constant concern in the pediatric setting. Many tumor types are treated with anthracyclines potentially at high doses including most sarcomas of childhood, neuroblastoma, and the leukemias. At biopsy, myocardial cell dropout and fibrosis are present. Young children are felt to be at particular risk for this morbidity. More recently, dexrazoxane has been given concomitantly with anthracyclines in an attempt to reduce cardiotoxicity. Of concern is mounting evidence of late congestive failure in many pediatric patients now over 10 years from the completion of chemotherapy.

11.2 Neurologic emergencies

Neurologic evaluation and intervention of the pediatric cancer patient can be complex. Many practitioners are relatively uncomfortable performing a neurologic examination in children and often fail to obtain reliable information. However, prompt recognition of neurologic complications related to cancer in the child is paramount so that long-term morbidity, or worse, mortality is avoided. Five complications are commonly seen in the pediatric setting: spinal cord compression, increased intracranial pressure, seizures, cerebrovascular accidents, and blindness.

11.2.1 Spinal cord compression

Spinal cord compression is a relatively common complication in the pediatric setting, largely accounting for the majority of the spinal cord complications reported in children with cancer. Tumor may encroach on the epidural space, subarachnoid space, or by neuraxis dissemination to the cord parenchyma. Sarcomas account for approximately 50 percent of the cases of epidural cord compression with neuroblastoma and the hematologic malignancies largely comprising the remaining cases. In contrast to the presentation seen in adults with direct extension of tumor from vertebral metastases, this presentation is uncommon in children. Presenting symptoms vary with back pain seen in 50–80 percent of patients depending on the series reported. The pain may be either local or radicular. Motor deficits are reported in 70 percent of cases with sensory deficits noted in approximately 30 percent of cases. A high index of suspicion is paramount and in general, back pain in a child with cancer should prompt an urgent evaluation to rule in or rule out the diagnosis of spinal cord compression. The diagnostic study of choice is magnetic resonance imaging (MRI) with administration of gadolinium. Axial imaging should be included. Where MRI is unavailable, lumbar myelography can be considered. Once the diagnosis has been established, prompt intervention is required. Steroids are routinely administered, although caution must be taken if a hematologic diagnosis is considered, since diagnostic specimens essential for establishing longitudinal risk factors for the patient might be compromised. For patients with an established diagnosis, the appropriate intervention is often defined and surgery, chemotherapy, or radiation therapy all have a potential role in treatment. For the newly presenting patient, specific intervention depends on the presumptive diagnosis. Every effort should be made to establish a tissue diagnosis. Hematologic tumors presenting with cord compression can sometimes be diagnosed by evaluation of the peripheral smear, bone marrow, or pathologic evaluation of a superficial node. The presence of an adrenal mass with extension strongly supports the diagnosis of neuroblastoma and may be confirmed by evaluation of urinary catecholamines. When the diagnosis is uncertain, surgical intervention serves the dual role of decompressing the spine and providing pathologic material for evaluation. Outcome is largely dependent on the prompt recognition of symptoms and effective decompression of the cord. Children who have become non-ambulatory can recover function, but only in about 50 percent of cases.

11.2.2 Increased intracranial pressure

Increased intracranial pressure (ICP) occurs fairly commonly in the pediatric setting. In contrast to adult patients where brain metastases are frequent, the majority of pediatric patients with raised intracranial pressure have primary CNS tumors causing obstruction of cerebral spinal fluid (CSF) outflow. Less common causes of raised ICP include venous thrombosis, CNS hemorrhage or infarction, and infection. Onset of raised ICP can be rapid, and often quite difficult to diagnose in young children. Presenting symptoms of headache and vomiting, commonly seen in older children and adults, may be replaced by irritability and lethargy with associated vomiting in the young child. Papilledema is often difficult to assess in the young child who may be unable to cooperate for the examination. Parinaud's syndrome (dorsal midbrain syndrome) may be noted in patients with obstruction in the region of the supranuclear pretectal or tectal region. Largely unique to young children is the ability to separate their sutures or have a bulging fontanelle as signs of increased ICP. Rapid acceleration in head circumference can often be documented in the young child and the practitioner is advised to carefully plot head circumference in patients with symptoms that might be suggestive of raised ICP. A variety of tumor types are associated with raised ICP in the pediatric setting (Table 11.1)

Treatment of raised ICP centers on rapid detection and intervention (see Chapter 2). Emergent imaging is indicated, and computed tomography (CT) scanning often suffices. Steroids are generally administered. Subsequent interventions are dependent on the stability of the patient. In emergent cases, intubation and osmotic diuresis are instituted. In less emergent cases, primary tumor removal, shunting, or ventriculoscopy can be considered.

11.2.3 Seizures

Seizures, while common in pediatrics, are rarely caused by primary CNS tumors. Primarily, this is due to the vast majority of tumors in children being infratentorial, as opposed to

Table 11.1 Tumors commonly associated with increased intracranial pressure in the pediatric setting

Medulloblastoma
Ependymoma
Cerebellar astrocytomas
Brain stem tumors
Tectal gliomas
Choroid plexus tumors

adults where supratentorial tumors predominate. Less than 1 percent of new onset seizures are due to brain tumors in pediatrics, and only 5 percent of pediatric patients with focal seizures have a brain tumor as the etiology of their seizure disorder. Much more common in the child with cancer is alternative explanations for seizures including: metastatic disease to the brain, CNS hemorrhage or infarction, infection, metabolic disturbances, and treatment-associated effects including radiation therapy (XRT) toxicity, chemotherapeutic toxicity, narcotics, anti-emetics, and antibiotics. Most seizures are brief and resolve spontaneously. For patients in status epilepticus, following appropriate airway and circulatory stabilization, anticonvulsants should be administered. Additional evaluation often includes CNS imaging and consideration of a lumbar puncture. Electroencephalography can assist in localization of the seizure focus.

11.2.4 **Cerebrovascular accidents**

Cerebrovascular accidents (CVA) are rare, but often devastating complications in the pediatric setting. The vast majority of cases are caused by thrombosis or hemorrhage. Embolic events are rare. Spontaneous hemorrhage of primary CNS tumors is rare, but may complicate removal at the time of surgery. It is the pediatric patient with systemic disease who may be at greatest risk of a CVA. The incidence has been reported to be as high as 3 percent of children with non-CNS malignancy. Causes include thrombocytopenia or coagulopathy, side effects of antineoplastic medications, infections, and metastatic spread of tumor. Hematologic malignancies, particularly acute promyelocytic leukemia (APML), pose substantial risk for disseminated intravascular coagulation (DIC) and hemorrhage. Fifteen percent of pediatric patients present with hyperleukocytosis and are at increased risk for hemorrhage. DIC may be insidious and the practitioner is cautioned to consider DIC in the setting of systemic signs of bleeding—even when thrombocytopenia may be additionally implicated. L-asparaginase therapy is commonly associated with thrombotic events in the brain. Treatment of the CVA is dependent on etiology. Often, despite rapid intervention, long-term sequelae occur. For pediatric patients with terminal disease metastatic to the CNS, a CVA is seen with some frequency. Decisions regarding intervention are complex.

11.2.5 **Visual loss**

Blindness, or progressive visual loss, is an unfortunate, but relatively rare complication of pediatric cancers. Retinoblastoma may present with insidious visual loss since the patients are generally quite young and symptoms may be subtle. Patients with unilateral disease often present with advanced disease with limited likelihood for preserved vision. In this setting, when disease is advanced, enucleation may be the preferred treatment. For bilateral disease, efforts are made to preserve both eyes when possible. A rare complication seen in these patients is glaucoma related to either compression of the trabecular meshwork or neovascularization following XRT. Optic pathway gliomas are another common cause of blindness in children. Selected populations (e.g. patients with neurofibromatosis) are at increased risk for the development of these tumors. When vision is retained on the affected side, attempts are made to spare the nerve. In settings where vision has been lost, removal of the glioma may be curative. Bilateral loss may occur when the tumor extends to the region of the optic chiasm or more extensively involves the hypothalamic region.

11.3 **Metabolic emergencies**

A variety of metabolic disturbances are seen in the pediatric patient with cancer. Timing of these complications varies, with certain problems (e.g. diabetes insipidus, hypercalcemia) evident at presentation. Others (e.g. tumor lysis syndrome (TLS)) tend to occur following the initiation of therapy or as complications of treatment (e.g. syndrome of inappropriate anti-diuretic hormone (SIADH)).

11.3.1 **Tumor lysis syndrome**

Tumor lysis syndrome is chemotherapy-induced cell lysis leading to hyperuricemia, hyperkalemia, and hyperphosphatemia. On rare occasions, the syndrome can be seen prior to the initiation of therapy in tumors that tend to be rapidly growing and presumably outstripping their nutritive supply. The syndrome is predominantly seen in the hematologic malignancies, with Burkitt's lymphoma and T-cell lymphoblastic lymphomas being the most common causes. Rarely, solid tumors such as neuroblastoma and the sarcomas will develop mild evidence of TLS upon initiation of therapy. For these tumors, minimal supportive care may be sufficient. Treatment for patients at risk for, or with evidence of, TLS centers on pristine fluid and electrolyte management as detailed in the chapter on metabolic complications (Chapter 3).

11.3.2 **Diabetes insipidus**

Diabetes insipidus is an unusual presenting symptom in the pediatric setting. Imaging may or may not demonstrate a definitive abnormality in the pituitary stalk or posterior pituitary on MRI. Certain tumors predominate with germinoma being the most common cause in the teenage patient. Other common causes include Langerhans' cell histiocytosis and presenting or resected craniopharyngioma.

11.3.3 Syndrome of inappropriate anti-diuretic hormone (SIADH) secretion

The SIADH secretion can be caused by a variety of conditions. In contrast to adults, where tumors such as small cell lung carcinoma are common causes of SIADH, few pediatric tumors have been implicated. It has been occasionally seen in children with craniopharyngioma and in a pediatric patient with nasopharyngeal carcinoma. More commonly, SIADH is seen in the setting of chemotherapeutic agents that impair the excretion of water by the kidneys. Common agents include cyclophosphamide, the vinca alkaloids, and occasionally cisplatin administration.

For guidelines on the treatment of SIADH see chapter 3.

11.3.4 Hypercalcemia

Hypercalcemia, while a common complication affecting 10–20 percent of adults with cancer, is a rare complication in children with malignancies. The most common causes in pediatrics include ALL, T-cell lymphoblastic lymphoma, and other NHL. Other tumors reported include neuroblastoma, Ewing's sarcoma, mesoblastic nephroma, alveolar rhabdomyosarcoma, small cell carcinoma of the ovary, and rhabdoid tumors of the kidney. Pathogenesis and treatment are discussed in chapter 3.

11.4 Hematologic emergencies

As with adult patients, hematologic complications are frequent in the pediatric patient. Hyperleukocytosis periodically presents in the child with hematologic malignancy and aplasia may be a presenting symptom of disease or an anticipated complication of myelotoxic therapy. Thrombosis has been discussed previously.

11.4.1 Hyperleukocytosis

Hyperleukocytosis is a presenting symptom in 10–15 percent of pediatric patients at diagnosis with ALL or AML. It is routinely seen in pediatric patients with chronic myelogenous leukemia (CML) in the chronic phase. Complications related to this presentation vary, with metabolic disturbances more commonly seen in patients with ALL, and hyperviscosity-associated symptoms more frequent in those with AML. Presenting symptoms can include: cardiopulmonary findings of dyspnea, hypoxemia, and right-ventricular heart failure; CNS symptoms of blurred vision, confusion, and stupor; and occasionally priapism in boys. These patients are at substantial risk for CNS or pulmonary hemorrhage and thrombocytopenia in the setting of hyperleukocytosis should be promptly treated. Fatal hemorrhage is frequently reported in children with AML and high white counts. Associated anemia can be problematic because simple transfusion may exacerbate hyperviscosity symptoms. In that setting, partial exchange transfusion may be indicated. Often, the practitioner may struggle with the choice of leukopheresis vs. initiation of chemotherapy. This decision may be complicated in the pediatric setting where establishment of large-bore venous catheters, required for leukopheresis, may be technically challenging in the youngest patients. Alternatively, chemotherapy can be initiated without white blood cell reduction. In both settings, the practitioner must anticipate development of TLS.

11.4.2 Aplasia

Aplasia of various lineages is a common presentation of hematologic malignancy in pediatrics. Anemia represents the most common cytopenia in children presenting with leukemia. In many cases, the anemia is modest, but in a subset of patients, anemia can be severe with clinical evidence of hemodynamic instability. Thrombocytopenia, as a singular cytopenia, is extremely rare in the pediatric setting with less than 1 percent of patients presenting with isolated thrombocytopenia. Children who present with isolated thrombocytopenia are more likely to have a diagnosis of idiopathic thrombocytopenic purpura (ITP) or aplastic anemia. Aplasia is also seen in the many solid tumors of childhood that can be metastatic to the bone marrow. These include neuroblastoma, Ewing's sarcoma, rhabdomyosarcoma, and retinoblastoma. CNS tumors, such as medulloblastoma, can metastasize to the marrow, but rarely is this noted at the time of initial diagnosis. Chemotherapy-associated aplasia is anticipated following myelotoxic therapy in children. Young children are at risk for prolonged aplasia in settings where they are exposed to the many common viruses of childhood.

11.5 Infectious emergencies

Infectious complications are the most common emergencies seen in the pediatric patient with cancer. A variety of immune defects heighten the risk of a severe infection. Central to these risks is the presence of neutropenia, sometimes present at diagnosis and for most patients, present at various times during their treatment due to chemotherapeutics and radiation therapy. Chemotherapy in the pediatric patient is often quite intensive and prolonged periods of neutropenia can be anticipated. Chemotherapy also negatively impacts B-cell and T-cell function that can be further compromised by the concomitant use of steroids included in many protocols. Splenectomy, historically required as part of the staging for pediatric patients with HD, is now less frequently performed. In patients where splenectomy has been performed (e.g. patients with transfusion-dependent hypersplenism) or in the setting of functional asplenia (e.g. post-radiation therapy), patients are at heightened risk for bacterial infection with encapsulated organisms. Gram-positive prophylaxis is indicated. Finally, disruption of skin and mucosal barriers plays a major role in heightening the risk of infection in the pediatric patient. With few exceptions, pediatric patients have central venous catheters placed to ease in the administration and monitoring of therapy. These catheters pose a major risk as a portal of infection and the synthetic catheter can be easily colonized with a variety of pathogens. Maintenance of catheters in children can be more problematic given the general tendency of younger children to be less conscientious with regard to hygiene. Sites of prior procedures (e.g. bone marrow aspirations, lumbar punctures) can allow for entry of skin pathogens. Mucosal disruption due to cytotoxic chemotherapy is a major problem for the pediatric patient. Mucositis can be severe and may be complicated by herpes simplex infection. Children are at increased risk for primary gingivostomatitis, which can markedly exacerbate mucosal injury.

Historical information useful at the time of presentation of a pediatric patient with a suspected infection or febrile neutropenia includes: date and time of last chemotherapy, previously documented infections, presence of a central line, prior splenectomy, and acute infectious exposures. Symptoms of concern include cough, dyspnea, chest pain, retrosternal pain, sore throat, dysphagia, abdominal pain, pain with defecation, vomiting, or diarrhea.

Physical examination must be thorough and the practitioner is cautioned to take the necessary time to thoroughly examine the young, often uncooperative, child. Findings in the pediatric patient may be remarkably subtle and a cursory examination will likely miss critical findings. Young children cannot articulate specific concerns and non-specific symptoms such as lethargy and irritability can be frequently misconstrued as non-infectious symptoms. All mucous membranes should be examined. Tympanic membranes should be viewed. Pulmonary examination should include inspection for tachypnea, flaring, or retractions as well as pulse oximetry in the patient with a suspected pulmonary process. Abdominal examination should assess for evidence of quadrant tenderness, which might suggest a diagnosis of typhilitis. The perirectal region should, at a minimum, be inspected for evidence of redness, swelling, or breakdown. Central line sites must be undressed to assess for erythema or drainage (in the case of an external catheter) as well as for evidence of tenderness along the tunnelled line. All sites of prior studies should be inspected. The entire skin surface should be examined for evidence of erythema, pustules, or vesicles.

Diagnostic evaluation is fairly standardized with blood cultures obtained from all central lumen, urine and throat cultures, and cultures of specific sites of potential infection (e.g. oral mucosa, perirectal region). A chest X-ray should be obtained if there is clinical evidence suggestive of a pulmonary process such as tachypnea, dyspnea, or hypoxemia. Lumbar puncture should be considered, but meningitis is rarely seen in the pediatric oncology patient. The exception is neuro-oncology patients, particularly in the perioperative period or in patients with ventriculo-peritoneal shunts or reservoirs.

Specific treatment choices in the febrile neutropenic patient are discussed in Chapter 12. Briefly, broad-spectrum antibiotic coverage should be instituted at the time of first fever, pending culture results. Various antibacterial combinations have been utilized and specific recommendations for the individual patient are dependent on indigenous flora, prior infections, and clinical findings at presentation. Additionally, infection control strategies may impact on the choice of agents utilized.

The spectrum of infections seen in the pediatric patient with cancer is largely similar to that seen in adults. Younger children have a higher incidence of upper respiratory and gastrointestinal infections that may complicate therapy with persistent fever and viral-associated myelosuppression. Distinguishing the patient with a viral illness from a patient with an invasive bacterial infection can be challenging to even the most astute clinician. Obligately, many children, likely infected with a virus, are over-treated for possible bacterial disease.

A cautionary word about the presentation of septic shock in the child. The clinician must be reminded that sepsis in the pediatric patient may be remarkably subtle initially. Hemodynamic compromise in pediatrics is heralded by tachycardia and poor perfusion. The characteristic finding of hypotension seen in the adult patient is a late, ominous finding in the pediatric setting.

11.6 Urologic emergencies

Urologic emergencies are seen in specific tumors at presentation, or during the course of therapy most frequently associated with specific antineoplastic therapy. Specific urologic emergencies include obstructive uropathies and hemorrhagic cystitis.

11.6.1 Obstructive uropathy

Obstructive uropathy of the upper tract most commonly occurs in children with bladder rhabdomyosarcomas or bulky retroperitoneal sarcomas including rhabdomyosarcomas. Less commonly, retroperitoneal lymphoid tumors also may lead to obstruction. Most cases present as a chronic obstruction that is symptomatically silent save for the symptoms of the tumor. The diagnosis is usually made by abdominal CT scan showing hydronephrosis. The condition is best managed by CT or ultrasound-guided percutaneous nephrostomy with or without placement of internal stents and should be done after consulting urologic surgeons. Once a percutaneous nephrostomy or a ureteral stent is placed, most cases are usually treated with combined modality therapy. Because these diseases tend to be relatively radiation- and chemo-sensitive, follow-up includes frequent radiologic evaluation of the tumor and stents, as well as the urine cultures. Ultimately, imaging studies and urologic evaluation can determine when to remove the percutaneous nephrostomy or internal stent.

Bladder outlet obstruction occurs infrequently in pediatric oncology but can be seen with spinal cord lesions, as well as secondary to narcotic or other medications. It is managed acutely by urethral catheter drainage.

11.6.2 Hemorrhagic cystitis

Fortunately, the incidence of hemorrhagic cystitis has decreased substantially with the now widespread use of mesna uroprotection during high-dose cyclophosphamide and ifosfamide therapy. With the introduction of mesna, the incidence of clinically significant hemorrhagic cystitis is now most frequently associated with allogeneic bone marrow transplantation, typically late onset after hematologic recovery. Several studies now implicate the BK human polyoma virus as a significant etiologic factor in this setting. These findings have led to recent attempts to include antiviral agents such as vidarabine as part of the uroprotective regimen given to selected bone transplant recipients.

Treatment of hemorrhagic cystitis is similar to standard approaches used in adult patients and primarily includes correction of thrombocytopenia and any coagulation abnormalities, hydration, and cessation of any ongoing bladder irradiation and/or chemotherapy. Often, insertion of a large bore urethral catheter into the bladder with lavage, followed by continuous bladder irrigation using a three-way Foley catheter may be necessary. These maneuvers should be initiated after consulting urologic surgeons. In general, if bladder irrigation is not successful in resolving the hemorrhage, direct visualization in the operating room may be necessary for electrocoagulation. Urologists may choose to instill 0.25 percent formalin through a Foley catheter while the patient is under anesthesia, which will control bleeding in the majority of cases. It should be mentioned that while radiation-induced cystitis may be common, especially when given in combination with cytotoxic therapy that may have independent bladder toxicity, this is rarely associated with true hemorrhagic cystitis.

11.7 **Gastrointestinal emergencies**

The major acute gastrointestinal complications of children with cancer include presentation of an acute abdomen, massive liver enlargement, and esophagitis. Each of these presentations occur in specific settings and require careful assessment and treatment.

A child presenting with acute abdominal tenderness must be evaluated immediately to determine whether surgical intervention is required. Involvement of the pediatric surgeon is necessary. Typically, it must be determined whether small bowel obstruction or ileus is present. Obstruction occurs when there is complete or partial mechanical occlusion of the bowel, whereas ileus refers to the loss of gastrointestinal motility without a mechanical cause. A careful history and physical examination, including supine and upright abdominal plain films, will usually help distinguish between these two conditions. In the child with cancer, ileus is typically associated with narcotics or vincristine. Treatment should be conservative and may require alteration of medication. Of particular note, another typical constellation occurring in this setting is the child treated with both vincristine and narcotics whose abdominal discomfort is secondary to severe constipation due to this combination of drugs. This can be clearly determined from the radiographs. Careful attention should be paid to maintaining regular bowel movements and usually stool softeners with or without bowel stimulants may be required to prevent this presentation. Patients with obstruction typically have abdominal or pelvic disease, or a history of abdominal surgery or radiation. Partial obstruction may be treated conservatively with bowel rest and gastric drainage, but may require surgical intervention if the obstruction cannot be reversed.

The child with cancer who presents with acute right lower-quadrant pain requires special attention. If this presentation occurs in the setting of neutropenia, particularly in a patient with leukemia, typhilitis or neutropenic enterocolitis must be a major concern.

This typically is a necrotizing colitis in the cecum caused by bacterial invasion of the cecum that may progress to full thickness bowel infarction and perforation. The most important key to diagnosing this life-threatening condition is early recognition. Patients may present with fever, diarrhea, nausea, vomiting, and abdominal pain, often localized to the right lower quadrant. This syndrome occurs in the setting of neutrophil counts below 500/μl. Clostridium septicum is the most common organism isolated but other organisms including gram negatives may be involved. Radiographic studies including plain films or CT scan may help confirm the diagnosis and may demonstrate pneumatosis of the intestine or bowel wall thickening with localized fluid collection. The overwhelming majority of patients can be managed medically with the prompt administration of appropriate antibiotics along with bowel rest and careful fluid and electrolyte management. Rarely, patients fail to respond to medical management and surgical intervention can be life saving although it carries a high risk.

Another unique presentation of childhood cancer is the infant with stage IV neuroblastoma who presents with massive hepatomegaly. This may be sufficient to cause respiratory compromise. Prompt initiation of a very short course of radiation therapy with lateral fields involving the liver usually is sufficient to relieve the respiratory distress and this can be followed with chemotherapy.

11.8 Summary of pediatric emergencies

Oncologic emergencies in children are both similar to those seen in adults as well as unique to pediatric oncology. The key to a favorable outcome is early recognition and intervention. As the cure rates of children with cancer continue to rise, successful recognition and treatment of pediatric oncologic emergencies will have a significant impact on overall survival in these tumors.

Suggested reading

Arthur, R.R., Shah, K.V., Baust, S.J., Santos, G.W., and Saral, R. (1986) Association of BK viruria with hemorrhagic cystitis in recipients of bone marrow transplants. *N Engl J Med*, 315, 230–4.

Bedi, A., Miller, C.B., Hanson, J.L., Goodman, S., Ambinder, R.F., Charache, P., Arthur, R.R., and Jones, R.J. (1995) Association of BK virus with failure of prophylaxis against hemorrhagic cystitis following bone marrow transplantation. *J Clin Oncol*, 13, 1103–9.

Chapman, C., Flower, A.J., and Durrant, S.T. (1991) The use of vidarabine in the treatment of human polyomavirus associated acute haemorrhagic cystitis. *Bone Marrow Transplant*, 7, 481–3.

Frick, M.P., Maile, C.W., Crass, J.R., Goldberg, M.E., and Delaney, J.P. (1984) Computed tomography of neutropenic colitis. *AJR Am J Roentgenol*, 143, 763–5.

Gonzales-Portillo, G. and Tomita, T. (1998) The syndrome of inappropriate secretion of antidiuretic hormone: an unusual presentation for childhood craniopharyngioma: report of three cases. *Neurosurgery*, 42, 917–21; discussion 921–2.

Kremer L.C., van Dalen, E.C., Offringa, M., Ottenkamp, J., and Voute, P. (2001) Anthracycline-induced clinical heart failure in a cohort of 607 children: long-term follow-up study. *J Clin Oncol*, 19, 191–6.

Krmar, R.T., Ferraris, J.R., Ruiz, S.E., Dibar, E., Morandi, A.A., and Ramirez, J.A. (1997) Syndrome of inappropriate secretion of antidiuretic hormone in nasopharynx carcinoma. *Pediatr Nephrol*, **11**, 502–3.

Lange, B., O'Neill, J., Goldwein, J., Packer, R., and Ross, A. (1997) In *Principles and Practice of Pediatric Oncology* (ed. P. Pizzo and D. Poplack) Lippincott-Raven, Philadelphia, pp. 1025–49.

Lipshultz, S.E., Colan, S.D., Gelber, R.D., Perez-Atayde, A.R., Sallan, S.E., and Sanders, S.P. (1991) Late cardiac effects of duxorubicin therapy for acute lymphoblastic leukaemia in childhood. *N Engl J Med*, **324**, 808–15.

Maghnie, M., Cosi, G., Genovese, E., Manca-Bitti, M.L., Cohen, A., Zecca, S., Tinelli, C., Gallucci, M., Bernasconi, S., Boscherini, B., Severi, F., and Arico, M. (2000) Central diabetes insipidus in children and young adults. *N Engl J Med*, **343**, 998–1007.

Mahboubi, S., Duckett, J.N., and Spackman, T.J. (1976) Ureteritis cystica after treatment of cyclophosphamide-induced hemorrhagic cystitis. *Urology*, **7**, 521–3.

Medary, I., Steinherz, L.J., Aronson, D.C., and La Quaglia, M.P. (1996) Cardiac tamponade in the pediatric oncology population: treatment by percutaneous catheter drainage. *J Pediatr Surg*, **31**, 197–9; discussion 199–200.

Quinn, J.A. and DeAngelis, L.M. (2000) Neurologic emergencies in the cancer patient [Review]. *Semin Oncol*, **27**, 311–21.

Rice, S.J., Bishop, J.A., Apperley, J., and Gardner, S.D. (1985) BK virus as a cause of hemorrhagic cystitis after bone marrow transplantation. *Lancet*, **2**, 844–5.

Shamberger, R.C., Weinstein, H.J., Delorey, M.J., and Levey, R.H. (1986) The medical and surgical management of typhlitis in children with acute nonlymphocytic (myelogenous) leukemia. *Cancer*, **57**, 603–9.

Wexler, L.H., Andrich, M.P., Venzon, D., Berg, S.L., Weaver-McClure, L., Chen, C.C., Dilsizian, V., Avila, N., Jarosinski, P., Balis, F.M., Poplack, D.G., and Horowitz, M.E. (1996) Randomized trial of the cardioprotective agen ICRF-187 in pediatric sarcoma patients treated with doxorubicin. *J Clin Oncol*, **14**, 362–72.

Chapter 12

Infectious Diseases Emergencies

Juan Gea-Banacloche, Stephen J. Chanock, and Thomas J. Walsh

Infection is frequently the immediate cause of death of the patient with cancer, and many times it constitutes a medical emergency. In this chapter, the main infectious disease syndromes in oncology are presented. Most commonly, the physician has to deal with a clinical problem without precise knowledge of the etiology, and that is why we have favored the syndromic approach. In some cases, most notably in bacteremia, the clinician is provided with some information, often incomplete, from the beginning. We attempt to present a guide that may help to formulate a differential diagnosis and therapeutic strategy under those circumstances. Specific coverage of particular pathogens can be found under the specific clinical entities.

12.1 Risk factors for infection in the oncologic patient

Several factors contribute to the increased risk for infection in the patient with cancer. The malignancy itself may compromise host defenses because of local anatomic abnormalities (obstruction, disruption of the integument) or through a systemic effect on host defenses (lymphomas and leukemias). The treatment may predispose to infection in several ways. Indwelling catheters or stents may facilitate colonization and infection. Chemotherapy and radiotherapy-induced mucositis allows invasion by colonizing microorganisms. Neutropenia is the single most important risk factor for bacterial and fungal infections. Steroids and other immunosuppressive agents depress cellular immunity. Lastly, the underlying condition that predisposed the patient to develop cancer may be associated with increased risk of infection (e.g. liver cirrhosis, chronic pulmonary disease, AIDS).

12.1.1 General approach according to host

A basic understanding of how different abnormalities in host defense contribute to different infections is of practical importance. Frequently several problems are present at the same time.

Neutropenia

The absolute neutrophil count (ANC) is the single most important risk factor for bacterial and fungal infection. The risk increases with decreasing counts, rapidity of the decrease and duration of neutropenia.

Splenectomy

The spleen is essential to eliminate opsonized pathogens and parasitized erythrocytes. Splenectomy also impairs the humoral response to new antigens. The defects in humoral immunity and phagocytosis predispose the patient to overwhelming sepsis with encapsulated organisms, particularly *Streptococcus pneumoniae*. Fulminant septicemia caused by *Capnocytophaga canimorsus* is more common. Hemolysis caused by *Babesia* may be more severe in the splenectomized patient.

Immunoglobulin defects

Quantitative and/or qualitative defects in immunoglobulins in chronic lymphocytic leukemia (CLL) and multiple myeloma predispose the patient to infections with encapsulated bacteria, like *Streptococcus pneumoniae*, *Haemophilus influenzae*, and *Neisseria meningitidis*.

Defects in cell-mediated immunity

T cells are essential for the immune response against viruses and many intracellular pathogens and they play a role in most other aspects of the immune response. Consequently, severe defects in T cell function will predispose the patient to the widest array of infections. AIDS is the prototype, but a similar situation is present in the recipient of a T cell-depleted hematopoietic stem cell transplant (HSCT). Milder defects in cell-mediated immunity occur with the use of corticosteroids, cyclophosphamide, fludarabine, and immunosuppressants like cyclosporin, methotrexate, FK-506, mycophenolate mofetil, anti-thymocyte globulin (ATG), and agents that block tumor necrosis factor (TNF) activity, Etanercept and anti-TNF monoclonal antibody (Infliximab/Remicade). Defects in cellular immunity predispose to viral infections, particularly cytomegalovirus (CMV) and other herpes viruses. There is also increased risk for bacteria like *Listeria* and *Nocardia*. Fungal infections are also more common: candidiasis, cryptococcosis and invasive infections with filamentous fungi like *Aspergillus*. *Toxoplasma gondii* and *Pneumocystis carinii* only cause disease in the presence of a significant defect in cell-mediated immunity. Anti-TNF monoclonal antibody (Infliximab/Remicade) has been associated with a particularly high frequency of disseminated mycobacterial disease.

12.2 **Specific infectious disease syndromes**

12.2.1 **Neutropenic fever**

Background

For operational purposes, fever is T $>38\,^{\circ}$C and neutropenia is an absolute neutrophil count (ANC) <500 per ml or expected to be below that threshold within 24 hours. Fever in the presence of neutropenia is a medical emergency. Studies performed in the 1970s showed that waiting to document an infection before starting treatment is associated with a 20–30 percent fatality rate, due mainly to overwhelming gram-negative sepsis.

Conversely, the initiation of empirical broad-spectrum antibiotics with good activity against *Pseudomonas aeruginosa* results in a much lower mortality, currently in the 3–5 percent range.

Microbiologically documented infection (most commonly bacteremia) is found only in approximately one third of the episodes of neutropenic fever. Another 25 percent of cases have clinically defined infection without microbiologic documentation. That leaves approximately 40 percent as fever of unknown origin, although most of these cases also respond to antibiotic treatment. The bacteria most commonly isolated in recent years are gram-positive organisms (*Staphylococcus epidermidis*, *Streptococcus viridans*) although gram-negative (*E. coli*, *Klebsiella*, *Enterobacter*) still account for a significant proportion of the episodes of bacteremia. *Pseudomonas aeruginosa* seems to be less common than in the past, although inter-institutional differences may be marked.

Neutropenia is a surrogate marker for risk. The presence of neutropenia frequently implies other defects in host defense, particularly breakdown of mucosal barriers. The successful management of fever and neutropenia rests on the ability to accurately gauge the changing risk in an individual patient. Decisions have to be re-examined and often changed.

Initial management

A swift approach to diagnosis and therapy is mandatory. A thorough history and physical examination should be performed (Table 12.1) but antibiotic therapy should not be delayed. Neutropenia blunts the inflammatory response so special attention to subtle abnormalities is required. The mouth should be examined for mucositis, marginal gingivitis and dental abscess. The perianal area has to be examined in search of cellulitis and fissures. Herpetic lesions may be present on either location. The catheter exit site has to be inspected and the tunnel tract palpated to rule out infection; any expressible material should be sent for culture. The skin should be inspected looking for cellulitis and

Table 12.1 Neutropenic fever: key features of the physical examination

Vital signs	Orthostatic hypotension, widened pulse pressure, hypoxemia
Skin/soft tissue	Rash, cellulitis, abscesses, nodules
	Consider: VZV, ecthyma gangrenosum
Mouth	Mucositis, thrush, herpes
	Necrotizing gingivitis, dental abscess
Catheter	
Exit site	Erythema, induration, exudates
Tunnel track	Erythema, induration, tenderness
Chest	Pleural rubs, adventitious heart sounds
Abdomen	Rebound, guarding, local tenderness
Perianal region	Ulceration, erythema, induration, abscess

other cutaneous manifestations of infection. The chest should be examined for adventitious sounds or pleural rubs. The abdomen should be evaluated for guarding or local tenderness. Blood cultures should be drawn (at least 20 ml in two different sets). Ideally, every port of a central line and a peripheral site should be sampled. Omitting the peripheral culture lowers the specificity of the test, but the sensitivity remains almost unchanged. Urinalysis and urine culture should be obtained. Stool culture and stool testing for *Clostridium difficile* toxin should be performed if the patient has diarrhea. A chest X-ray should be always part of the initial evaluation, as it will serve as an important baseline study.

Broad-spectrum antibiotics should be started promptly (Table 12.2). If there are no localizing signs of infection, the initial choice should take into account the institution's patterns of antimicrobial resistance to select one of the following options:

1. Monotherapy with ceftazidime, cefepime, imipenem or meropenem.
2. Dual therapy with an extended-spectrum beta-lactam and an aminoglycoside.

Vancomycin may be included in the initial regimen only in special circumstances, as discussed below.

Although the initial success in the treatment of fever and neutropenia was observed with combination therapy, most studies have shown that monotherapy with the agents listed above is equally effective and less toxic. The concept of dual therapy is rooted in the original studies on the management of fever and neutropenia, when the combination of an aminoglycoside and a carboxy- or ureidopenicillin was used in an effort to attain synergy against gram-negative bacteria, particularly *Pseudomonas*. It is unclear that this approach is of benefit with current third-generation cephalosporins and carbapenems. There is no convincing evidence that combined therapy is better than single agent, although many authorities would still recommend two antibiotics particularly in the setting of complicated *Pseudomonas* infections. As monotherapy, ceftazidime is probably the reference standard, and no single agent has been proved consistently superior. The other three recommended antibiotics provide better gram-positive coverage, but all four are equally ineffective against coagulase-negative staphylococci. Ceftazidime or cefepime are used in many centers as first line therapy. Given their broad anti-anaerobic spectrum, meropenem and imipenem are usually reserved for cases of suspected anaerobic or resistant infections (Figure 12.1).

The inclusion of vancomycin as part of the initial regimen is not associated with improved outcome but may select for emergence of resistant pathogens and so it is not routinely recommended. If a gram-positive bacteremia is identified, vancomycin should be added at that point pending susceptibility testing. However, vancomycin should be included in the initial regimen when there is evidence of catheter exit site infection, tunnel infection, soft tissue infection, or when alpha-hemolytic streptococcal infections are likely. Known carriers of methicillin-resistant *Staphylococcus aureus* and penicillin-resistant *Streptococcus pneumoniae* also receive vancomycin empirically.

Table 12.2 Neutropenic fever: initial management and modifications

Initial therapy: Monotherapy

Ceftazidime	2 g q 8 hourly	Standard. Median time to defervescence 4–5 days.
Cefepime	2 g q 8 hourly	Equivalent to ceftazidime against gram-negative, better coverage of gram-positive bacteria, including *Streptococcus* spp. and *Staph. aureus*
Imipenem	500 mg q 6 hourly	Broader spectrum: gram-positive, gram-negative, anaerobes. Preferred if intra-abdominal source likely. Equivalent efficacy to ceftazidime but more toxic
Meropenem	1 g q 8 hourly	Spectrum similar to imipenem; possibly less GI intolerance; possibly less neurotoxicity (seizures)

Modifications

Vancomycin + aztreonam	1 g q 12 hourly 2 g q 6–8 hourly	Penicillin-allergic patient
Vancomycin	1 g q 12 hourly	Empiric use limited to the following: • Obvious intravascular device infection (exit site, tunnel infection) • High risk of alpha-hemolytic streptococcal infection (see text) • Known carrier of oxacillin-resistant *Staph. aureus* or *Strep. pneumoniae* Empirical addition to monotherapy for persistent fever is not effective
Aminoglycosides Gentamicin Tobramycin Amikacin	Once-daily dosing effective in neutropenia	Include in the initial regimen if: • Patient is hemodynamically unstable • High suspicion of multiresistant gram-negative bacilli, e.g. ecthyma gangrenosum
Metronidazole	500 mg q 6 hourly	Add to ceftazidime or cefepime for enhanced anaerobic coverage (particularly Bacteroides fragilis group); less effective for microaerophilic bacteria (e.g. many anaerobes from the oral cavity)

Rescue regimen

Meropenem (imipenem) + tobramycin (gentamicin)		If clinical deterioration (e.g. hypotension, new pulmonary infiltrate) occurs Persistent fever alone is not a reason to switch

Antifungal addition

Antifungal coverage indicated for persistent fever after day 5–7 and for new pulmonary infiltrates during broad-spectrum antibiotic treatment

Amphotericin B deoxycholate	0.6 mg kg^{-1}/day	Standard; consider 1 mg kg^{-1} when the suspicion for *Aspergillus* is higher
Liposomal Amphotericin B (AmBisome)	3 mg kg^{-1}/day	At least as effective as amphotericin B and less toxic; high acquisition cost probably offset by decreased severe toxicities
Fluconazole	400 mg/day	Only in selected low-risk patients (solid tumors, short duration of neutropenia, no previous antifungal prophylaxis)

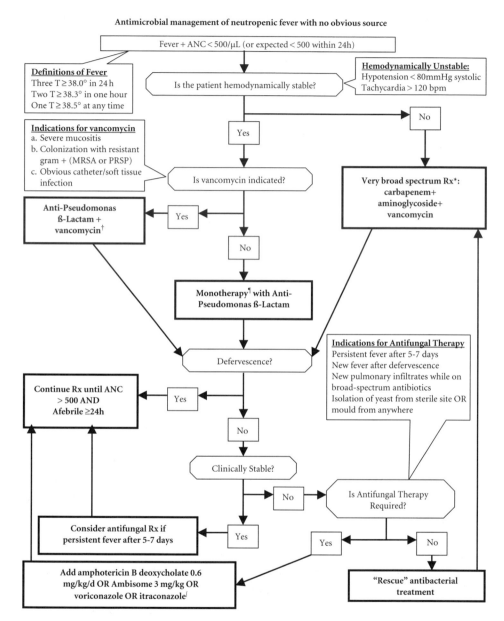

Fig. 12.1 This figure represents the general approach to patients with fever and neutropenia without a clinically or microbiologically documented infection. For specific infections, see text and table 12.2. As emphasized in the text, daily reassessment is mandatory.

Fig. 12.1 (notes)

*This 'rescue antibacterial regimen' will vary between institutions depending on the local patterns of antibiotic resistance. Sometimes (e.g., patients at high risk of aminoglycoside nephrotoxicity) the combination carbapenem + quinolone + vancomycin is substituted. In our institution we typically use meropenem + tobramycin + vancomycin.

†Vancomycin should be discontinued after 48h if there is no bacteriological documentation of a pathogen requiring its use, except in soft tissue or tunnel infections.

¶Monotherapy is preferred, as no combination regimen has proved superior. Anti-Pseudomonas ß-lactam refers to ceftazidime, cefepime, imipenem and meropenem only. Other ß-lactams have activity against *Pseudomonas*, but they have not shown to be adequate monotherapy for fever and neutropenia. We routinely treat the penicillin-allergic patient with aztreonam + vancomycin.

ʃFor a detailed discussion of antifungal therapy options, see text. The standard approach has been the addition of amphotericin B deoxycholate at a dose of 0.6 mg/kg/d. Liposomal amphotericin B 3 mg/kg/d has been shown to be at least as effective and less toxic in this setting. Other approaches are discussed in the text. Recently published randomized controlled trials of itraconazole and voriconazole in this setting indicate these antifungal triazoles are other options at the following dosages: voriconazole 6 mg/kg q 12h i.v. x2 doses loading, followed by 3 mg/kg q 12h i.v. (4 mg/kg i.v. in children) maintenance; itraconazole injection 200 mg q 12h i.v. x4 doses loading, followed by 200 mg i.v. qd.

Abbreviations: MRSA: Methicillin (oxacillin)-resistant *Staphylococcus aureus*; PRSP: Penicillin-resistant *Streptococcus pneumoniae*.

Special situations

1. The hypotensive patient should receive broader spectrum coverage, including an extended-spectrum beta-lactam, an aminoglycoside and vancomycin.

2. In the presence of perianal cellulitis, marginal gingivitis or suspected intra-abdominal infection (e.g. typhilitis) adequate anaerobic coverage should be provided (imipenem or meropenem, or addition of metronidazole). One should also initiate empirical antibacterial therapy with anaerobic coverage in those patients with abdominal symptoms but no fever.

3. The presence of pulmonary infiltrates warrants coverage against the agents of community-acquired pneumonia, including *Streptococcus pneumoniae, Legionella, Chlamydia* and *Mycoplasma*. Azithromycin or a newer fluroquinolone such as levofloxacin should be added to the regimen.

4. In hospitals with high incidence of extended-spectrum beta-lactamase (ESBL)- or stably derepressed beta-lactamase-producing gram-negative bacteria (see below) carbapenems (imipenem and meropenem) should be preferred over cephalosporins (ceftazidime and cefepime).

5. In the penicillin-allergic patient, the combination of aztreonam and vancomycin should be used.

Re-evaluation and antibiotic changes

The successful management of fever and neutropenia requires constant monitoring and re-evaluation. Modification of therapy is required in 10–40 percent of cases. Daily physical examinations are mandatory, with special attention devoted to mouth, skin and perianal region.

Persistent fever is not, *per se*, an indication for changing or adding antibiotics. The median time to normalization of temperature with ceftazidime has been 4–5 days in many studies spanning more than 20 years. If the patient is persistently febrile but otherwise clinically stable, the current regimen should be continued. Appropriate changes should be made based on new clinical findings and/or microbiology lab results. Most positive cultures become so within 48 hours. Antibiotics should be adjusted accordingly, although the standard broad-spectrum coverage should be maintained.

In cases of clinical worsening, defined as hemodynamic instability without focal findings a "rescue" regimen with enhanced coverage for resistant gram-negative and gram-positive bacteria should be used (e.g. meropenem or imipenem + aminoglycoside (chosen according to institutional susceptibility patterns) ± vancomycin). After 5 days of unresponsive neutropenic fever, consideration should be given to the empirical initiation of antifungal therapy.

Empirical antifungal therapy

Profound, prolonged neutropenia is associated with significant risk of invasive fungal infection. These infections have high mortality when treatment is initiated after they have been unequivocally diagnosed. The rationale for empirical antifungal therapy is the early treatment of occult fungal infections and prevention of mycoses in high-risk patients. Randomized studies published in the 1980s showed that the empirical addition of amphotericin B after 4–7 days of persistent fever unresponsive to broad-spectrum antibiotics decreased the number of proven invasive fungal infections and the number of deaths caused by fungal infections. Practice Guidelines published by the Infectious Diseases Society of America (IDSA) recommend the addition of empirical antifungal treatment to the initial regimen if fever persists after 5–7 days. The optimal day on which antifungal coverage should be initiated has not been determined, and it is likely to be different for different groups of patients. A systematic effort to find the presumed fungal infection should be carried out. When possible, CT scans of sinuses and lungs should be obtained. PCR and galactomannan detection to identify *Aspergillus* have been reported to be useful in early diagnosis. However, their precise role warrants further study.

The addition of antifungal therapy is considered a standard of care but it is useful to differentiate the following clinical situations:

1. In selected low-risk patients who have not received antifungal prophylaxis, it may be acceptable to empirically start fluconazole 400 mg/day, as this approach has been

shown to be as effective as low-dose amphotericin B in some randomized controlled trials. This approach may be used only for low-risk patients who are expected to be neutropenic for a relatively short time.

2. The current approach in high-risk neutropenic patients is the addition of amphotericin B at 0.6 mg kg^{-1} or liposomal amphotericin B at 3 mg kg^{-1}. This dose will be enough to treat the majority of *Candida* infections and it might prevent progression of an occult mould infection until recovery from neutropenia. This dose, however, may not be optimal to treat systemic candidiasis caused by *Candida glabrata* or *Candida krusei* and is clearly inadequate to treat established invasive aspergillosis.

3. For patients who have received antifungal prophylaxis with fluconazole, azole resistant, non-*albicans Candida* (*C. glabrata, C. krusei*) or filamentous fungi (mainly *Aspergillus* spp.) are the most likely fungal pathogens. When the suspicion for these organisms is high, it may be preferable to administer amphotericin B at a dose of 1 mg kg^{-1}/day or lipid formulations of amphotericin B at 5 mg kg^{-1}/day.

Amphotericin B lipid formulations Part of the controversy regarding the empirical use of amphotericin B derives from its toxicity. The newer lipid-based formulations (liposomal amphotericin B, amphotericin B lipid complex, amphotericin B colloidal dispersion) are definitely less toxic and allow dose escalation above what was possible with amphotericin B deoxycholate. However, their acquisition cost is much higher. Regarding efficacy, liposomal amphotericin B (AmBisome) 3 mg kg^{-1}/day has been shown to be at least as effective as 0.6 mg kg^{-1}/day of conventional amphotericin B in a randomized controlled trial of fever and neutropenia and it significantly reduced the frequency of proven invasive fungal infections. Regarding cost there is mounting evidence that the decreased toxicity associated with these drugs may offset their steep acquisition cost. We favor the use of lipid formulations in patients who are in significant risk of renal toxicity (see below).

Treatment duration

In general, antibiotics should be continued for the duration of neutropenia or to complete the standard course for the documented infection (whichever is longer). Before stopping therapy, the patient should be non-neutropenic and afebrile for at least 24 hours.

When the antifungal therapy was started empirically, without any evidence of fungal infection, it can be discontinued once the patient is afebrile and with ANC >500 per ml. If there was some documentation of fungal infection, the treatment duration varies (see specific infections).

Outpatient therapy

Not all patients with neutropenic fever are at the same risk of significant morbidity or mortality. There have been efforts by several investigators to identify the subgroup of patients with very low risk of complications. Uncontrolled cancer, presence of other significant medical conditions and development of the fever during hospitalization define a high-risk group. Outpatients without co-morbidities and with cancer in remission constitute the low-risk group. Randomized studies have shown that low-risk patients without significant mucositis, no end-organ infections and projected short neutropenia may be managed safely with oral antibiotics as inpatients. The outpatient management of neutropenic fever, however, should be considered investigational at this time.

12.2.2 **Bacteremia/fungemia**

A report of positive blood cultures from the laboratory may represent a true medical emergency or contamination. Blood cultures should always be repeated. Antibiotic therapy should be initiated or not depending on the clinical situation. If the patient is neutropenic, bactericidal antibiotics with activity against the isolated organism should always be started or added. The same is true for the febrile and/or clinically unstable patient. If the patient is not neutropenic, the management will differ according to the pathogen. When the isolate is a virulent, common pathogenic organism, like *Staphylococcus aureus*, *Pseudomonas* and enteric gram-negative bacilli, empirical treatment should be initiated even if the patient is afebrile and clinically stable. If the isolate is coagulase-negative *Staphylococcus,* the diagnosis should be confirmed before starting antibiotics.

It is important to try to identify the source of the bacteremia, as it may require specific treatment. During neutropenia, the gastrointestinal tract is the most common portal of entry. At other times, catheter-associated bacteremia is probably most common. Continuous bacteremia is uncommon and suggests an intravascular source. Finally, it is essential to document that the bacteremia has cleared during therapy and after.

The initial information from the microbiology laboratory has important implications for management. Some pathogen-specific considerations follow.

Gram-positive cocci (GPC)

Gram-positive bacteria have replaced gram-negative bacilli as the most common blood isolates in the neutropenic patient. The common pathogens include coagulase-negative staphylococci, *Streptococcus*, *Staphylococcus aureus* and *Enterococcus*. The Gram stain morphology may help as clusters suggest staphylococci, long chains *Strep. Viridans,* and pairs and short chains suggest *Enterococcus* (or, rarely, *Streptococcus pneumoniae*). Coagulase-negative staphylococci are the most common isolates. Most commonly, they are contaminants but they are also the most common cause of catheter-related infections. *Staphylococcus lugdunensis* is a coagulase-negative staphylococcus that has caused abscesses and severe, destructive endocarditis in previously normal valves, similar to *Staph. aureus.* Other GPC that have caused disease in the immunocompromised patient with an intravascular catheter include *Micrococcus, Leuconostoc* and *Pediococcus. Leuconostoc* and *Pediococcus* are intrinsically resistant to vancomycin, but susceptible to penicillin G, ampicillin and clindamycin. *Stomatococcus mucilaginosus* has been isolated with increasing frequency in immunocompromised patients with bacteremia and/or CNS infection.

In general, pending definitive identification and susceptibility testing, vancomycin should be started when the blood cultures grow GPC. Antibiotic treatment should be adjusted after reviewing susceptibilities.

***Staphylococcus aureus* bacteremia**   *Staph. aureus* bacteremia is associated with an extremely high likelihood of metastatic complications if it is not adequately treated. In general, any intravascular device should be removed. Routine transesophageal echocardiogram has been recommended in *Staph. aureus* bacteremia to rule out occult endocarditis. Fludoxacillin, oxacillin or nafcillin are the drugs of choice. Vancomycin should be used for penicillin-allergic patients and in case of methicillin resistance (MRSA). The duration of treatment varies with the clinical circumstances. If the likely source of the bacteremia is removed and there is no evidence of metastatic complications two weeks of intravenous antibiotics are sufficient. Commonly four to six weeks will be necessary.

***Streptococcus* viridans**   *Streptococcus* viridans (α-hemolytic *streptococcus*) is part of the normal flora of the gastrointestinal tract. They have been known to cause subacute bacterial endocarditis for decades, and they have always been isolated as agents of gram-positive bacteremia during neutropenia. More recently, a syndrome of overwhelming infection with acute respiratory distress syndrome (ARDS), shock and high mortality during intensive cytotoxic therapy and mucositis has been described. The most frequent isolate in this clinical entity has been *Streptococcus mitis*. Risk factors for this disease include severe mucositis (particularly following treatment with Ara-C), use of H_2 blockers or antacids and use of prophylactic antibiotics with good activity against gram-negative bacteria such as ciprofloxacin and trimethoprim-sulfamethoxazole (TMP/SMX). Given that these organisms are not predictably susceptible to penicillin or cephalosporins, vancomycin should be used pending susceptibility testing. In institutions where this infection is common and in patients at high risk, vancomycin should be included as part of the initial regimen for neutropenic fever. The use of prophylactic penicillin G or ampicillin around the time of the transplant to prevent this complication has not been consistently successful because of penicillin-resistant strains.

Vancomycin-resistant enterococcus (VRE)   The increasing prevalence of vancomycin-resistant enterococci is a significant problem, and it underscores the importance of promoting a rational antibiotic policy. VRE is usually a nosocomial pathogen. Risk factors for the VRE carrier state include exposure to antibiotics, particularly cephalosporins, vancomycin and metronidazole.

VRE is usually *Enterococcus faecium*, but *Enterococcus faecalis* can occasionally be resistant to vancomycin. The organism typically appears in debilitated patients who have been hospitalized for some time and have received multiple antibiotics. VRE most commonly produces bacteremia, but urinary tract infections, intra-abdominal and wound infections have been reported. It is unclear if the resistance to vancomycin is an independent risk factor for increased mortality, but it makes management more difficult. Any carrier of VRE should be placed in contact isolation. The need for medical treatment should be assessed. As treatment of carriers is largely ineffective, antibiotic therapy should be reserved for active infection. Any devices (intravenous catheters, Foley catheters) that may be associated with the infection should be removed, and cultures repeated. If a urine culture was positive, it needs to be ascertained if it was urinary tract infection or just asymptomatic bacteriuria.

Once it is determined that treatment is necessary, the two available options are quinupristin-dalfopristin (Synercid) and linezolid. Susceptibility testing to these agents should be conducted, because in some countries there is a high background resistance to Synercid and linezolid-resistant VRE has been described. Synercid is active only against *E. faecium*, but not *E. faecalis*. Both antibiotics are only bacteriostatic, and treatment failures with and without the development of resistance during therapy have been well documented.

Gram-positive bacilli

Both the clinical presentation and the Gram stain morphology are important in arriving at a tentative diagnosis of an etiologic agent. For example, *Listeria monocytogenes* should be considered as the agent in a patient with altered mental status and gram-positive bacilli in the blood cultures. Several gram-positive bacilli are resistant to vancomycin so it is essential to analyze carefully the clinical picture before choosing an empirical regimen.

***Clostridium* bacteremia**   *Clostridium septicum* bacteremia is strongly associated with malignancy, typically leukemia and colon carcinoma. Occasionally the bacteremia precedes the diagnosis of cancer. Frequently the bacteremia is accompanied by spontaneous myonecrosis or non-traumatic gas gangrene. In this syndrome patients present with severe, acute pain in the affected muscles. The pain may initially seem out of proportion to the physical findings. Dusky discoloration, crepitus and hemorrhagic bullae may ensue with rapid extension of the necrosis accompanied by hypotension. *Clostridium septicum* is isolated from the blood cultures and the tissue. The most common underlying malignancies are leukemia and colon cancer, but neutropenia of any cause is known to be a predisposing factor. *Clostridium septicum* bacteremia may also occur in necrotizing enterocolitis (typhlitis) in the neutropenic patient. Penicillin G is active against *C. septicum*.

Clostridium perfringens may occasionally represent transient, innocuous bacteremia, but it has also been associated with massive intravascular hemolysis, fulminant sepsis and death. Penicillin G is the treatment of choice.

Clostridium tertium has been associated with bacteremia in neutropenic patients with gastrointestinal symptoms, typically watery or bloody diarrhea, and perirectal cellulitis. *Clostridium tertium* is significant because it is commonly resistant to penicillin, clindamycin, third-generation cephalosporins and sometimes metronidazole. Vancomycin is typically effective.

Listeria monocytogenes   Malignancy is a predisposing factor for listeriosis. *Listeria monocytogenes* bacteremia may occur isolated or accompanying central nervous system infection (see below). The treatment of choice is ampicillin; gentamicin is frequently added in combination. Trimethoprim-sulfamethoxazole is an alternative in the penicillin-allergic patient. Vancomycin has only marginal efficacy against *Listeria* and should not be used.

Bacteremia caused by other gram-positive bacilli   *Bacillus* spp. are large, boxcar-shaped aerobic rods. They are common contaminants of blood cultures, but they may cause catheter infection and even a septic picture. As causes of bacteremia, they usually require removal of infected vascular catheters.

Corynebacterium ("diphteroids") are part of the normal skin flora and are commonly contaminants, but in the neutropenic patient with a IV catheter they may represent true infection, (particularly *Corynebacterium jeikeium). Corynebacterium jeikeium* is usually resistant to multiple antibiotics and it may require treatment with vancomycin and sometimes removal of the catheter. Several species from the genus corynebacterium (*Corynebacterium striatum, Corynebacterium pseudodiphteriticum*) have caused disease in immunocompromised hosts, particularly pneumonia sometimes with abscess formation.

Lactobacillus spp. is another anaerobic gram-positive that more commonly represents contamination but can cause serious infection in neutropenic patients. *Lactobacillus rhamnosum* is frequently resistant to vancomycin and third-generation cephalosporins, but susceptible to penicillin, ampicillin, erythromycin and clindamycin.

Propionibacterium in the blood is usually a contaminant, but *Propionibacterium* infections of intraventricular reservoirs and plastic devices have been well documented.

Gram-negative bacilli

As a rule, gram-negative bacilli in the blood should not be considered contaminants. Gram-negative bacteremia can evolve rapidly into sepsis and shock, and empirical antibiotic treatment should be started immediately. As discussed below, the susceptibility of a particular gram-negative bacterium may be difficult to predict, and it is entirely reasonable to initiate treatment with two antimicrobials to ensure adequate coverage until the results of the susceptibility testing are available. Once the antibiogram is known, the need for "double-coverage" is questionable. The empirical choice of antimicrobials may be facilitated by information derived from the Gram-stain morphology and the oxidase reaction. Although the list of possible pathogens is staggering it is useful to decide early if the isolate belongs to the family Enterobacteriaceae ("enteric" gram-negative bacilli) or if it is more likely a *Pseudomonas* or another non-fermenting bacterium.

Enteric gram-negative bacilli   Bacteria belonging to the family Enterobacteriaceae are the most common gram-negative isolates. *E. coli* and *Klebsiella* are the most prevalent, but the use of prophylactic antibiotics such as ciprofloxacin or TMP/SMX may increase the relative prevalence of more resistant enteric organisms *Enterobacter, Citrobacter* and *Serratia.*

Klebsiella and *E. coli* were once predictably susceptible to third generation cephalosporins, but this is no longer the case. For example, the prevalence of strains that synthesize extended-spectrum beta-lactamases (ESBL-producers) is increasing. ESBLs are plasmid-encoded enzymes with activity against most third-generation cephalosporins and aztreonam. Resistance to aminoglycosides and fluoroquinolones seems to be more common among ESBL-producers. Carbapenems (imipenem and meropenem) are the drugs of choice; piperacillin-tazobactam is not predictably effective.

Other species, most notably *Enterobacter cloacae* (but also *Serratia* spp., *Morganella morganii* and *Citrobacter freundii*) have inducible chromosomal cephalosporinases. Resistance to third-generation cephalosporins during treatment may develop due to the presence of stably derepressed mutants. For these organisms, carbapenems or fluoroquinolones may be better alternatives.

Pseudomonas aeruginosa *Pseudomonas* infection may be suggested by the typical morphology of a slender gram-negative rod in pairs and a positive oxidase reaction. *Pseudomonas aeruginosa* is among the most lethal agents of gram-negative bacteremia in the neutropenic patient. *Pseudomonas* used to be considered a nosocomial pathogen but it may also present as a community-acquired infection (up to half the cases in some recent series).

Pseudomonas infection has been traditionally considered an indication for combination antibiotic treatment, as resistance develops frequently during treatment and there is experimental evidence suggesting synergy between beta-lactams and aminoglycosides. However, the evidence that combination therapy improves the outcome in clinical practice is very limited. A particularly challenging problem is the management of *Pseudomonas* resistant to all commonly available antimicrobial agents. Strategies that have been employed successfully in this situation include the use of colistin or polymixin, combination of agents and administration of beta-lactams (ceftazidime, aztreonam) by continuous infusion at high doses that ensure levels continuously above the MIC.

Other gram-negative bacilli *Stenotrophomonas maltophilia* is a long, slender gram-negative bacillus, usually oxidase-negative. It appears typically in debilitated patients who have received multiple antibiotic courses, including imipenem. The presence of cellulitis may be a significant clue. The mortality is high. *Stenotrophomonas* is characteristically resistant to imipenem and other beta-lactams with the notable exception of ticarcillin. It is also frequently resistant to fluoroquinolones. The antibiotic that is more consistently effective is trimethoprim-sulfamethoxazole (TMP/SMX). Susceptibility testing should be performed by the broth/microdilution technique and not by agar diffusion tests.

Acinetobacter is a cocco-bacillary, oxidase-negative gram-negative bacillus. *Acinetobacter baumanii* is frequently resistant to multiple antibiotics, including imipenem.

Capnocytophaga is a fastidious fusiform gram-negative rod that has caused bacteremia in neutropenic patients with mucositis and fulminant sepsis in splenectomized patients.

Anaerobic gram-negative bacteremia Bacteremia due to anaerobic gram-negative bacilli is uncommon in neutropenic patients. Its presence in any patient may signify a source arising from the abdomen or alimentary tract. The presence of gram-negative bacilli that grow only in anaerobic bottles should make the clinician consider the possibility of anaerobic bacteremia. *Fusobacterium necrophorum* has been associated with Lemierre's syndrome (jugular vein thrombophlebitis with pulmonary septic emboli). *Bacteroides* bacteremia usually originates from the colon, and its isolation in blood cultures strongly suggests an intra-abdominal source, including pelvic septic thrombophlebitis. Bacteroides produces a beta-lactamase and it has become increasingly resistant to clindamycin and cefoxitin. Metronidazole is the agent of choice, although carbapenems and beta-lactam+beta-lactamase inhibitor combinations are usually effective.

Fungemia

Candidemia   The clinical spectrum of Candidemia extends from patients who are asymptomatic to critically ill patients with fever, hypotension and distributive shock indistinguishable from gram-negative sepsis. In any case, a positive blood culture for candida cannot be ignored and requires specific treatment, usually including removal of intravascular catheters. The patient should be examined for subcutaneous nodules. An ophthalmic evaluation with fundoscopic exam is indicated in non-neutropenic patients.

Identification of the species of candida has therapeutic implications. *Candida albicans* is the species isolated most frequently. The germ tube test should allow the laboratory to provisionally identify a candida isolate as *albicans* or non-*albicans* in a few hours. For the treatment of *Candida albicans* in the non-neutropenic host, amphotericin B 0.5–0.6 mg kg^{-1}/day or fluconazole 400 mg/day seem to be equivalent. The evidence that fluconazole is equally effective for candidemia in the neutropenic host is less firm.

The frequency of non-*albicans* candidemia seems to be increasing, particularly in centers where fluconazole prophylaxis is widely used. The treatment of non-*albicans* candidemia is less well defined. The susceptibility of different species to different antifungals is variable. *Candida krusei* is intrinsically resistant to fluconazole and *Candida glabrata* may have intermediate resistance and become completely resistant during treatment with fluconazole. *C. glabrata* and *C. krusei* may also have reduced susceptibility to amphotericin B. From the practical standpoint, this means that if the patient is critically ill and the species of *Candida* is unknown the safest treatment option is amphotericin B at 1 mg kg^{-1}/day. For a stable patient who has not received azoles recently the initial treatment may be fluconazole 400 mg/day. Once the species is known, treatment may be adjusted. The treatment of choice for *C. lusitaniae* is fluconazole, as this species is frequently resistant to amphotericin B.

Other fungi

Trichosporon   *Trichosporon* is a yeast that can cause severe disease in immunocompromised patients, particularly during neutropenia. It can cause disseminated infection with fungemia, funguria and deep-seated invasion (lungs, kidneys, eyes, skin). Purpuric papules and nodules with necrotic central ulceration are characteristic in disseminated infection. A falsely positive serum cryptococcal antigen determination may be present in 30–40 percent of cases. This yeast is resistant to the fungicidal effect of amphotericin B. Antifungal triazoles are especially active against this pathogen. Fluconazole 400–800 mg/day is the preferred therapy.

12.2.3 **Respiratory infections**

Upper respiratory infections

Upper respiratory infections may be emergencies in the setting of profound neutropenia and allogeneic stem cell transplantation (allo-HSCT). These patients carry a high risk of developing viral pneumonia in infections caused by respiratory syncytial virus (RSV), influenza, parainfluenza and adenovirus. Nasopharyngeal (NP) washing is the initial diagnostic procedure of choice in the absence of lower respiratory tract involvement. The results of rapid testing (typically by immunoblot or ELISA) may be available within a few hours, but their sensitivity is only approximately 50 percent when compared with viral culture. Bronchoalveolar lavage (BAL) is appropriate if repeated NP washings are non-diagnostic and symptoms persist.

Oseltamivir, an inhibitor of the neuraminidase of influenza virus A and B, has been shown to be effective as empirical treatment (75 mg bid) in immunocompetent patients with fever and symptoms of influenza if the prevalence of influenza is high (i.e., during an influenza outbreak). Zanamivir 2 inhalations twice a day (10 mg bid), can also be used. As the drug is well tolerated and relatively non-toxic, it is used empirically in HSCT patients during the influenza season pending the results of viral culture. In the setting of an allogeneic HSCT patient, treatment with aerosolized ribavirin is indicated for RSV upper respiratory infection to try to prevent the development of pneumonia, which is associated with significant mortality (>50%). The best regimen has not been determined. Ribavirin may be administered as a total dose of 6 g/day either at a concentration of $20\,\mu g\,ml^{-1}$ over 18 hours or at $60\,\mu g\,ml^{-1}$ over 2 hours three times a day. In some studies, intravenous immunoglobulin at a dose of $500\,mg\,kg^{-1}$ every other day has been added but evidence of its efficacy is lacking. The efficacy of ribavirin for infections caused by parainfluenza or adenovirus is only anecdotal.

Sinusitis

The presence of obstruction (e.g. nasopharyngeal carcinoma or lymphoma) predisposes to the development of acute and chronic sinusitis. The common etiologic pathogens of acute sinusitis in the absence of significant immune compromise are *Streptococcus pneumoniae*, *H. influenzae* and *Moraxella catarrhalis*. For the non-neutropenic patient treatment with levofloxacin 500 mg/day or amoxicillin-clavulanic 875/125 mg bid is administered.

Sinusitis in the neutropenic patient requires broad-spectrum antibiotics with activity against *Streptococcus pneumoniae* and *Pseudomonas aeruginosa* and prompt ENT examination. CT scan should be obtained for diagnosis if possible, as this test is more sensitive and specific than sinus radiography and allows the detection of early bony erosion or orbital involvement.

Fungal sinusitis is a medical emergency in the neutropenic patient. A high index of suspicion must be maintained, as some of the typical signs and symptoms of sinusitis may be absent. If the CT shows bony erosion, it is essential to obtain a tissue sample (sinus aspirate or biopsy). The same is true if a presumed bacterial sinusitis does not improve after 48–72 hours of aggressive medical treatment with antibiotics and decongestants. Minimal crusting of the turbinates may indicate invasive fungal infection. *Aspergillus* and moulds from the order Mucorales (*Mucor, Rhizopus, Absidia*) are the more common causative agents, but other fungi-like *Fusarium* may cause sinusitis. Invasion of the orbit or the brain may ensue and progress relentlessly. The appearance of signs of cranial nerve involvement may represent cavernous sinus thrombosis. Surgical intervention is critical to reduce the bulk of disease. *Aspergillus* sinusitis requires the use of amphotericin B at maximum doses (1–1.5 mg kg^{-1}/day). Lipid preparations of amphotericin allow the administration of higher doses and may be preferable. Granulocyte transfusions (preferably G-CSF-mobilized) are probably of benefit in this situation to sustain the patient until the resolution of neutropenia. However, once brain-blood vessel invasion has occurred even normal neutrophil counts may be ineffective.

Pneumonia

Localized or diffuse pulmonary infiltrates in the immunocompromised host may be secondary to infectious or non-infectious causes. Possible infectious etiologies vary depending on the predisposing defect in host defenses. The timing of the infiltrates (early versus late during neutropenia) and the radiologic pattern (generalized versus focal) can be helpful to decide the most appropriate and expeditious workup.

Pulmonary infiltrates in the neutropenic patient   When a patient presents with febrile neutropenia and focal pulmonary infiltrates adequate coverage for the most common causes of community-acquired pneumonia should be included in the antibiotic regimen. In this regard, none of the first-line antibiotics has any activity against *Legionella*, and ceftazidime has very little activity against *Strep. pneumoniae*. The combination ceftazidime + newer-generation fluoroquinolone (levofloxacin, gatifloxacin, moxifloxacin) is appropriate. As gram-negative bacilli including *Pseudomonas* are still the most likely pathogens, the standard beta-lactam with anti-pseudomonal activity should be maintained. Bronchoalveolar lavage (BAL) should be performed early. Diffuse pulmonary infiltrates and/or respiratory insufficiency are indications for emergent BAL.

If the pulmonary infiltrates appear during broad-spectrum antibiotic treatment of febrile neutropenia the likelihood of fungal infection is very high, and empirical amphotericin B should be started. Bronchoalveolar lavage should be obtained immediately, keeping in mind that a negative result does not exclude fungal infection. The presence of severe thrombocytopenia and/or coagulopathy has to be taken into account, but the need to obtain a definitive diagnosis cannot be overemphasized. A CT of the chest should be obtained before proceeding to the BAL. The CT allows selection of the lung segments to be sampled and it may show patterns typical of fungal infection (halo sign) or other pathogens, although the radiologic findings are only suggestive and never pathognomonic.

Fungal pneumonia

Aspergillosis   *Aspergillus* spp. is the most common filamentous mould causing disease in cancer patients. *Aspergillus fumigatus* is the most common species, but *A. flavus* and

A. terreus are also frequently pathogens. *Aspergillus niger* is usually a contaminant, although it can cause disease. *Aspergillus* conidia are inhaled into the respiratory tract, where they can germinate and cause disease in the paranasal sinuses and the lung. Subsequent dissemination may occur, and any organ may be involved, most notably the CNS, liver, skin and heart. Neutropenia is the most important risk factor, followed by high-dose corticosteroids. It should be stressed that more than half of the cases of aspergillosis in the HSCT setting take place when the patients are not neutropenic in the post-engraftment period.

The typical presentation of aspergillosis during neutropenia is persistent or recurrent fever and a new pulmonary infiltrate during antibiotic treatment. Aspergillosis may develop during low-dose amphotericin B treatment. Chest pain and hemoptysis may occur, occasionally with a new pleural rub. This syndrome requires high-dose amphotericin B ($1–1.5$ mg kg^{-1}/day), amphotericin B lipid complex ($5–10$ mg kg^{-1}/day) or liposomal amphotericin B ($5–10$ mg kg^{-1}/day). Every effort should be made to confirm the diagnosis. In this situation, a respiratory specimen (induced sputum, BAL) culture positive for Aspergillus has a strong positive predictive value for invasive aspergillosis. The definitive diagnosis requires demonstration of septate branching hyphae invading the tissues, but frequently the presence of thrombocytopenia and coagulopathy precludes obtaining a transbronchial biopsy or a fine-needle aspirate (FNA).

Invasive aspergillosis is generally fatal unless the underlying defect in host defenses resolves. Surgical resection of pulmonary lesions has been performed successfully during neutropenia. Granulocyte transfusions have been used in an attempt to slow down the progression of the disease until marrow recovery. Comprehensive guidelines for the treatment of *Aspergillus* have been published recently. The progression of disease despite maximally tolerated doses of amphotericin B (deoxycholate or lipid formulations) is not uncommon. The combination of amphotericin B with itraconazole has not consistently shown antagonism in uncontrolled case series. The newer azoles, in particular voriconazole, offer promise as future options for the treatment of aspergillosis. Caspofungin acetate, a member of the new family of antifungal drugs echinocandins, has been recently approved in the U.S. for patients with invasive aspergillosis who were unresponsive to or intolerant of other antifungal agents. G-CSF should be administered to patients with persistent neutropenia. Whether cytokine therapy with GM-CSF or IFN-γ is as beneficial as adjunctive therapy in non-neutropenic patients is investigational.

Zygomycosis   This disease is a life-threatening infection requiring urgent intervention. It is caused by moulds belonging to the class Zygomycetes. The core common genera include *Mucor*, *Rhizopus*, *Absidia* and *Cunninghamella*. These organisms are angioinvasive, and the disease is characterized by infarct and necrosis. Several classic forms (rhinocerebral, pulmonary, gastrointestinal, primary cutaneous and disseminated) have been described. Surgical resection is frequently the most important part of treatment. High-dose amphotericin B is required.

Fusariosis   Fusariosis is a systemic fungal infection caused by members of the genus *Fusarium*. It usually appears during profound, persistent neutropenia. The disease may be similar to aspergillosis, with pulmonary infiltrates, sinusitis and skin nodules that develop necrosis. Blood cultures are frequently positive. The disease may develop or progress during amphotericin treatment. Successful outcome is usually contingent on neutrophil recovery.

Dematiaceous fungi (*Phaeohyphomycosis*)   These moulds are characterized by a brown to black color in the cell walls of their hyphae and conidia. In the neutropenic or otherwise immunocompromised patient sinusitis, pneumonia and disseminated infection may ensue. The activity of amphotericin against some of these organisms is limited, and itraconazole or voriconazole may be the treatment of choice. *Alternaria, Bipolaris, Cladosporium* and *Wangiella* are some of the genera.

Pulmonary infiltrates in patients with defects in cell-mediated immunity   Defects in cellular immunity are common in patients with lymphoma, and in any patient who has received corticosteroids, fludarabine, anti-TNF therapies and other immunosuppressing agents. Besides the common bacterial pathogens, patients with defects in cell mediated immunity are at risk for infections by *Nocardia*, mycobacteria, fungi, *Pneumocystis carinii* and viruses. A BAL should be obtained with specific requests for acid-fast, modified acid-fast (to detect *Nocardia*), fungal stains, *Pneumocystis* stain and viral culture. A test for *Legionella* antigen in the urine should be obtained.

The empirical antibiotic regimen in this situation typically includes trimethoprim-sulfamethoxazole (for *Pneumocystis*) and a newer quinolone with activity against *Legionella*. Depending on the degree of immunosuppression, the radiologic findings and epidemiological considerations, antiviral and antifungal agents may be added pending the results from the BAL.

***Nocardia* species**   *Nocardia* species are gram-positive branching rods, ubiquitous in the soil. They are opportunistic pathogens particularly in the setting of depressed cellular immunity. Pneumonia is the most common manifestation but the infection is commonly disseminated to the brain and the skin. Formation of suppurative lesions is characteristic. Blood cultures are usually negative. In the lung, a dense lobar infiltrate is more frequent, but multiple pulmonary nodules with or without cavitation are also common. The diagnosis will frequently require bronchoscopy with BAL or fine-needle aspiration.

Identifying the species of Nocardia may be important for treatment purposes, as antibiotic susceptibilities vary. Typically, long-term (6 months to a year) treatment with TMP/SMX, alone or combined with ceftriaxone, is required. Imipenem combined with amikacin has also shown in vivo efficacy. For long-term oral treatment in patients unable to tolerate TMP/SMX, minocycline is recommended. Nocardia infections have occurred despite the use of TMP/SMX prophylaxis for PCP.

Pneumocystis carinii   Molecular taxonomy has shown *Pneumocystis* to be closely related to fungi. The characteristic presentation is subacute with dry cough, fever, dyspnea and hypoxemia. The radiologic picture is usually a diffuse bilateral interstitial infiltrate, but atypical localized forms may be seen. In the HIV-negative patient, BAL is typically required for the diagnosis. Treatment is with high-dose TMP/SMX (TMP 5 mg kg^{-1} q 6 hourly). Prednisone is routinely added if pO$_2$ is <70 mm Hg.

Viral pneumonia

Community-acquired respiratory virus. Community-acquired respiratory virus (RSV, influenza, parainfluenza, adenovirus) can cause pneumonia in the immunocompetent as well as the immunocompromised host. Pneumonia is more common and more severe in the presence of significant defects in cell-mediated immunity, particularly post-allo-HSCT.

Herpesviridae   Herpes simplex, varicella-zoster virus, human herpesvirus 6 (HHV-6) and cytomegalovirus (CMV) can all cause pneumonitis in the immunocompromised patient.

CMV pneumonia   CMV pneumonitis was very common in the allo-HSCT recipient before the use of current prophylactic or pre-emptive strategies. It usually appeared around day 40–60 post-transplant. Now the standard of care to prevent this complication is to either treat all recipients prophylactically until day 100 post-transplant, or to monitor CMV by antigenemia (expression of the viral protein pp65 in white blood cells) or PCR in the blood and treat if there is evidence of reactivation. This pre-emptive strategy is based on the fact that reactivation typically precedes clinical disease by 1–2 weeks. Although occasional cases without prior laboratory evidence of reactivation still occur, they are exceptional. These preventive modalities have resulted in the appearance of "late" CMV pneumonitis. It presents 100 days after the transplant as a diffuse interstitial infiltrate with hypoxemia. Fever may or may not be present. The diagnosis is made by the identification of CMV in the BAL, either by immunostaining, shell vial culture or cytology (cytopathic effect). Although it is usually thought that CMV is only a significant pulmonary pathogen after hematopoietic stem cell transplantation, it is also a cause of pneumonia and ARDS in other immunodeficient states. However, interpretation of a positive CMV culture in the BAL is not clear outside of the allo-HSCT setting. The presence of positive immunostaining or cytopathic effect in the cytologic analysis from the BAL, or a lung biopsy may be required to confirm the diagnosis. Treatment consists of ganciclovir 5 mg kg^{-1} q 12 hourly for 2–3 weeks and IVIG 500 mg kg^{-1} q 48 h for 10 doses. Maintenance suppressive treatment with ganciclovir 5 mg kg^{-1} q 24 hourly for 5 days/week is required afterwards for a variable period.

12.2.4 **Central nervous system infections**

General approach

In the immunocompromised patient it is important to consider early the possibility of CNS infection. The presentation may be atypical, and abnormal mentation is more common than overt meningitis. Mild changes in the level of consciousness, headache or photophobia should be investigated promptly by imaging (preferably MRI) and usually lumbar puncture. The cerebrospinal fluid (CSF) should be sent for routine Gram stain and bacterial culture, cryptococcal antigen, fungal culture and viral PCR.

Intraventricular reservoir infections

Cancer patients may have intraventricular reservoirs that may become infected. Infection of an Ommaya may present with fever, headache and meningismus or may be asymptomatic. The organisms responsible are usually *Propionibacterium acnes*, *Staph epidermidis*, α-hemolytic streptococci and gram-negative bacilli. A trial of antibiotics with the reservoir in place may be attempted. Intraventricular vancomycin (10 mg/24 hours) has been used for susceptible bacteria, although it may not be necessary if there is meningeal inflammation.

Listeriosis

Listeria monocytogenes meningo-encephalitis with or without bacteremia is more frequent in cancer patients, particularly when there are associated defects of cellular immunity. The disease usually presents subacutely with fever and encephalitic changes (headache, confusion, disorientation, memory loss) and, sometimes, focal neurologic signs. Rhomboencephalitis is an uncommon clinicopathological entity in which *Listeria* infects the brainstem. The presentation includes cranial nerve palsies and cerebellar signs. MRI may show brainstem involvement. Although this syndrome may be caused by many other pathogens, it should suggest *Listeria* infection. The CSF in listeriosis may show normal glucose and increased cell number (PMN or mononuclear cells) with gram-positive coccobacilli. Blood cultures are frequently positive even when the CSF culture is not. Ampicillin or penicillin is the treatment of choice, typically in combination with gentamicin. TMP/SMX may be an alternative in the penicillin-allergic patient.

Cryptococcal meningitis

Cryptococcal meningitis should be considered when a defect in cellular immunity is present. AIDS patients are especially at risk, but patients on corticosteroid treatment for lymphoid malignancies are also at risk. The presentation may be subtle with subacute headache, fever and abnormal level of consciousness. India ink preparations of the CSF will commonly be negative; the diagnostic modality of choice is detection of cryptococcal antigen in the CSF.

Brain abscess

Brain abscess infrequently presents with the classic triad of fever, headache and focal neurologic signs. It may occur as a complication of a local infection (sinusitis, otitis media) or as part of systemic dissemination of infection. In the absence of a local focus of infection, fungi (notably *Aspergillus*, but also *Candida*) and *Nocardia* are common causes in the immunocompromised patient. A biopsy and culture is necessary for the diagnosis, but sometimes there will be other lesions outside the CNS more amenable to biopsy.

12.2.5 Soft tissue infections

Skin findings are common in oncology, and they may represent infectious disease emergencies. It has been emphasized that the specificity of skin findings may be less in immunocompromised patients due to the limited ability to mount an inflammatory response. The practical implication is that a skin biopsy should be performed early.

Ecthyma gangrenosum presents typically in neutropenic patients as an erythematous patch or papule that then develops a necrotic center, although it may be quite polymorphic in appearance. It may be single or multiple. It is usually a manifestation of *Pseudomonas aeruginosa* bacteremia, but similar lesions may be seen with other gram-negative bacteremias, as well as with fungal infections (particularly angioinvasive fungi like *Aspergillus* and Zygomycetes). Pathology shows invasion of the blood vessels and ischemic necrosis, very limited inflammation and numerous organisms. Although primary bacteremia with subsequent seeding of the skin may be the most common mechanism, the lesion can also follow local inoculation, with subsequent bacteremia particularly in the neutropenic patient. When such a lesion is observed, antibiotic therapy with optimal coverage of *Pseudomonas* should be started and a biopsy or aspirate of the margin of the lesion should be obtained. This is typically a local manifestation of a systemic problem, and systemic therapy is the most important aspect of management. However, tissue invasion can progress and spread extremely fast in the absence of neutrophils, so early surgical consultation and close monitoring are mandatory.

Perianal cellulitis can develop during the course of neutropenia. Prolonged neutropenia during induction chemotherapy for acute leukemia is the classic setting. Perianal fissures alone are common and respond well to ceftazidime without anaerobic coverage. However, the presence of perianal cellulitis, induration or perirectal involvement warrants anaerobic coverage. Treatment should initially be conservative with antibiotics, stool softeners and sitz baths. In the presence of a perirectal infection, true abscess and unremitting infection, incision and drainage may be required, but ideally, any intervention should be delayed until after resolution of neutropenia.

Cellulitis may be primary when the skin constitutes the portal of entry or secondary to bacteremic spread. In the normal host, 90 percent of cases are caused by *Streptococcus* and *Staphylococcus*. In the patients with cancer gram-negative cellulitis, commonly secondary to hematogenous spread has been well documented. Patients with liver disease are particularly prone to this complication. *E.coli*, and other enterobacteriaceae like *Enterobacter* and *Morganella* are most common. *Stenotrophomonas maltophilia* infection may present with cellulitis and bacteremia. *Helicobacter cinaedi* has been described as a cause of bacteremia, multifocal cellulitis and arthritis in immunocompromised patients, particularly in HIV infection.

Cancer patients appear to be at increased risk for streptococcal toxic shock syndrome and severe soft tissue infections caused by *Streptococcus pyogenes* (Group A *Streptococcus*). The classic presentation includes nonspecific symptoms (malaise, nausea, vomiting) and pain out of proportion to any visible skin abnormality, followed by rapidly progressive necrotizing fasciitis, multiorgan failure and shock. Treatment includes aggressive surgical debridement and antibiotics. Clindamycin or clindamycin plus penicillin G seem to result in a better clinical outcome than penicillin alone. The addition of IVIG ($0.5 \, \text{mg kg}^{-1}$ once) was associated with reduced mortality in a case-control study.

Reactivation of Varicella-Zoster Virus (VZV) in the form of zoster is most common, but multi-dermatomal and disseminated infection is also frequent. Typically, the lesions have vesicles, but the rash may also be maculopapular. Any vesicular rash may be caused by VZV or HSV; confirmatory diagnostic tests should be performed. In the case of VZV, the direct fluorescent assay (DFA) is more sensitive than virus culture, and allows rapid diagnosis. HSV may be diagnosed by shell vial culture in 24–48 hours. Visceral involvement in the organs corresponding to the affected dermatomes has been described. Abdominal pain simulating an acute abdomen has been well documented, as well as hematuria and dysuria. Occasionally visceral involvement may appear in the absence of skin lesions. The treatment of choice for VZV in the immunocompromised patient is IV acyclovir at 10 mg kg^{-1} q 8 hourly. Although oral famciclovir at a dose of 500 mg q 8 hourly has shown to be equally effective for the treatment of VZV in the normal host, there are no studies documenting equivalence in the immunocompromised patient. The high plasma levels achievable with IV acyclovir are not comparably achieved with oral therapy. Treatment prevents dissemination, shortens the duration of the disease and seems to prevent post-herpetic neuralgia.

12.2.6 Intravascular device-associated infections

Catheter-related infections include local infections and bloodstream infections. Recent guidelines by the IDSA, the American College of Critical Care Medicine (for the Society of Critical Care Medicine), and the Society for Healthcare Epidemiology of America attempt to provide definitions. Exit site infections are diagnosed clinically by the presence of erythema, induration and tenderness within 2 cm of the catheter exit site. A tunnel infection is characterized by erythema along the subcutaneous tract of a tunneled (e.g. Hickman or Broviac) catheter that extends beyond 2 cm of the exit site. Blood cultures may be positive or not. A catheter-associated bloodstream infection implies the presence of positive blood cultures.

When a catheter infection is suspected a swab of any exudate should be obtained. The need for antibiotic therapy varies. Site infections usually can be managed with local care and oral antibiotics (typically oxacillin), but if there is significant cellulitis around the catheter IV vancomycin may be necessary. The catheter can usually be kept in place. Tunnel infections typically require removal of the catheter and giving systemic antibiotics. Bloodstream infections require systemic antibiotics, and sometimes catheter removal. The antibiotic coverage should be determined by the results of blood cultures or cultures of the exit site. Since coagulase-negative staphylococci, *Staph. aureus* and *Enterococcus* account for 80 percent of the positive blood cultures, vancomycin is the empirical agent of choice if gram-positive cocci are reported from positive blood cultures. Amongst the gram-negative rods, *Pseudomonas, Stenotrophomonas* and *Acinetobacter* are particularly common. However, a wide variety of low-virulence organisms is able to colonize the catheter and eventually produce clinical infection (Table 12.3).

Table 12.3 Selected emerging microorganisms responsible for infectious diseases in oncology

	Syndrome	Comment	Treatment
Bacteria			
Gram-positive			
Gram-positive cocci			
α-hemolytic streptococcus	Bacteremia and shock	Hematologic malignancy, HSCT	Vancomycin
Stomatococcus mucilaginosus	Bacteremia, meningitis/encephalitis	Hematologic malignancy + neutropenia + mucositis	? Vancomycin +
Leuconostoc	Catheter-associated bacteremia, gastroenteritis, meningitis	Neutropenia, total parenteral nutrition Resistant to vancomycin	Clindamycin
Gram-positive bacilli			
Corynebacterium JK	Catheter-associated bacteremia, sepsis, endocarditis	Sometimes the catheter has to be removed	Vancomycin
Rhodococcus equi	Pneumonia + Brain abscess	Defects in cell-mediated immunity: HIV, lymphoma, leukemia	? Vancomycin + erythromycin
Bacillus	Catheter-associated bacteremia	The catheter should be removed	Vancomycin
Listeria monocytogenes	Bacteremia Meningoencephalitis	Neoplasia, defects in cell-mediated immunity	Ampicillin + gentamicin
Spore-forming gram-positive anaerobes			
Clostridium septicum	Bacteremia/sepsis Necrotizing enterocolitis Distant myonecrosis	Acute leukemia in relapse, colon carcinoma	Penicillin G
Clostridium difficile	Colitis	Antineoplastic agents, antibiotics	Metronidazole Oral vancomycin
Clostridium tertium	Bacteremia (often polymicrobial), diarrhea	Neutropenia + bowel mucosa damage + previous cephalosporins	Vancomycin

Organism	Clinical syndrome	Risk factors/comments	Treatment
Non spore-forming gram-positive anaerobes			
Lactobacillus rhamnosus	Bacteremia	Resistant to vancomycin	Penicillin, Clindamycin
Propionibacterium	Ommaya reservoir infection	Often the reservoir may remain in place	Ampicillin
Gram-negative			
Vibrionacea			
Aeromonas hydrophila	Bacteremia, peritonitis, cellulitis, necrotizing fasciitis	Malignancy, liver disease	Third-generation cephalosporins
Non-fermentative gram-negative bacilli			
Acinetobacter calcoaceticus-baumanii	Catheter-associated bacteremia, Pneumonia	Multiple prior antibiotics Often resistant to imipenem/meropenem	Imipenem/meropenem or ciprofloxacin
Achromobacter (formerly *Alcaligenes*) *xylosoxidans*	Catheter-associated bacteremia		Imipenem/meropenem
Burkholderia cepacia	Catheter-associated bacteremia, cellulitis	Nosocomially acquired	Meropenem, TMP/SMX, fluoroquinolones
Chryseobacterium meningosepticum	Meningitis in neonates Bacteremia, lung infection in adults	Multiple prior antibiotics, neutropenia	Minocyclin, TMP/SMX, ciprofloxacin
Moraxella	Catheter-associated bacteremia		Third-generation cephalosporin
Ralstonia paucula (previously CDC group IV c-2)	Catheter-associated bacteremia, peritonitis	HSCT, acute leukemia Peritoneal dialysis	Third-generation cephalosporins
Sphingomonas paucimobilis	Catheter-associated bacteremia		Ciprofloxacin
Stenotrophomonas maltophilia	Bacteremia with cellulitis, pneumonia	Multiple prior antibiotics	TMP/SMX, ticarcillin-clavulanate

Table 12.3 (continued)

	Syndrome	Comment	Treatment
"Fastidious" gram-negative bacilli			
Capnocytophaga	Bacteremia, septic shock	Neutropenia (± Mucositis)	Clindamycin (increasing frequency of beta-lactamase producers)
Legionella pneumophila, *Legionella micdadei*	Pneumonia	Defects in cell-mediated immunity	Azythromycin, fluoroquinolones
Gram-negative anaerobes			
Fusobacterium nucleatum	Bacteremia, pharyngitis, jugular vein thrombosis with septic pulmonary emboli	Cancer, neutropenia, oral mucositis	Clindamycin, metronidazole
Leptotrichia buccalis	Bacteremia	Cancer, leukemia, mucositis	Penicillin, clindamycin, cephalosporins
Nocardia			
Nocardia asteroides, *Nocardia nova* *Nocardia farcinica*	Pneumonia, brain abscess, skin	Defects in cell-mediated immunity	Sulfonamides (TMP/SMX) imipenem + amikacin
Non-tuberculous mycobacteria *Mycobacterium fortuitum,* *Mycobacterium chelonei,* other	Catheter-associated bacteremia, disseminated infection, pulmonary, subcutaneous nodules	Catheter has to be removed in cases of bacteremia	Treatment varies for different species; it is advisable to obtain I.D. consultation

Fungi
Yeasts

	Disease	Comments	Treatment
Non-albicans Candida			
Candida glabrata	Fungaemia, candiduria, intra-abdominal infections	May be resistant to fluconazole or develop resistance to fluconazole during treatment	Amphotericin B ≥ 0.7 mg/kg/day
Candida krusei	Fungemia	Intrinsically resistant to fluconazole	Amphotericin B ≥ 1.0 mg/kg/day
Candida lusitaniae	Breakthrough fungemia	May be resistant to amphotericin B	Fluconazole 400 mg/day
Trichosporon	Fungemia and funguria, pneumonia, cutaneous lesions, chorioretinitis	Profound neutropenia. Amphotericin B only inhibitory, not fungicidal Fluconazole is more active *in vivo*	Fluconazole + amphotericin B

Moulds

	Disease	Comments	Treatment
Hyaline moulds (Hyalohyphomycosis)			
Non-fumigatus Aspergillus Aspergillus flavus Aspergillus terreus	Pneumonia, sinusitis, CNS, skin disease	*Aspergillus terreus* may be more susceptible to itraconazole than to amphotericin B	Amphotericin B (1–1.5 mg/kg) or Itraconazole
Zygomycetes Mucor, Rhizopus, Rhizomucor, Absidia, Cunninghamella	Pulmonary, rhinocerebral, gastrointestinal, cutaneous	Blood vessel invasion with extensive infarction	Amphotericin B (1–1.5 mg/kg) + surgery
Fusarium	Pneumonia, sinusitis, cutaneous lesions "Black nail"	Blood cultures are frequently positive; often refractory to standard doses of amphotericin B	Amphotericin B (1–1.5 mg/kg)
Dematiaceous moulds (Phaeohyphomycosis)			
Pseudoallescheria boydii	Pulmonary infection, sinusitis, disseminated	Intrinsically resistant to amphotericin B	Itraconazole + amphotericin B
Scedosporium inflatum	Fungemia, CNS, soft tissue	Resistant to all available antifungal agents	? Amphotericin B
Bipolaris	Sinusitis, pneumonia, CNS infection	Blood cultures may be positive	Itraconazole

Indications for long-term indwelling catheter removal

Numerous different recommendations regarding removal of long-term indwelling catheters may be found. The following recommendations are based on the experience at the National Cancer Institute over the last 25 years and are not always in agreement with the IDSA/SCCM guidelines. We usually recommend removal of the catheter in the following situations:

1. The patient does not need the catheter any longer.

2. Tunnel infections.

3. Any pathogen if the blood cultures are persistently positive after 72 hours of adequate antibiotics.

4. Specific pathogens:

    (a) Mycobacteria

    (b) *Candida* infections

    (c) *Staphylococcus aureus*

    (d) Bacillus spp

We have been able to clear infections caused by all other pathogens, including *Corynebacterium jeikeium, Pseudomonas, Stenotrophomonas* and *Acinetobacter*. We routinely administer the antibiotics through the different lumens when a multi-lumen catheter is in place, either splitting the dose or alternating the lumens.

12.2.7 **Gastrointestinal/intra-abdominal infections**

The oncologic patient with fever and abdominal pain is at risk for all common intra-abdominal catastrophes and some others that are unique to the underlying condition. The presence of biliary tract cancer and/or stenting, intestinal obstruction secondary to adhesions or tumor involvement as well as chemotherapy-induced chemotherapy and mucositis put the patient at grave risk.

Mucositis

Chemotherapy-induced mucositis may be complicated by superinfection with herpes simplex (HSV) or *Candida* spp. Viral cultures to rule out herpes should be obtained routinely, as in the presence of chemotherapy or radiation-induced mucositis may not produce typical lesions. Treatment of severe oral herpetic mucositis in the immuno-compromised host consists of IV acyclovir 5 mg kg^{-1}/8 hours. For less severe disease and if the patient can tolerate the oral route valaciclovir 1000 mg q 12 hourly or famci-clovir 250 mg q 12 hourly is adequate. Acyclovir-resistant herpes does occur, particularly in HIV positive patients or after multiple relapses and courses of acyclovir. Large lesions that do not respond to standard doses of acyclovir are suggestive of resistance to the drug. Resistance is caused by mutation of the viral thymidine kinase; the mutation makes the virus resistant to valaciclovir, famciclovir and ganciclovir but not to foscarnet, which becomes the treatment of choice. The fact that a patient is known to harbor acyclovir-resistant virus does not imply that subsequent relapses are caused by the resistant strain. The combination of acyclovir and foscarnet has been shown to be successful in some cases that had shown resistance to both agents.

Esophagitis

Odynophagia and dysphagia may be secondary to herpetic esophagitis instead of, or in addition to, candidiasis and treatment-induced mucositis. The diagnosis requires endoscopy with biopsy, but if this is not feasible due to thrombocytopenia, a therapeutic trial with fluconazole for candidiasis and acyclovir for herpes infection is in order.

Gangrenous cholecystitis

Cholecystitis (some time acalculous), may occur in the immunocompromised patient. Malignant obstruction is a predisposing factor. During neutropenia, the signs and symptoms may be subtle until gangrenous cholecystitis develops. Subsequent invasion of the full thickness of the gallbladder by enteric gram-negative bacilli and other intestinal flora (most characteristically *Clostridium* spp.) may result in gas formation and extension of the necrosis to the abdominal wall (emphysematous cholecystitis). Some cases of gangrenous cholecystitis caused by *Candida* have been reported.

Typhlitis (necrotizing enterocolitis)

This syndrome was described initially in the setting of prolonged neutropenia after induction therapy for acute leukemia, but it may be seen in any neutropenic patient. Abdominal pain starts typically in the right lower quadrant and is accompanied by fever and bloody diarrhea. The most severe form of the disease is characterized by necrotizing inflammation of the cecum caused by aerobic and anaerobic gram-negative rods and *Clostridium*, with *Pseudomonas aeruginosa* and *Clostridium septicum* bacteremia. A whole spectrum of disease probably exists, with less severe forms being more common. The management should be conservative initially, with fluids, hematologic support, and broad-spectrum antibiotics with activity against *Pseudomonas* and anaerobes. Barium enema and endoscopy should be avoided during neutropenia. Abdominal CT or MRI should be performed to monitor for processes that require early intervention to resect necrotic bowel or drain abscesses.

Clostridium difficile-associated colitis

C. difficile is a common pathogen in the hospitalized patient. The use of chemotherapeutic agents and antimicrobials (particularly clindamycin, cephalosporins and imipenem) may be the triggering event. The diarrhea may be non-specific. Leucocytes may not be present in the stool, even if the patient is not neutropenic. The presence of *C. difficile* colitis increases the probability of VRE bacteremia. The diagnosis may be made by detection of toxin in the stool by ELISA or cytotoxicity assay (the gold standard) or by isolation of the microorganism. Treatment is with metronidazole 500 mg q 6 hourly (p.o. or IV) or, in refractory or particularly severe cases, oral vancomycin 125–250 mg q 6 hourly. The association of *C. difficile* colitis with graft-versus-host disease of the bowel carries a mortality up to 70 percent.

Peritonitis

Spontaneous infection of malignant ascites is uncommon. Peritonitis, however, may occur secondary to tumor involvement of the bowel and microperforation. A specific syndrome of clostridial peritonitis and bacteremia with involvement of the abdominal wall has been described.

Hepatosplenic candidiasis

Hepatic or hepatosplenic candidiasis presents during the recovery of neutropenia with spiking fevers and a rise in alkaline phosphatase. Typical bulls-eye lesions in the liver and spleen may be demonstrated by ultrasound or CT scan. A prolonged course of antifungal treatment (fluconazole 400 mg daily in stable patients) is required. Patients may continue to receive chemotherapy, but the antifungal treatment has to be maintained throughout the course of neutropenia.

12.2.8 **Urinary tract infections**

Bacteruria

Bacteruria ($>10^5$ colonies ml^{-1}) in the presence of neutropenia should be treated even in the absence of symptoms. In non-neutropenic patients, asymptomatic bacteruria does not require treatment. The presence of ureteral stents or nephrostomy tubes increases the risk of colonization. Therapy should be administered only for symptomatic episodes, to avoid selection of resistant bacteria.

Candiduria

Candiduria is a common finding in the oncologic patient with an indwelling urinary catheter who is receiving broad-spectrum antibiotics. Candida colonization does not require treatment. Removal of the catheter is frequently sufficient to eliminate the problem. Persistent candiduria may be significant because in the immunocompromised patient it can progress to *Candida* pyelonephritis and systemic dissemination. In addition, candiduria may sometimes be the only manifestation of disseminated candidiasis. If the decision is to treat, Fluconazole 400 mg/day for 1–2 weeks is the treatment of choice for *Candida albicans*. In the case of non-*albicans* candida, amphotericin B is the drug of choice.

12.3 **Antimicrobial toxicity and drug interactions**

12.3.1 **Toxicity**

Some basic knowledge of the toxicity of antimicrobials and the possibility of interactions in complex patients taking multiple drugs is important.

Toxicity plays a significant role in the choice of antimicrobial agent. A brief outline of the more common toxicities of the different classes of agents follows.

Penicillins, cephalosporins and other beta-lactams

The penicillins and cephalosporins have bactericidal effect and have the best efficacy/toxicity profile, and in general should be preferred when available. The most common toxicities are development of drug rash and diarrhea. Between 10 and 20 percent of patients admitted to the hospital will give a history of penicillin allergy. A history of morbilliform (not urticarial!) rash to penicillin or amoxicillin is common; these patients are considered to be at low risk for developing an immediate hypersensitivity reaction when exposed to beta-lactams and can receive these drugs without undergoing testing. If there is a history of anaphylaxis or other manifestations of immediate hypersensitivity the entire class of beta-lactam drugs should be avoided. If there are no alternative agents, skin testing with major and minor determinants of penicillin should be performed. If the skin test is negative, the probability of anaphylaxis is very low. If the skin test is positive, desensitization is required. Imipenem and meropenem can cross-react with penicillins, but the proportion of patients with a self-reported allergy to penicillin who develop a possible reaction with meropenem is only 2–6 percent. Aztreonam (a monobactam) is usually assumed to have no cross-reactivity with beta-lactams, but it does have structural similarities with ceftazidime and cross-reactivity has been shown in vivo. Nevertheless, most studies support the safety of aztreonam in patients with IgE-mediated reaction to penicillins.

Most beta-lactams require dosage-adjustment in the presence of significant renal dysfunction. Ceftriaxone is preferentially eliminated in the bile, and it has been associated with the development of biliary sludge and biliary colic.

All beta-lactams are epileptogenic. Imipenem is the most commonly implicated although seizures are rare when used at 500 mg/6 hours. Meropenem may have less epileptogenic potential than imipenem (it can be used to treat meningitis).

Vancomycin

Vancomycin, in its present purified formulation, is not nephrotoxic. It may, however, potentiate the nephrotoxicity of other drugs that are frequently used at the same time: aminoglycosides, amphotericin, acyclovir, cyclosporin. In the presence of renal insufficiency and the concomitant use of some of these agents, it may be useful to adjust the dosing using peak and trough levels. The standard recommendation is to maintain the trough between 5 and 10 and peak $<40 \mu g \, ml^{-1}$. Routine level determinations and dosing adjustments are not indicated in the absence of renal failure or other potentially nephrotoxic drugs.

The "red man syndrome" is a non-immunologically mediated histamine release seen with rapid infusion of vancomycin and characterized by flushing and pruritus in the face and trunk, and occasionally angioedema and hypotension. Management consists of lengthening the duration of the infusion to two hours and premedicating with antihistamines.

Aminoglycosides

Aminoglycosides are associated with a significant risk of nephrotoxicity and ototoxicity particularly in the elderly, with preexisting renal insufficiency, hypotension, concomitant use of other nephrotoxic drugs or ototoxic drugs (for instance, frusemide) and prolonged courses. Once-daily dosing is associated with less nephrotoxicity without loss of efficacy even in the neutropenic patient. The effect of extended-interval dosing in ototoxicity is less clear, and there are data that suggest increased ototoxicity. Aminoglycosides should never be used as monotherapy, as resistance develops quickly. Differences in toxicity are not well established between the different drugs in this class, and institution-specific susceptibility data should play the main role in the selection.

Fluoroquinolones

Ciprofloxacin, levofloxacin, moxifloxacin and gatifloxacin are generally safe. Neurotoxicity has been an issue with ciprofloxacin, particularly in the elderly patient with other conditions that may predispose to seizures. The hepatotoxicity of trovafloxacin, albeit extremely rare, has all but eliminated the use of this drug.

Metronidazole

Common metronidazole toxicities include a disulfiram effect, dysgeusia, neuropathy and seizures.

Clindamycin

Clindamycin is associated with a high risk of pseudomembranous colitis.

Quinupristin-dalfopristin

Quinupristin-dalfopristin (Synercid) main toxicity is phlebitis that frequently requires administration through a central venous line. Common side effects include myalgia and arthralgia.

Linezolid

Linezolid belongs to a new class of antimicrobials, the oxazolidinones. Clinical experience is limited, but leukopenia and thrombocytopenia may occur frequently when the drug is used for more than 2 weeks.

Amphotericin B

Amphotericin B deoxycholate is associated with a predictable plethora of toxicities. Infusion-related toxicities include chills, fever, nausea and vomiting. Hypotension and hypertensive reactions have been described. In most instances, these effects may be minimized by the judicious use of antihistamines and acetaminophen before the infusion. Chills may be treated with meperidine.

Amphotericin B causes nephrotoxicity directly by its effects on the proximal and distal tubules and indirectly by reducing renal blood flow. Either mechanism may result in additive or synergistic toxicity in combination with other drugs. Nephrotoxicity may be prevented by salt loading (administered as normal saline before and after amphotericin). The action of amphotericin in the kidney consistently produces potassium and magnesium wasting, increasing the risk of toxicity with other drugs like diuretics or cyclosporin A.

The lipid formulations of amphotericin B have shown to be less nephrotoxic. A randomized controlled trial has shown that liposomal amphotericin B is associated with less infusion-related toxicity and less nephrotoxicity than amphotericin B lipid complex with similar efficacy. However, an infusion reaction characterized by decreased oxygen saturation and back pain during the infusion seems to be characteristic of the liposomal form. This reaction can be prevented by the use of diphenhydramine before the infusion.

The best strategy for the use of amphotericin B lipid formulations with optimal efficacy and minimal toxicity at a reasonable cost remains to be defined. Amphotericin B-related toxicity can be minimized by the judicious use of premedication and salt loading, and it develops over several days. For stable patients without other risk factors for nephrotoxicity we favor using conventional amphotericin B as a first-line choice and switching to the lipid formulation only in cases of treatment failure or development of nephrotoxicity. If the risk of nephrotoxicity is high (previous renal dysfunction, concomitant use of other nephrotoxic agents such as aminoglycosides, cyclosporin or cisplatinum) we start with lipid formulations.

12.3.2 Interactions

Additive nephrotoxicity

Several antimicrobial agents may result in additive nephrotoxicity when used with other drugs. Cisplatinum and ifosfamide cause irreversible renal dysfunction in a significant proportion of patients and will render the kidneys more susceptible to subsequent drug-related injuries. Extreme caution should be exercised when administering nephrotoxic antimicrobials to patients who have received these agents.

In the case of HSCT patients, the presence of cyclosporin A or tacrolimus potentiates the toxicity of amphotericin B and aminoglycosides. Acyclovir may also be nephrotoxic in high doses, and some patients may require foscarnet for treatment of CMV. This is the kind of situation where vancomycin may contribute to worsening renal function. In these patients, it is common to use lipid formulations if amphotericin B is required. The list of medications should be reviewed daily and the doses adjusted according to the estimated creatinine clearance. Cyclosporin levels should be monitored routinely every 48–72 hours. If aminoglycosides are required, once-daily dosing should be used.

Other drug–drug interactions

Two drug classes have enough interactions to double-check the medication list before prescribing them: the azoles and the fluoroquinolones.

Systemic azoles   Fluconazole and itraconazole may cause interactions by several mechanisms. Itraconazole absorption is pH-dependent. Consequently, anti-H_2 agents and proton pump inhibitors will decrease its absorption. To optimize absorption, itraconazole capsules should be taken with meals. Conversely, itraconazole oral solution should be taken on an empty stomach.

Both itraconazole and fluconazole are substrates and inhibitors of cytochrome P-450 (CYP) isoforms, which are important in the metabolism of many drugs. By inhibition of CYP3A4, itraconazole will cause increased levels of cyclosporin, tacrolimus, methylprednisolone, busulfan, and many benzodiazepines, dihydropiridine calcium channel blockers, warfarin and HMG-CoA reductase inhibitors. All these interactions have been clinically significant. On the other hand, inducers of CYP3A4 (phenytoin, carbamazepine) will counteract this effect and will decrease the levels of itraconazole. Itraconazole has caused digoxin toxicity by inhibition of digoxin tubular secretion in the kidney. The combination of vinca alkaloids and itraconazole may lead to acute autonomic neuropathy including hypotension and respiratory arrest.

Fluconazole absorption is not pH-dependent, and its effect on the P-450 system in the liver may be less than itraconazole. However, the interactions with benzodiazepines, cyclosporin and warfarin remain significant. Fluconazole increases the level of phenytoin. Rifampin may increase fluconazole metabolism enough to cause sub-therapeutic levels of the antifungal; the dose of fluconazole should be increased.

Fluoroquinolones   Antacids inhibit the absorption of all quinolones, but other interactions differ for different members of the family. Some of them have been associated with prolonged Q–T interval (moxifloxacin, sparfloxacin). Most quinolones increase the levels of cyclosporin and theophylline and may increase the prothrombin time of patients on warfarin. Ciprofloxacin increases the risk of seizures with foscarnet and may interact in variable ways with phenytoin (levels should be measured).

Suggested reading

Bodey, G.P. (2000) Management of persistent fever in the neutropenic patient. *Am J Med*, **108**, 343–5.

Bodey, G.P., Rodriguez, S., Fainstein, V., and Elting, L.S. (1991) Clostridial bacteremia in cancer patients. A 12-year experience. *Cancer*, **67**, 1928–42.

Cagnoni, P.J., Walsh, T.J., Prendergast, M.M., Bodensteiner, D., Hiemenz, S., Greenberg, R.N., Arndt, C.A., Schuster, M., Seibel, N., Yeldandi, V., and Tong, K.B. (2000) Pharmacoeconomic analysis of liposomal amphotericin B versus conventional amphotericin B in the empirical treatment of persistently febrile neutropenic patients. *J Clin Oncol*, **18**, 2476–83.

Chatzinikolaou, I., Abi-Said, D., Bodey, G.P., Rolston, K.V., Tarrand, J.J., and Samonis, G. (2000) Recent experience with Pseudomonas aeruginosa bacteremia in patients with cancer: Retrospective analysis of 245 episodes. *Arch Intern Med*, **160**, 501–9.

Chernik, N.L., Armstrong, D., and Posner, J.B. (1977) Central nervous system infections in patients with cancer. Changing patterns. *Cancer*, **40**, 268–74.

Elting, L.S., Bodey, G.P., and Keefe, B.H. (1992) Septicemia and shock syndrome due to viridans streptococci: a case-control study of predisposing factors. *Clin Infect Dis*, **14**, 1201–7.

EORTC International Antimicrobial Therapy Cooperative Group (1989) Empiric antifungal therapy in febrile granulocytopenic patients. *Am J Med*, **86**, 668–72.

Gomez, L., Martino, R., and Rolston, K.V. (1998) Neutropenic enterocolitis: spectrum of the disease and comparison of definite and possible cases. *Clin Infect Dis*, 27, 695–9.

Gopal, A.K., Fowler, V.G. Jr., Shah, M., Gesty-Palmer, D., Marr, K.A., McClelland, R.S., Kong, L.K., Gottlieb, G.S., Lanclos, K., and Li, J., Sexton, D.J., and Corey, G.R. (2000) Prospective analysis of Staphylococcus aureus bacteremia in nonneutropenic adults with malignancy. *J Clin Oncol*, 18, 1110–5.

Hughes, W.T., Armstrong, D., Bodey, G.P., Brown, A.E., Edwards, J.E., Feld, R., Pizzo, P., Rolston, K.V., Shenep, J.L., and Young, L.S. (1997) 1997 guidelines for the use of antimicrobial agents in neutropenic patients with unexplained fever. Infectious Diseases Society of America. *Clin Infect Dis*, 25, 551–73.

Klastersky, J., Paesmans, M., Rubenstein, E.B., Boyer, M., Elting, L., Feld, R., Gallagher, J., Herrstedt, J., Rapoport, B., Rolston, K., and Talcott, J. (2000) The Multinational Association for Supportive Care in Cancer risk index: A multinational scoring system for identifying low-risk febrile neutropenic cancer patients. *J Clin Oncol*, 18, 3038–51.

Marron, A., Carratala, J., Gonzalez-Barca, E., Fernandez-Sevilla, A., Alcaide, F., and Gudiol, F. (2000) Serious complications of bacteremia caused by Viridans streptococci in neutropenic patients with cancer. *Clin Infect Dis*, 31, 1126–30.

Mermel, L.A., Farr, B.M., Sherertz, R.J., Raad, I.I., O'Grady, N., Harris, J.S., and Craven, D.E. (2001) Guidelines for the Management of Intravascular Catheter-Related Infections. *Clin Infect Dis*, 32, 1249–72.

Murray, B.E. (2000) Vancomycin-resistant enterococcal infections. *N Engl J Med*, 342, 710–21.

Nelson, R.R. (1999) Intrinsically vancomycin-resistant gram-positive organisms: clinical relevance and implications for infection control. *J Hosp Infect*, 42, 275–82.

Pizzo, P.A., Hathorn, J.W., Hiemenz, J., Browne, M., Commers, J., Cotton, D., Gress, J., Longo, D., Marshall, D., McKnight, J., *et al.* (1986) A randomized trial comparing ceftazidime alone with combination antibiotic therapy in cancer patients with fever and neutropenia. *N Engl J Med*, 315, 552–8.

Pizzo, P.A., Robichaud, K.J., Gill, F.A., and Witebsky, F.G. (1982) Empiric antibiotic and antifungal therapy for cancer patients with prolonged fever and granulocytopenia. *Am J Med*, 72, 101–11.

Rex, J.H., Walsh, T.J., Sobel, J.D., Filler, S.G., Pappas, P.G., Dismukes, W.E., and Edwards, J.E. (2000) Practice guidelines for the treatment of candidiasis. Infectious Diseases Society of America. *Clin Infect Dis*, 30, 662–78.

Stevens, D.A., Kan, V.L., Judson, M.A., Morrison, V.A., Dummer, S., Denning, D.W., Bennett, J.E., Walsh, T.J., Patterson, T.F., and Pankey, G.A. (2000) Practice guidelines for diseases caused by Aspergillus. Infectious Diseases Society of America. *Clin Infect Dis*, 30, 696–709.

Walsh, T.J., Finberg, R.W., Arndt, C., Hiemenz, J., Schwartz, C., Bodensteiner, D., Pappas, P., Seibel, N., Greenberg, R.N., Dummer, S., Schuster, M., and Holcenberg, J.S. (1999) Liposomal amphotericin B for empirical therapy in patients with persistent fever and neutropenia. National Institute of Allergy and Infectious Diseases Mycoses Study Group. *N Engl J Med*, 340, 764–71.

Wolfson, J.S., Sober, A.J., and Rubin, R.H. (1985) Dermatologic manifestations of infections in immunocompromised patients. *Medicine* (Baltimore), 64, 115–33.

Chapter 13

Hematologic Emergencies

Niamh O'Connell and Shaun R. McCann

13.1 Introduction

Many advances and new treatments are becoming available for patients with cancer. Hematologic complications in cancer patients are most often due to the therapy administered and occasionally due to the malignancy itself. This chapter suggests guidelines to the management of these problems in patients undergoing treatment for cancer.

13.2 Thrombocytopenia

Thrombocytopenia (a platelet count $<150 \times 10^9 \, l^{-1}$), is most commonly encountered in oncology as a result of treatment of the patient's underlying disease, that is, it is a reflection of myelotoxicity secondary to chemotherapy or much less frequently, radiotherapy. Thrombocytopenia may also be seen in association with disseminated intravascular coagulation (DIC) or with bone marrow metastases. In addition, certain malignant conditions are associated with immune-mediated thrombocytopenia. The degree of thrombocytopenia is the primary determinant of the investigations and interventions, which are indicated, but other factors such as active bleeding, anemia, concurrent medications and the type and site of the tumor need to be considered. Multiple causes of thrombocytopenia may co-exist in a given patient.

13.2.1 Treatment-related thrombocytopenia

In the majority of cases the chemotherapy, which has been administered to the patient, will cause myelosuppression and result in thrombocytopenia. In these instances neutropenia almost invariably accompanies the low platelet count. The interval from the time of administration until the onset of thrombocytopenia is usually seven to ten days and the degree of thrombocytopenia will reflect the dose of the chemotherapeutic agent given. Other factors such as the number of courses of myelosuppressive agents previously administered and the interval between them may also influence the degree of thrombocytopenia as will pelvic radiotherapy. Certain chemotherapeutic agents invariably produce thrombocytopenia (Table 13.1). Drugs such as BCNU may produce a delayed second fall in the platelet count at 6 weeks and this may overlap with the

Table 13.1 Chemotherapeutic agents commonly causing thrombocytopenia

Drugs causing thrombocytopenia in a dose-dependent manner	
Alkylating agents	
Mustards	Chlorambucil
	Melphalan
	Cyclophosphamide
	Ifosfamide
	Busulphan
	Metchlorethamine
Nitrosoureas	BCNU
	CCNU
Tetrazines	Dacarbazine
Aziridines	Thiotepa
	Mitomycin C
Antimetabolites	Methotrexate
	Cytarabine
	Gemcitabine
	5 azacytidine
	6 thiopurines
	Hydroxyurea
	5 Fluorouracil (bolus dosing)
Topoisomerase interactive agents	Epipodophyllotoxins
	Topotecan
	Anthracyclines
Miscellaneous	Carboplatin
	Vinblastine (but not vincristine)
	Procarbazine
	Fludarabine
	Cladribine (2CDA)
Drugs causing delayed thrombocytopenia	
Nitrosoureas (BCNU, CCNU)	Thrombocytopenia occurs 3–6 weeks post drug administration
Drugs causing idiosyncratic thrombocytopenia	
Busulphan	Idiosyncratic bone marrow hypoplasia Recovery often prolonged

myelosuppression of the next course of treatment. For this reason the interval between treatments with BCNU is usually 6 weeks. Therefore, knowledge of the type, dose and timing of the chemotherapy and its potential to cause a low platelet count is essential when evaluating a patient with thrombocytopenia. If the degree of thrombocytopenia occurs more rapidly or is more severe or more prolonged than anticipated, then a second mechanism should be suspected and the dose of the chemotherapeutic agent given should be checked.

13.2.2 **Cancer-related thrombocytopenia**

Bone marrow metastases

The presence of bone marrow metastases should be suspected if anemia or thrombo-cytopenia is observed prior to treatment or if chemotherapy induces a sudden or excessive fall in the hemoglobin or platelet count (Fig. 13.1). A leukoerythroblastic blood film, if present, should also alert the clinician to the possibility of bony metastases. Table 13.2 lists

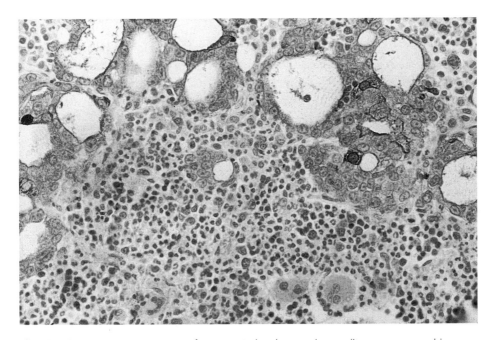

Fig. 13.1 Bone marrow metastases from prostatic adenocarcinoma (bone marrowrephine biopsy, x 40, H and E).

Table 13.2 Cancers which commonly metastasize to bone marrow

Breast
Lung
Prostate
Thyroid
Kidney
Bladder
Endometrial
Cervical
Pancreatic

Note: Breast, lung and prostate cancer account for 50 percent.

tumors which commonly metastasize to bone. In many cases occult bone marrow metastases may be present without clinical symptoms or abnormalities in the full blood count.

13.2.3 Immune-mediated thrombocytopenia

Immune-mediated destruction of platelets may occur as the sole mechanism causing thrombocytopenia or may co-exist with other mechanisms, such as myelosuppression following chemotherapy. As a general rule patients with autoimmune thrombocytopenia experience less bleeding for a given platelet count when compared to patients whose thrombocytopenia is secondary to chemotherapy or other mechanisms which cause bone marrow failure. Autoimmune thrombocytopenia may occur in association with autoimmune hemolytic anemia (Evans' syndrome) and in this case will be accompanied by a positive direct antiglobulin test (Coombs' test). Table 13.3 provides a list of malignant diseases associated with immune-mediated platelet destruction.

13.2.4 Disseminated intravascular coagulation (DIC)

Thrombocytopenia may accompany a clinical or subclinical DIC. Investigation and management of this condition are discussed.

Assessment of patient

Three key questions are vital in determining the management of the thrombocytopenic patient.

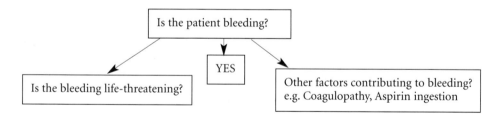

Table 13.3 Malignant diseases which are associated with autoimmune thrombocytopenia

Chronic lymphocytic leukemia
Non-Hodgkin's lymphoma
Hodgkin's disease
Lung cancer
Breast cancer
Gastrointestinal cancer

Immune-mediated platelet destruction is much more commonly seen with lymphoid malignancies than solid tumors.

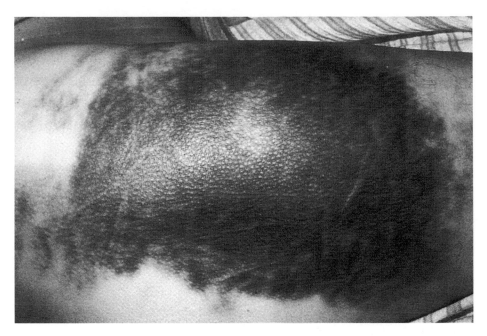

Fig. 13.2 Massive thigh haematoma secondary to an intra muscular injection in a patient with thrombocytopenia and DIC.

Note that massive bleeding may occur in response to minor trauma, for example, intramuscular injection in patients who have thrombocytopenia and/or DIC (Fig. 13.2).

Clinical assessment:

1. Full clinical examination including examination of the fundi for retinal hemorrhage and blood pressure (hypertension in association with severe thrombocytopenia may predispose to intracerebral hemorrhage).

2. A history of the type of tumor, prior chemotherapy, blood and platelet counts before treatment.

3. A history of ingestion of other drugs such as aspirin, non-steroidal anti-inflammatory drugs and anticoagulants is relevant as these agents will enhance bleeding and this may prompt action at a higher platelet count.

Laboratory investigations:

1. Blood film examination to assess platelet numbers. In addition, the presence of schistocytes (red blood cell fragments) may indicate concurrent DIC (Fig. 13.3).

2. Full blood count. Comparison of the present and pre-treatment haemoglobin may indicate if significant blood loss has occurred. Note that patients with a low hemoglobin are more likely to bleed for a given platelet count.

3. Coagulation screen to include PT, APPT, Fibrinogen and D-Dimers.

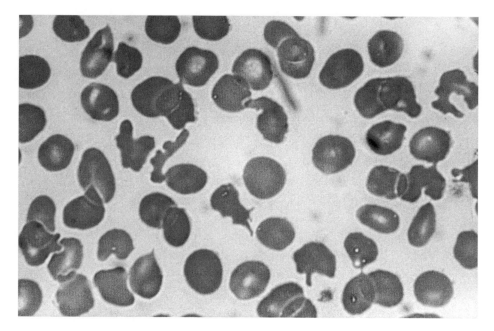

Fig. 13.3 Blood film demonstrating schistocytes secondary to DIC.

If there is no obvious relationship between platelet count and administration of chemotherapy or the presence of DIC then other mechanisms should be suspected and a bone marrow aspirate and trephine examination may be indicated. In immune-mediated thrombocytopenia, plentiful megakaryocytes are expected since platelet destruction occurs in the peripheral circulation. If bone marrow metastases are the primary mechanism of thrombocytopenia, the bone marrow trephine is the most sensitive diagnostic tool (Fig. 13.1).

Action based on assessment

An algorithm for the management of thrombocytopenia is shown in Fig. 13.4.

Observation alone

Patients who have a platelet count of $>10 \times 10^9\,1^{-1}$ and who are not bleeding may be managed conservatively, provided that they have a full clinical examination daily including fundal examination. If the patient is clinically stable, not bleeding and has no evidence of sepsis or coagulopathy, with a hemoglobin $>8\,g\,dl^{-1}$, then observation is adequate.

Platelet transfusion

If the platelet count is $<10 \times 10^9\,1^{-1}$ or the patient is bleeding (e.g. mucosal bleeding, petechiae) give random donor platelets. Each five donor units or one single donor

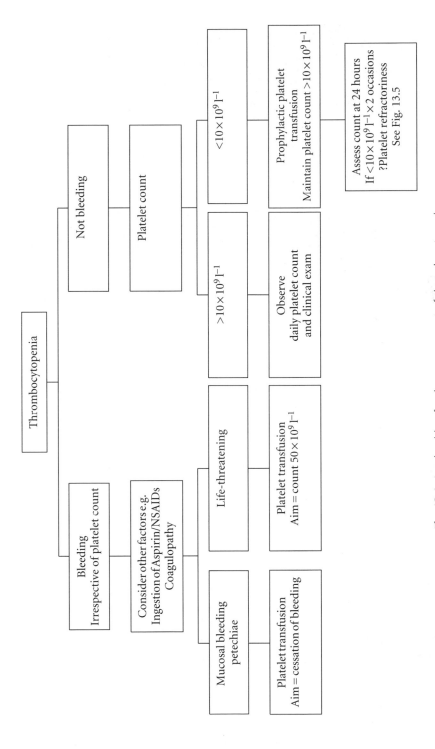

Fig. 13.4 An algorithm for the management of thrombocytopenia.

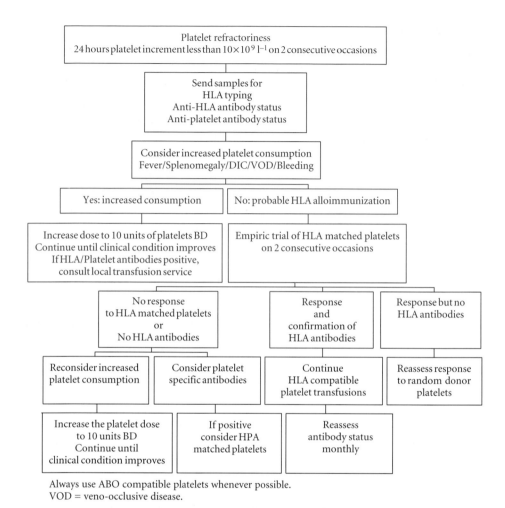

Fig. 13.5 An algorithm for the management of platelet refractoriness.

apheresis pack should raise the platelet count by approximately $10 \times 10^9 1^{-1}$ at 24 hours post-transfusion. If bleeding is life-threatening, increase the platelet count to $50 \times 10^9 1^{-1}$. If bleeding is not life-threatening, a platelet count of $>10 \times 10^9 1^{-1}$ will suffice. Remember the key end point is arresting the bleeding and this may occur without a significant platelet rise. However, failure to obtain the expected platelet rise after two consecutive transfusions (platelet refractoriness) may be due to conditions which cause increased platelet consumption (e.g. fever, splenomegaly) or may be related to human leukocyte antigen (HLA) alloimmunization from previous transfusions or pregnancies. An algorithm for the management of platelet refractoriness is given in Fig. 13.5.

Red cell transfusion

If the hemoglobin is $<8 \, g \, dl^{-1}$ transfuse with two units of packed RBCs.

Cytokine therapy

Thrombopoietin is a cytokine which increases platelet production from megakaryocytes in the bone marrow. Two forms of recombinant human thrombopoietin have been developed, a full length molecule rhTPO and a truncated molecule, rHuMGDF (recombinant human megakaryocyte growth and development factor). It was hoped that these agents would decrease the thrombocytopenia caused by chemotherapy, thereby decrease bleeding and the requirement for platelet transfusions. Early results showed that rHuMGDF could produce severe thrombocytopenia and it is currently not available for clinical use in the setting of chemotherapy-induced thrombocytopenia. rhTPO is well tolerated and does produce dose dependent increases in the platelet count thus attenuating chemotherapy-induced thrombocytopenia and reducing the need for platelet transfusions. Recombinant Interleukin 11 has also been evaluated in randomized controlled trials and has received FDA approval for the prevention of severe chemotherapy-induced thrombocytopenia at a dose of $50\,\mu g\,kg^{-1}$ s.c. daily starting the day after chemotherapy ends until the platelet count is $>50 \times 10^9\,l^{-1}$ and the expected nadir has passed.

Irradiated blood products

Irradiated blood products should be given if the patient has received a peripheral stem cell (PBSC) or bone marrow allograft or autograft, has Hodgkin's disease or has received purine analogues due to the risk of transfusion associated graft-versus-host disease in these conditions.

Coagulopathy

Coagulopathy is usually seen in the context of sepsis or "tumor lysis syndrome".

Depending on the patient's age and circulatory status, correct the coagulopathy with FFP and fibrinogen concentrate or cryoprecipitate (see section on the management of DIC).

Concurrent sepsis

This should be suspected in a neutropenic patient in the presence of coagulopathy and broad spectrum antibiotics should be commenced, for example, gentamicin and piperacillin/tazobactem (substitute a quinolone for gentamicin if there is renal impairment). If the patient has an indwelling right atrial catheter consider gram positive sepsis and teicoplanin or vancomycin may be appropriate.

Repeated clinical evaluation following support care is vital, that is has the bleeding stopped, is sepsis resolving? If thrombocytopenia is primarily due to chemotherapy, then platelet support will be required until bone marrow function recovers. Consider other mechanisms of thrombocytopenia if the platelet count does not recover when expected.

13.3 **Thrombocytosis**

13.3.1 **Cancer-related thrombocytosis**

A high platelet count ($>450 \times 10^9\,l^{-1}$) may be found in association with occult malignancy and may precede the diagnosis or may be present with well-established disease.

Tumors which metastasize to bone are more commonly associated with high platelet counts. Patients who have had a prior splenectomy will have a higher baseline platelet count and this may enhance the elevated platelet count in association with malignancy.

The clinical implications of an elevated platelet count in association with malignancy are controversial and definitive data on the risks of adverse events secondary to thrombocytosis in these patients are lacking. The probability of a thrombotic event is related to the patient's age and other risk factors for arterial and venous thrombosis, such as atherosclerosis, cardiac arrhythmias or local venous stasis. Older patients with pre-existing risk factors, therefore, warrant intervention at a lower absolute platelet count while high platelet counts are less likely to be associated with morbidity in younger patients. Thrombocytosis has been shown to be an adverse prognostic factor in a number of malignant conditions, including locally advanced cervical carcinoma, renal cell carcinoma and primary lung carcinoma but not vulval carcinoma. Data on the prognostic significance of thrombocytosis in ovarian carcinoma are conflicting.

The possibility of an underlying myeloproliferative disorder should also be considered as this may co-exist with malignancy. Examination of the blood film and a bone marrow aspirate and biopsy with cytogenetic analysis are required to rule out these conditions.

13.3.2 Therapeutic options

An algorithm for the management of thrombocytosis may be found in Fig. 13.6.

The optimal therapy to normalize the platelet count is to treat the underlying disease. In many cases, however, a complete response of the malignancy to therapy may be delayed or may not be possible. In these situations, the decision to treat a patient with an elevated platelet count will depend not only on the absolute platelet count but also on the presence or absence of risk factors for arterial or venous thrombosis and any prior history of thrombosis. Recommendations on the absolute platelet count, at which to treat, and the type of treatment, derive mainly from studies of patients with myeloproliferative disorders. In a randomized study by Cortelazzo in 1995, of high risk patients with essential thrombocythemia who had a median platelet count of $788 \times 10^9 \, l^{-1}$, 85 percent of whom were aged >60 years, and 46 percent of whom had a history of previous thrombosis, control of the platelet count to $<600 \times 10^9 \, l^{-1,}$ reduced the incidence of thrombotic events from 24 percent (untreated group) to 3.6 percent (group treated with hydroxyurea). In an analysis of 129 patients by Buss in 1985, with both myeloproliferative and reactive thrombocytosis, thrombotic events occurred with equal frequencies in both groups. In general, a platelet count of $>1000 \times 10^9 \, l^{-1}$, in addition to other risk factors for thrombosis warrants intervention.

13.3.3 Platelet lowering agents

Drugs which are commonly used to control the platelet count in myeloproliferative disorders are hydroxyurea and anagrelide. Note that hydroxyurea can cause profound

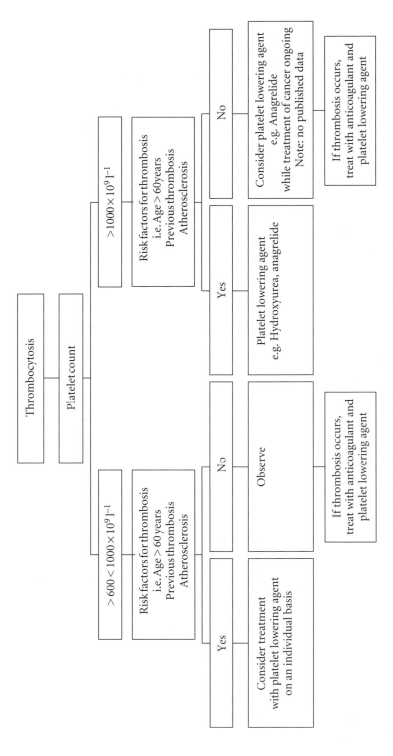

Fig. 13.6 An algorithm for the management of thrombocytosis.

myelosuppression in a dose-related manner and in the elderly, can also result in a precipitous fall in blood counts. Therefore, monitoring of the full blood count, fortnightly initially and monthly thereafter is mandatory. It should be noted that hydroxyurea causes a marked elevation in the mean cell volume (MCV) which is not clinically significant. Anagrelide is a selective platelet lowering agent and therefore will not cause pancytopenia but it has positive inotropic and vasodilatory properties. The most common adverse effects are palpitations and fluid retention. Anagrelide is contra-indicated in patients with known or suspected cardiac disease.

Platelet lowering agents	Suggested doses
Hydroxyurea	Initiate treatment with 15 mg kg/day Titrate to maintain platelet count $<600 \times 10^9 \, l^{-1}$
Anagrelide	Initiate treatment with 0.5 mg QDS daily
	Increase by 0.5 mg per day every 7 days as tolerated until platelet count $<600 \times 10^9 \, l^{-1}$

Platelet pheresis is a useful temporary measure to reduce the platelet count acutely if there are symptoms of impending serious thrombosis such as a transient ischaemic attacks. The use of aspirin is controversial. In myeloproliferative disorders, a platelet function defect exists in addition to an increase in absolute platelet numbers. Excess bleeding episodes can occur with aspirin therapy, especially if the platelet count is not controlled. Similar data are not available on the risks of bleeding or the prevention of thrombosis associated with the use of aspirin in the patient with malignancy and thrombocytosis. It is prudent to use aspirin only in those patients whose platelet count is $<1000 \times 10^9 \, l^{-1}$ and who do not have other risk factors for bleeding.

13.4 Disseminated intravascular coagulation (DIC)

Disseminated intravascular coagulation is a clinical syndrome characterized by systemic activation of coagulation leading to intravascular deposition of fibrin and thrombosis of small and medium sized vessels. Depletion of natural anticoagulants such as protein C and antithrombin and suppression of fibrinolysis also add to the pro-thrombotic state. In addition, there may be consumption of multiple coagulation factors and platelets leading to bleeding. The delicate balance between factors which promote thrombosis and factors which lead to bleeding will determine the clinical presentation of the patient.

13.4.1 Cancer-related DIC

Clinical evidence of DIC is seen in 10–15 percent of patients with disseminated cancer. Laboratory markers of activation are found in 50–70 percent of patients with cancer and include increased levels of fibrinogen, fibrin degradation products and coagulation factors V, VIII, IX and XI. More specialized tests of coagulation activation such as fibrinopeptide A, prothrombin activation fragments 1+2 and thrombin–antithrombin complexes are also elevated. Certain malignant conditions such as mucin-secreting adenocarcinomas are particularly associated with DIC. However, many tumors express molecules such as tissue factor or cancer procoagulant which initiate the coagulation cascade by activating factors VII and X respectively.

The clinical outcome depends on the degree of activation of the coagulation system and on compensatory activation of the fibrinolytic pathway. In the majority of patients, laboratory evidence of coagulopathy is not associated with clinical symptoms. If clinical symptoms exist, thrombosis or hemorrhage may occur depending on the balance between prothrombotic and antithrombotic factors.

Thrombotic events in the arterial or venous system may be a manifestation of an occult carcinoma. High levels of fibrinogen and factor VIII are associated with thrombosis even in the non-malignant state and are often elevated as an acute phase response to underlying malignancy. In these cases the coagulation times (PT, APTT) may be shorter than normal due mainly to elevated levels of factor VIII and fibrinogen. Trousseau's syndrome is a recurrent, migratory thrombophlebitis originally described in association with gastric carcinoma. This classical manifestation of occult malignancy is most commonly associated with carcinoma of the pancreas but it may also be seen with other adenocarcinomas such as lung, prostate and stomach.

In other patients, depletion of multiple coagulation factors including fibrinogen and factor VIII occurs and leads to bleeding. Platelet numbers are decreased because of "consumption" and platelet function is abnormal due to adverse interactions with FDPs. This results in diffuse bleeding with prolonged coagulation time and a low platelet count. The fibrinogen is often low but may be normal since the baseline fibrinogen is elevated in patients with cancer. Therefore, a "normal" fibrinogen does not rule out DIC.

13.4.2 **Treatment-related DIC**

As has been stated, many patients with cancer have an activated coagulation and fibrinolytic system without clinical signs. In certain situations treatment of the underlying cancer, usually when the treatment results in significant lysis of tumor cells, shifts the delicate balance rapidly in favor of fibrinolysis. Sepsis may also be present in these critically ill patients, especially if they are neutropenic and this contributes to the DIC. The bleeding is often diffuse and the first clue is commonly bleeding at venepuncture sites or at the exit site of indwelling right atrial catheters.

Investigation of a patient suspected of having a DIC

Clinical examination:

1. Clinical examination including fundoscopy to check for retinal hemorrhage.
2. Look specifically for evidence of thrombosis or bleeding, that is, inspect upper and lower limbs for edema or tenderness. Loss of the normal concavity in the supra-clavicular fossa may indicate a subclavian vein thrombus. Inspect venepuncture or marrow aspiration sites and indwelling catheter exit sites for bleeding.

Laboratory investigation:

1. Full blood count to include platelet count and examination of a blood film.
2. Coagulation screen to include PT, APPT, D-dimers and fibrinogen.

13.4.3 Diagnosis of DIC

There is no single diagnostic test for DIC. The presence of a prolonged PT and APTT with elevated levels of D-dimers and a low or low-normal fibrinogen in a clinical setting known to be associated with DIC will confirm the diagnosis in a bleeding patient. A blood film may show fragmented red blood cells (Fig. 13.3). Patients with thrombosis may have a shortened PT and APTT, a high or high-normal fibrinogen and elevated D-dimers. All features may not be present in every patient.

Serial tests are required to monitor progression of the condition and response to therapy and to direct further treatment.

13.4.4 Treatment of DIC

An algorithm for the treatment of DIC is given in Fig. 13.7.

The essence of action is supportive care. Removal of the underlying precipitant is advised. Therefore, the tumor should be treated where possible and if concomitant sepsis is present, it should be managed aggressively.

13.4.5 The bleeding patient

Platelet transfusion

Random donor platelets should be given until the platelet count is $>20 \times 10^9 \, l^{-1}$ or until bleeding has stopped. If bleeding is life-threatening then raise the platelet count to $50 \times 10^9 \, l^{-1}$.

13.4.6 Coagulation factor replacement

Fresh frozen plasma (FFP) contains all coagulation factors including fibrinogen and von Willebrand's factor. The usual dose is 12–15 mls kg^{-1} and it is indicated in patients who are bleeding with a prolonged PT and APTT. It should correct multiple factor deficiencies. Solvent detergent treated (SD) FFP which is virally inactivated has been developed and where available, its use is preferable to non-virally inactivated FFP. There are a number of problems associated with the use of FFP. Large volumes may be needed to correct the PT and APTT which may lead to fluid overload. FFP is unlikely to fully correct the PT and APTT in severely deficient patients since the maximum coagulation factor level after FFP is approximately 20 percent of normal in these patients. A common cause of fluid overload is excessively fast rates of infusion of FFP. Table 13.4 gives suggested rates of infusion for FFP. Transfusion transmitted disease from known and unknown agents is always a risk, especially with non-virally inactivated products. Other serious complications associated with FFP include anaphylaxis and transfusion-associated acute lung injury (TRALI). Therefore, as with all blood products, the risk–benefit ratio should be considered for each individual patient.

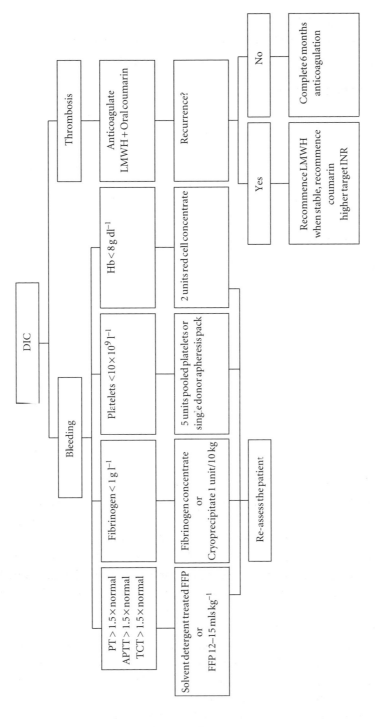

Fig. 13.7 An algorithm for the management of DIC.

Table 13.4 Fresh frozen plasma or SD plasma prescription and rate per hour

Patient weight (kg)	Units required	Duration of transfusion (hours)
20	1	3–4
30	2	3–4
40	3*	4
50	3	3.5
60	4	3–4
70	5*	4
80	5	3–4
90	6	3–4
100	7	3–4

*Suggest thawing one unit less initially.

The recommended infusion rate of plasma is a unit over 30 min to an uncompromised adult. In the elderly, the very small or the patient with cardiac compromise in the non-bleeding situation, transfusion rates for plasma should not exceed 2–4 mls kg per hour. The recom-

13.4.7 Replacement of fibrinogen

If a bleeding patient with DIC has a fibrinogen level of $<1\,g\,l^{-1}$, replacement of fibrinogen should be given in addition to FFP. Two products are available: Fibrinogen concentrate (virally inactivated, pooled donor plasma) and cryoprecipitate (not virally inactivated but limited donor exposure). Best practice suggests that the virally inactivated product is preferable but local availability will determine the choice of product.

13.4.8 Red cell transfusion

Red blood cell transfusion should be given if bleeding is present and the hemoglobin is $<8\,g\,dl^{-1}$.

13.4.9 Other replacement therapies

Natural anticoagulants such as protein C and antithrombin may become depleted due to consumption secondary to the generalized activation of coagulation in DIC. In addition, levels of these proteins may fall further due to decreased synthesis in the presence of liver failure and certain drugs such as heparin and L-Asparaginase. Plasma derived, virally inactivated concentrates of antithrombin and Protein C have been developed. At present, there is some evidence that replacement therapy in DIC can stabilize the coagulopathy where deficiencies of these proteins are demonstrated. However, it is currently recommended that the use of these products be confined to clinical trials.

If DIC has occurred as a manifestation of the underlying malignancy then appropriate treatment with chemotherapy should be given. DIC will continue unless the underlying tumor is treated. If the DIC has arisen as a consequence of chemotherapy, then supportive care should be given until the chemotherapy begins to become effective. With appropriate support care the DIC should stabilize in 2–3 days.

13.4.10 The patient with thrombosis

Thrombosis is a common manifestation of chronic compensated DIC in the patient with cancer. Approximately 15 percent of patients present with thrombosis in the course of their disease but as many as 30–50 percent of patients have evidence of thrombosis at post-mortem examination.

In some cases, thrombosis may be the presenting feature which leads to the diagnosis of cancer. In other cases, thrombosis arises as a late event. The temporal relationship of the thrombosis to the diagnosis of malignancy can be a prognostic indicator. A recent study has found that thrombosis which occurs as the presenting symptom of cancer is associated with advanced disease and a poor prognosis. Thrombosis associated with malignancy may arise in unusual sites, for example, arterial thrombosis, non-bacterial endocarditis and hepatic and portal veins.

Where the thrombosis has been confirmed, anticoagulation is indicated. Initial therapy with low molecular weight heparin (LMWH) is the treatment of choice since this is not affected by interactions with acute phase proteins. Care should be taken with patients with renal failure and dosing should be altered according to the anti Xa level or unfractionated heparin should be used. Once the patient has been stabilized on LMWH for at least 24 hours oral anticoagulation can be commenced with coumarin. Long-term anticoagulation may be considered if the underlying malignancy is not in remission. Approximately 10 percent of patients with cancer suffer recurrence of venous thromboembolism despite adequate anticoagulation. In these situations, treatment with LMWH will allow stabilization of the thrombus with subsequent transfer back to an oral coumarin with a higher target INR. Inferior vena caval filters have a role to play in patients with a contraindication to anticoagulation.

13.4.11 Thromboprophylaxis

Clearly, patients with cancer have a predisposition to thrombosis and should receive thromboprophylaxis with LMWH postoperatively and during periods of immobility. In addition, recent reports of thrombosis associated with long haul flights suggest that LMWH prophylaxis is advisable for patients with cancer who are travelling long distances.

Suggested reading

Anagrelide Study Group (1992) Anagrelide, a therapy for thrombocythaemic states: experience in 577 patients. *Am J Med*, **92**, 69–76.

Arfvidsson, B., Eklof, B., Kistner, R.L., Massuda, E.M., and Sato, D.T. (2000) Risk factors for venous thromboembolism following prolonged air travel. Coach class thrombosis. *Hematol Oncol Clin North Am*, **14**, 391–400.

BCSH Blood Transfusion Task Force (1996) Guidelines on gamma irradiation of blood components for the prevention of transfusion-associated graft-versus-host disease. *Transfus Med*, 6, 261–71.

Beutler, E. (1993) Platelet transfusions: The 20,000/μl trigger. *Blood*, 81, 1411–13.

Buss, D.H., Stuart, J.J., and Lipscomb, G.E. (1985) The incidence of thrombotic and hemorrhagic disorders in association with extreme thrombocytosis: an analysis of 129 cases. *Am J Hematol*, 20, 365–72.

Colman, R.W. and Rubin, R.N. (1990) Disseminated intravascular coagulation due to malignancy. *Semin Oncol*, 17, 172–86.

Colvin, B.T. (1998) Management of disseminated intravascular coagulation. *Br J Haematol*, 101(Suppl 1), 15–17.

Contrino, J., Hair, G., Kruetzer, D.L., and Rickles, F.R. (1996). In situ detection of expression of tissue factor in vascular endothelial cells: correlation with the malignant phenotype of human breast disease. *Nat Med*, 2, 209–15.

Cortelazzo, S., Finazzi, G., Ruggeri, M., Vestri, O., Galli, M., Rodeghiero, F., and Barbui, T. (1995) Hydroxyurea for patients with essential thrombocythemia and a high risk of thrombosis. *N Engl J Med*, 332, 1132–6.

Falanga, A. and Rickles, F.R. (1999) Pathophysiology of the thrombotic state in the cancer patient. *Seminn Thromb Hemost*, 25, 172–82.

Goad, K.E. and Gralnick, H.R. (1996) Coagulation disorders in cancer. *Hematol Oncol Clin North Am*, 10, 457–84.

Hernandez, E., Donohue, K.A., Anderson, L.L., Heller, P.B., and Stehman, F.B. (2000) The significance of thrombocytosis in patients with locally advanced cervical carcinoma: a gynecologic oncology group study. *Gynecol Oncol*, 78, 137–42.

Hillen, H.F.P. (2000). Thrombosis in cancer patients. *Ann Oncol*, 11(Suppl 3), 273–6.

Isaacs, C., Robert, N.J., Bailey, F.A., Schuster, M.W., Overmoyer, B., Graham, M., Cai, B., Beach, K.J., Loewy, J.W., and Kaye J.A. (1997) Randomized placebo-controlled study of recombinant human interleukin-11 to prevent chemotherapy-induced thrombocytopenia in patients with breast cancer receiving dose-intensive cyclophosphamide and doxorubicin. *J Clin Oncol*, 15, 3368–77.

Kaye, J.A. (1998) FDA licensure of NEUMEGA to prevent severe chemotherapy-induced thrombocytopenia. *Stem Cells*, 16 (Suppl 2), 207–23.

Kyrle, P.A., Minar, E., Hirschl, M., Bialonczyk, C., Stain, M., Schneider, B., Weltermann, A., Speiser, W., Lechner, K., and Eichinger, S. (2000) High plasma levels of factor VIII and the risk of recurrent venous thromboembolism. *N Engl J Med*, 343(7), 457–62.

Lavie, O., Comerci, G., Daras, V., Bolger, B.S., Lopes, A., and Monaghan, J.M. (1999) Thrombocytosis in women with vulvar carcinoma. *Gynecol Oncol*, 72, 82–6.

Levi, M., and ten Cate, H. (1999) Current concepts: Disseminated Intravascular Coagulation. *N Engl J Med*, 341, 586–92.

Menczer, J., Schejter, E., Geva, D., Ginath,S., and Zakut, H. (1998) Ovarian carcinoma associated thrombocytosis. Correlation with prognostic factors and with survival. *Eur J Gynaecol Oncol*, 19, 82–4.

Pedersen, L.M. and Milman, N. (1996) Prognostic significance of thrombocytosis in patients with primary lung cancer. *Eur Respir J*, 9, 1826–30.

Rebulla, P., Finazzi, G., Marangoni, F., Avvisati, G., Gugliotta, L., Tognoni, G., Barbui, T., Mandelli, F., and Sirchia, G. (1997) The threshold for prophylactic platelet transfusions in adults with acute myeloid leukaemia. *N Engl J Med*, 337, 1870–75.

Schinzel, H. and Weilemann, L.S. (1998) Antithrombin substitution therapy. *Blood Coagul Fibrinolysis*, **9** (Suppl 3), 17–22.

Smith, O.P., White, B., Vaughan, D., Rafferty, M., Claffey, L., Lyons, B., and Casey, W. (1997) Use of protein-C concentrate, heparin, and haemodiafiltration in meningococcus-induced purpura fulminans. *The Lancet*, **350**, 1590–3.

Sorensen, H.T., Mellemkjaer, L., Olsen, J.H., and Baron, J.A. (2000) Prognosis of cancers associated with venous thromboembolism. *N Engl J Med*, **343**, 1846–50.

Symbas, N.P., Townsend, M.F., El-Galley, R., Keane, T.E., Graham, S.D., and Petros, J.A. (2000) Poor prognosis associated with thrombocytosis in patients with renal cell carcinoma. *BJU Int*, **86**, 203–7.

Tepler, I., Elias, L., Smith, J.W. II, Hussein, M., Rosen, G., Chang, A.Y., Moore, J.O., Gordon, M.S., Kuca, B., Beach, K.J., Loewy, J.W., Garnick, M.B., and Kaye, J.A. (1996) A randomised placebo-controlled trial of recombinant human interleukin-11 in cancer patients with severe thrombocytopenia due to chemotherapy. *Blood*, **87**, 3607–14.

Vadhan-Raj, S. (2000) Clinical experience with recombinant human thrombopoietin in chemotherapy-induced thrombocytopenia. *Semin Hematol*, **37**, 28–34.

Zeimet, A.G., Marth, C., Muller-Holzner, E., Daxenbichler, G., and Dapunt, O. (1994) Significance of thrombocytosis in patients with epithelial ovarian cancer. *Am J Obstet Gynecol*, **170**, 549–54.

Chapter 14

Dermatologic Emergencies

Martin M. Eatock

14.1 Introduction

Whilst there are few true oncologic emergencies affecting the skin, patients receiving treatment for cancer are exposed daily to potentially serious hazards to the skin as a result of drug extravasation following chemotherapy or as a result of an acute dermatologic radiation reaction. These problems are not life-threatening, however their early recognition and management are important in order to prevent significant morbidity and functional impairment.

Paraneoplastic phenomena with cutaneous involvement are relatively common, for example acanthosis nigricans, however these do not constitute an oncologic emergency. Some cutaneous paraneoplastic phenomena are often associated with multi-organ involvement and may be life-threatening. These conditions, although rare, are important as they often occur in potentially curable malignancies such as lymphoma and leukemia.

This chapter will identify these paraneoplastic dermatologic emergencies and treatment-related dermatologic emergencies and will discuss their recognition and management.

14.2 Dermatologic emergencies as a consequence of cancer treatment

14.2.1 Chemotherapy-related emergencies

The principal dermatologic problem related to chemotherapy is one of drug extravasation during administration. In the 1970s, reports of cytotoxic drug extravasation suggested that this occurred in 1–6 percent of patients receiving anthracycline chemotherapy. In the 1980s, however, the incidence of cytotoxic extravasation was reported to be less than 0.01 percent by the Clinical Oncology Association of Australia. The decrease in the incidence of cytotoxic drug extravasation is largely due to improved awareness of the problem and also to the adoption of improved methods of drug administration. These will not be reviewed here, but it should suffice to say that the best treatment of cytotoxic extravasation is its prevention, which depends on the administration of chemotherapy by appropriately trained personnel.

Patients receiving chemotherapy by infusion into a peripheral vein are at increased risk of drug extravasation and, for this reason, vesicant drugs should be administered using a central venous catheter where possible. Vesicant drugs administered peripherally should be administered as a bolus injection over 5–10 min concurrently with a fast flowing saline infusion through the same venous cannula.

The management of extravasation where this has occurred is dependent on the drug administered. An algorithm for the management of cytotoxic extravasation along with an "extravasation pack" should be available in all clinical areas where such drugs are administered. Examples of these are shown in Fig. 14.1 and Table 14.1. Table 14.2 classifies cytotoxic drugs according to their vesicant potential.

Anthracyclines

The anthracyclines, doxorubicin, daunorubicin and epirubicin, are amongst the most commonly used cytotoxic drugs and also result in the most serious extravasation reactions. These drugs are highly lipophilic and may be retained in subcutaneous tissues for protracted periods of time. Histopathologic studies from animal models show that extravasation of doxorubicin results in necrosis of involved tissues and this process is independent of an inflammatory response.

Ulceration and necrosis may occur as an ongoing process up to 5 months after an extravasation of these drugs and is significant in around 30 percent of patients experiencing such an extravasation. In the case of doxorubicin, clinically significant ulceration is most likely where greater than 3 mg of drug has extravasated. Such ulceration not only involves the skin but may also involve underlying tissues and structures such as tendon and muscle and such patients may require surgical debridement and reconstructive surgery before wound healing can occur.

Table 14.1 Contents of the extravasation pack

Extravasation reporting form

Hot pack

Cold pack (stored in freezer)

4×10 ml sodium chloride 0.9% injection

Hydrocortisone injection $100 \, mg \times 2$

4×2 ml water for injections

1% hydrocortisone cream

Hyaluronidase 1500 IU injection

Chlorpheniramine injection 10 mg

Sodium chromoglycate 100 mg caps $\times 10$

$2 \times$ sodium thiosulfate 50% injection

Mepyramine cream

Some packs will also include DMSO solution for topical application and 1.4% sodium bicarbonate.

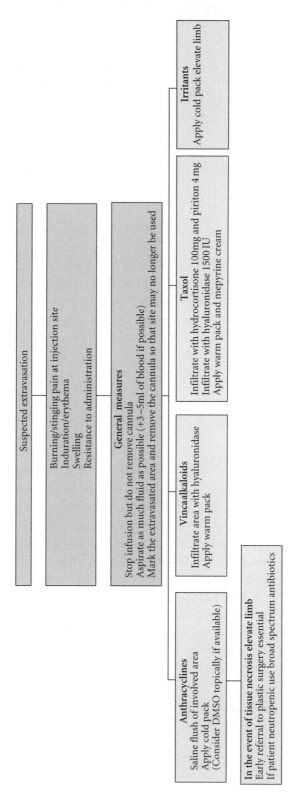

Fig. 14.1 Management algorithm for suspected cytotoxic extravasation.

Table 14.2 Chemotherapeutic agents classified according to vesicant potential

Vesicants	Irritants	Non-Irritants
Doxorubicin	Carboplatin	Cyclophosphamide
Epirubicin	Cisplatin (concentration	Gemcitabine
Daunorubicin	$<0.5\,\mathrm{mg\,ml^{-1}}$)	Ifosfamide
Vincristine	Etoposide	Raltitrexed
Vinblastine	Mitozantrone	Fludarabine
Vindesine	Docetaxel	Cytarabine
Vinorelbine	Methotrexate	Thiotepa
Mitomycin	5-fluorouracil	
Taxol	Liposomal daunorubicin	
Mustine	Melphalan	
Carmustine		
Dacarbazine		
Treosulphan		
Amsacrine		
Cisplatin (but only in concentrations $>0.5\,\mathrm{mg\,ml^{-1}}$ and therefore not clinically relevant in most situations)		

Clinical features of anthracycline extravasation

Extravasation is characterized by pain or a burning sensation along the course of the vein associated with erythema and often itching. This may be difficult to distinguish from a flare reaction, which may also cause erythema and a burning sensation along the course of the vein and occurs in around 3 percent of patients receiving anthracyclines. A flare reaction usually settles spontaneously after around 30–45 min and may be minimized by increasing the rate of the simultaneous fast flowing saline infusion.

The natural history of an anthracycline extravasation is dependent on the quantity and concentration of the extravasated drug. With a significant extravasation the initial symptoms persist and are followed within 48–72 hours by skin blistering, swelling and induration. An eschar then forms with underlying subcutaneous necrosis after 2–3 weeks followed by overt ulceration after 3–4 weeks. Small ulcers may heal spontaneously but larger ulcers do not.

Management of anthracycline extravasation The prompt management of an extravasation injury may prevent or minimize the extent of the injury. In the first instance one should:

1. Attempt to aspirate as much of the extravasated drug as possible as soon as the extravasation is recognized.

2. This should be followed by skin cooling of the affected area. This is supported by randomized trial evidence.

A number of specific treatments have been suggested, however the basis for many of these is anecdotal as there are few randomized clinical trials of the pharmacologic treatment of extravasation. The use of many agents such as corticosteroids or sodium bicarbonate are probably based on false premise and are unlikely to be effective as they have shown no benefit in animal models. A number of reports suggest that topical dimethylsulphoxide (DMSO) may be helpful in preventing skin ulceration related to anthracycline extravasation, however these reports are usually of 2 or 3 patients and the largest reported study to date is of 20 patients. In this study no patients developed skin ulceration, however no report is made of the estimated extravasated drug dose. Animal studies are equivocal. DMSO may in itself result in a burning sensation and result in skin desquamation and is not licensed for usage in this indication. Its use may be considered for large anthracycline extravasations, but cannot be routinely recommended and there is a need for well-conducted clinical studies to resolve this question.

Vinca alkaloids

Like anthracyclines these drugs, particularly vincristine and vinblastine, are highly vesicant. Following extravasation, they typically produce pain, swelling and erythema within minutes. Skin blistering occurs after several days and this then usually resolves over a period of weeks. Skin ulceration has been reported, however this is unusual. Some patients report persistent symptoms of pain and swelling for up to 6 months after the initial injury and this may be sufficiently debilitating to warrant excision of the affected area of skin. More commonly, patients report delayed paraesthesia and superficial sensory loss, which may persist after the skin lesions have healed.

Management of vinca alkaloid extravasation   As for anthracycline extravasation the immediate management of vinca alkaloid extravasation involves:

1. Attempted aspiration of drug through the original cannula.

2. In the case of vinca alkaloid extravasation, skin cooling results in worsening of the skin toxicity. Therefore, in contrast to the management of anthracycline extravasation, patients should be treated with mild skin warming.

3. There is good evidence from laboratory studies that the administration of hyaluronidase by subcutaneous injection into the involved area enhances the clearance of extravasated drug from the skin and this is routinely recommended.

Other putative antidotes have been investigated in clinical and laboratory studies, such as corticosteroids or glutamic acid. These either exacerbate the situation (i.e. corticosteroids) or make little difference to the outcome.

Mitomycin C

Like the vinca alkaloids and anthracyclines, mitomycin is a potent vesicant and may produce severe soft tissue necrosis on extravasation. Reactions to extravasation are often delayed and cases are reported of ulceration occurring at the site of a previous injection after the administration of a subsequent dose weeks later. When clinically apparent, extravasation is characterized by severe pain and swelling in the affected area. A high proportion of patients will require surgical management if ulceration develops. Laboratory studies have suggested that DMSO or sodium thiosulphate may be protective against skin ulceration, however there are few reports of the use of these in patients.

Other agents

The agents described above represent the commonly used cytotoxic drugs, which result in the most severe extravasation reactions. Many other agents are moderately vesicant, but rarely result in significant functional impairment following extravasation. Cisplatin has been reported to produce skin ulceration, however this is extremely unlikely with the concentrations of drug used in normal clinical practice. The epipodophyllotoxins have been associated with phlebitis and local swelling, but only rarely result in ulceration, however with the relatively dilute drug concentrations used in clinical practice this is unlikely to occur. It is recommended, however, that with large etoposide extravasations subcutaneous administration of hyaluronidase is used to prevent further problems.

A management algorithm for cytotoxic extravasation is shown in Fig. 14.1.

14.2 **Surgical management of extravasation injuries**

A significant proportion of patients will require surgical intervention following cytotoxic extravasation, particularly following extravasation of anthracyclines. All patients who develop skin ulceration as a consequence of extravasation will require debridement of all necrotic tissue. Surgical reconstruction following this may be immediate for superficial ulcers or staged depending on the condition of the wound following debridement. Surgical reconstruction may also be required for involved nerves or tendons.

It is recommended that all patients experiencing significant extravasations of vesicant drugs are referred for a plastic surgical opinion at an early stage to allow early intervention should this become required.

14.3 **Dermatologic emergencies as a complication of cancer**

14.3.1 **Paraneoplastic phenomena**

Paraneoplastic pemphigus (PNP)

Paraneoplastic pemphigus is a recently recognized syndrome first described in 1990. It is characterized clinically by the presence of blisters or erosions involving primarily mucous membranes but may also present with a skin eruption which eventually produces typical bullae. This is an autoimmune process and is characterized further by histologic findings of epidermal acantholysis and keratinocyte necrosis in association with epidermal basement membrane deposition of IgG and complement, the detection of serum antibodies to various epithelial antigens, including desmoplakin I and II, and the immunoprecipitation of a protein complex from keratinocytes with serum antibodies. This disease is associated with a variety of neoplasms, however, most cases reported occur in association with hematologic malignancies such as non-Hodgkin's lymphoma, Castlemans disease or chronic lymphocytic leukemia although some cases have been reported in association with soft tissue sarcoma, bronchial carcinoma and renal cell carcinoma. It usually presents in patients who already have a diagnosis of malignant disease but it may be the presenting feature.

Clinical findings

1. Mucous membrane involvement—The majority of patients present with oral erosions and ulceration (Fig. 14.2). Other mucous membranes such as the conjunctivae may also be affected and nasal ulceration may present with epistaxis.

2. Ocular involvement—usually manifest by conjunctivitis, however corneal ulceration and scarring may also occur.

3. Cutaneous features—erythema and vesiculobulous lesions. A minority of patients will present with these as the primary features, however they will all develop mucous membrane disease during the course of the illness.

This is a serious complication of malignancy and may result in death. The skin barrier function for infection is impaired and this may lead to localized infection. However, in patients who are immunosuppressed as a result of their underlying malignancy, or treatment for this, may rapidly develop systemic sepsis which may be life-threatening.

Paraneoplastic pemphigus is a systemic autoimmune disorder involving the respiratory and gastrointestinal tracts. Respiratory tract involvement is of particular concern as it may lead to bronchiolitis obliterans and death.

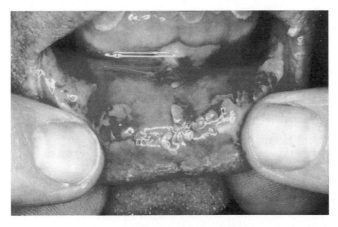

Fig. 14.2 Paraneoplastic pemphigus with marked labial ulceration and erosion. (Please see color section between pages 116 and 117.)

Diagnosis   The diagnosis of PNP is usually established following biopsy of a lesion and also of non-involved skin.

1. Histopathologic features include epidermal necrosis, suprabasal acantholysis, vacuolar interface dermatitis. These features are associated with a lymphocytic response. The presence of dyskeratotic keratinocytes is highly suggestive of PNP and may be helpful in distinguishing this from other pemphigus subtypes.

2. Biopsies of non-involved skin should be assessed by direct immunofluorescence. This typically shows intercellular binding of IgG as well as binding of IgG and/or IgM along the dermal–epidermal junction.

Treatment and prognosis   The prognosis of PNP is poor with death occurring in 75–90 percent of patients usually within 6–12 months of presentation. The mainstay of treatment for this is the use of immunosuppressive therapy such as high dose corticosteroids with or without other agents such as cyclosporine, along with treatment of the underlying malignancy. The recommended initial treatment in the acute situation is with prednisolone $1–2$ mg kg^{-1} per day.

Sweet's syndrome (acute febrile neutrophilic dermatosis)

Sweet's syndrome is characterized by the association of fever, leukocytosis and a cutaneous eruption. This may occur as a complication of a number of autoimmune diseases, such as rheumatoid arthritis and inflammatory bowel disease. It also may occur as a drug reaction, following viral infection and in pregnancy. Around 25 percent of cases of Sweet's syndrome are associated with an underlying malignancy.

Clinical findings   Sweet's syndrome is characterized by:

1. Sudden onset of well-demarcated tender erythematous cutaneous papules or plaques favoring the face and upper body (Fig. 14.3).

2. Fever, usually preceding the onset of the rash.

3. Arthritis or arthralgia is described in about one-third to one-half of patients.

4. The involvement of other organs such as the lungs, kidney, liver and central nervous system has been described.

Hematologic findings are typically a leukocytosis associated with a raised erythrocyte sedimentation rate; however, in Sweet's syndrome associated with malignancy anemia and thrombocytopenia are also common. Around 50 percent of patients will have abnormal liver function tests, particularly a raised alkaline phosphatase.

Treatment and outcome   Unlike PNP, Sweet's syndrome is self-limiting with a median duration of around 4 weeks, however around 15 percent of patients will develop chronic relapsing disease. Corticosteroids are the mainstay of treatment, the usual initial dose of prednisolone being $1–2$ mg $^{-1}kg^{-1}$ per day. The fever and malaise usually respond rapidly to the initiation of treatment within hours. Mucosal lesions usually respond within

(a) (b)

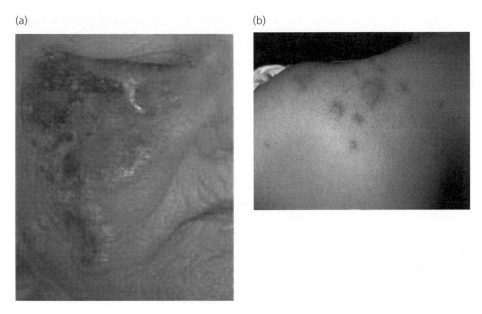

Fig. 14.3 Typical cutaneous features of Sweet's syndrome showing violaceous papules or plaques studded with pustules affecting the face (a) and torso (b). (Please see color section between pages 116 and 117.)

a few days of starting treatment, however skin lesions may take several weeks to resolve. Non-steroidal anti-inflammatory agents are useful in the management of arthralgia.

Suggested reading

Bertelli, G. (1995) Prevention and management of extravasation of cytotoxic drugs. *Drug Saf*, 12, 245–55.

Bourke, J.F., Keohane, S., Long, C.C., Kemmett, D., Davies, M., Zaki, I., and Graham-Brown, R.A.C. (1997) Sweet's syndrome and malignancy in the UK. *Br J Dermatol*, 137, 609–13.

Dorr, R.T. (1990) Antidote to vesicant chemotherapy extravasations. *Blood Rev*, 4, 41–60.

Heitmann, C., Durmus, C., and Ingianni, G. (1998) Surgical management after doxorubicin and epirubicin extravasation. *J Hand Sur*, 5, 666–8.

Lear, J.T., Athertopn, M.T., and Byrne, J.P. (1997) Neutrophilic dermatoses: pyoderma gangrenosum, and Sweet's syndrome. *Postgrad Med J*, 73, 65–8.

Shenaq, S.M., Abbase, E.H., and Friedman, J.D. (1996) Soft tissue reconstruction following extravasation of chemotherapeutic agents. *Surg Oncol Clin North Am*, 5, 825–45.

Sklavounou, A. and Laskaris, G. (1998) Paraneoplastic pemphigus: a review. *Oral Oncol*, 34, 437–40.

Takahashi, M., Shimatsu, Y., Kazama, T., Otsuka, T., and Hashimoto, T. (2000) Paraneoplastic pemphigus associated with bronchiolitis obliterans. *Chest*, 117, 603–7.

Chapter 15

Radiation Emergencies

Timothy Kinsella

15.1 Introduction

The management of patients with cancer is generally a multi-modality proposition. Rarely are patients treated with one intervention alone, whether surgery, chemotherapy or radiation therapy. The role of radiation in the treatment of cancer patients has therefore grown tremendously in the past few decades. It has been estimated that more than fifty percent of all cancer patients will receive radiation at some point in their management. Although radiation may remain the sole treatment of choice for some early cancers, for example, basal cell skin cancers and early stage vocal cord cancers, its role has dramatically expanded. Ionizing radiation is used in both a definitive fashion and as adjuvant therapy. Technological advances using three-dimensional computer driven planning has allowed higher doses to be delivered in a fashion that is better tailored to treating neoplasms in locations where previously treatment could not be given due to normal tissue toxicity. New combinations of radiation and chemotherapy have enhanced the oncologist's ability to cure, or at least more effectively treat a number of cancers. This increased application of radiation and the combination of chemotherapy and radiation make it absolutely essential that the various treating physicians involved in the management of the patient with cancer have knowledge of the expected side effects of treatment and their effective management. Occasionally the morbidity is more than anticipated and timely assessment and therapeutic intervention may be required to satisfactorily relieve the problem. Radiation oncologists generally are aware of the side effects and complications of their prescribed treatment, but this basic knowledge must also be shared with numerous other health care professionals. Adequate knowledge of the benefits, side effects and complications of radiation therapy will help streamline the care of these patients and result in better outcomes, both acutely and in the long term.

Whether used alone, in combination with chemotherapy or following surgery, the major role of the radiation oncologist is to achieve local–regional control of the tumor by using ionizing radiation. The goal may be either total eradication of the macroscopic (or microscopic) malignancy, or it may simply be the palliation of a particular symptom by reducing the amount of tumor present. In any case there is damage that is perpetrated by the radiation, affecting both the tumor and the normal peri-tumoral tissue, as well as any tissue through which the radiation passes. The injury can be divided into early, intermediate, or late stages, depending upon when the radiation effects are manifested. There are some well-accepted definitions of these various stages.

1. *Early* radiation effects and damage occur during the actual treatment (usually after a few weeks of therapy) or within a few weeks of the completion of therapy. Common examples of these side effects are mucositis or esophagitis, alopecia, skin erythema and diarrhea.

2. *Intermediate* effects are noted a few weeks to a few months following therapy. Radiation pneumonitis can be classified in this category.

3. *Late* effects occur several months to, occasionally, several years following radiation therapy. Radiation-induced bowel fibrosis and stricture, dementia in some older patients undergoing whole brain irradiation and peripheral neuropathies are examples of late effects.

There are a number of technical and radiation delivery factors that determine the effect radiation has on the normal tissue. These include:

1. the total dose of radiation delivered;
2. the energy of the radiation;
3. the length of time over which it is delivered (fractionation);
4. the inherent sensitivity of the organ tissue;
5. volume of the organ treated.

Higher doses, frequently administered doses and large volume of the organ in the field of treatment cause greater morbidity. The radiation oncologist may have to risk a certain defined morbidity in order to achieve his or her goal, especially in the case of definitive, potentially curable situations. In no way should a decision be made to compromise cure in order to avoid toxicity. Limiting the side effects by treating them promptly if they occur is imperative. Clinical morbidity needs to be adequately assessed in regard to the organs affected and their importance to survival. Irreparable damage to some organs may lead to death or severe morbidity, while damage to other structures may be associated with moderate to minimal morbidity. Underlying disorders such as lupus erythematosis, and Crohn's disease may introduce other patient-specific factors that may enhance the risk for serious side effects and complications. Some side effects may be very annoying to patients and may impact on the quality of life, but may not be life-threatening. Attention, however, both to longevity and life quality must be maintained.

One other factor that will affect toxicity has already been mentioned, and that is the combination of chemotherapy and radiation. Even if the chemotherapy is not administered concurrently with the radiation there may be enhanced toxicity compared to the toxicity of either modality alone. Subclinical damage caused by one or the other modality may be recalled by subsequent exposure to the other agent. The damaging effects of the two modalities may be similar, thus increasing the target organ injury expected by either modality alone. The two modalities may interact in a manner that results in tissue injury not usually expected from either modality alone. The wide variety of chemotherapeutic agents available and the uniqueness of each radiation plan require constant surveillance for potential problems.

The desire to define "dose-limiting tissues" led to the classification of organs into three categories grouped in terms of life-threatening potential. Minimal and maximal tissue tolerance doses were defined by Rubin and Casarett by 5 percent and 50 percent rates of complications at 5 years.

1. **Class I organs** (heart, brain, spinal cord, bone marrow, liver, kidney, stomach and intestines) were those in which radiation injury resulted in death or severe morbidity.

2. **Class II organs** (eye, ear, endocrine glands, ovary, testes, esophagus, oral cavity and pharynx, skin, rectum, bone and cartilage, bladder and ureters) results in moderate to mild morbidity. Damage to these organs is usually compatible with survival.

3. **Class III organs** (muscle, uterus, vagina, breast lymph nodes, large vessels) sustain injury which is usually transient, reversible and without clearly defined morbidity.

Although radiation oncologists use this information as a basic guideline to define therapy, the possible interaction with other agents may in fact lower the threshold for significant organ damage.

Morbidity can best be discussed, and the side effects of different regimens can be better compared, if a standardized scoring system is used. The most commonly used scoring schemes have been devised by the Radiation Therapy Oncology Group (RTOG) and the European Organization for Research and Treatment of Cancer (EORTC). A Late Effects of Normal Tissue (LENT) scoring scheme has also been developed.

Although some radiation complications are preventable by meticulous treatment planning, many are not. The practitioner should be able to anticipate the unavoidable side effects of treatment and should prepare the patient for them. Many of the side effects will occur during the course of treatment and therefore successful management is necessary in order to complete treatment in a timely fashion. Because some effects will not be encountered until a few weeks to a few months after treatment, close follow-up for an extended period is essential after treatment cessation. The following sections will discuss the most common toxicities and the recommended management.

15.2 **Hematopoetic stem cells**

Whether or not radiation effects can be seen in regard to the hematopoetic stem cell compartment depends considerably on the volume of marrow in the field of radiation. Large volumes of treatment many result in neutropenia, seen within a week or so of the initiation of irradiation. Preceding or concomitant chemotherapy exposure may accelerate or aggravate this response. Thrombocytopenia may occur a week or two after the neutropenia. Rarely is radiation-induced anemia seen, but if large volumes of marrow have been treated there is the possibility of anemia occurring. In situations where patients have undergone multiple courses of radiation to sites of bone metastases this may become a problem. It is generally felt that hemoglobin levels of $10\,\mathrm{g\,dl^{-1}}$ or greater be preserved during treatment (if necessary, by transfusion) in order to maintain adequate neoplastic tissue oxygenation which may be a factor in maintaining tumor radiosensitivity. In addition to transfusion, growth factors can be administered to patients with red or white cell deficiencies.

15.3 Oral cavity/pharynx

Many neoplasms of the head and neck area are treated with radiation either as definitive therapy or in combination with chemotherapy and/or surgery. The effects of radiation in this region result in a number of acute and long-term side effects that can greatly affect the patient's well being. Treatment to the oral cavity and pharyngeal areas affects mucosa, taste and salivary glands. These effects result in the major toxicities associated with radiation in this area: mucositis, taste disturbances and xerostomia. Within a few weeks of commencing radiation, oral mucositis and pharyngitis develop. Initially the mucosa may only appear inflamed, later patchy desquamation can develop which often leads to confluent desquamation involving all the surfaces within the field of treatment. This condition may be worsened by the development of candidiasis. This fungal infection is characterized by a thick whitish cheese-like coating over the tongue and mucosal surfaces. Both the damaged mucosal surfaces and the diminished serous component of the salivary glands production of saliva encourage the overgrowth of this fungus. Significant taste disturbances may ensue due to these changes as well as due to direct effects on the taste buds.

Oral mucositis is a distressing toxic effect of radiation and many agents and methods have been used to try to ameliorate these symptoms. During the acute phases of the mucositis some degree of soothing relief can be obtained by the use of oral rinses. The most effective intervention may be obtained by frequent oral lavage using a dilute salt solution made by dissolving a teaspoon of bicarbonate and a teaspoon of table salt in a quart of warm tap water. In addition topical anesthetics such as 2 percent viscous xylocaine can be used by mixing a teaspoon of the viscous xylocaine with a tablespoon of liquid antacid and using the solution as a mouth rinse (which can be swallowed) just prior to eating or drinking. Patients however need to be forewarned of the numbing effects of the viscous xylocaine so that care can be taken in avoiding hot temperature foods and liquids. Patients should also be cautioned to avoid coarse or spicy foods and alcohol (including alcohol-containing mouthwashes). An additional intervention is the use of a mucosal protecting agent such as sucralfate suspension. Clinical and histopathologic demonstration of reduction in oral mucositis with sucralfate suggests that it may be recommended not only for the treatment but also the prevention of oral mucositis induced by radiation therapy. Two teaspoonfuls administered four times daily (one hour before meals and at bedtime) may slow the development of mucositis and promote healing. Despite these interventions pain may be severe enough to warrant analgesic therapy, including narcotics. Based on the findings of the role of the inflammatory cascade in the response of normal tissues to radiotherapy, anti-inflammatory drugs might be efficacious. Many patients, especially those on chemotherapy or with a history of gastritis or ulcer disease, may not be candidates for anti-inflammatory drugs.

Maintenance of adequate nutrition and hydration is a primary concern during radiation to the head and neck area and in some circumstances it may be necessary to insert a feeding tube to ensure adequate hydration and caloric intake. This intervention is best undertaken sooner rather than later. Patients who are nutritionally unsound at the initiation of treatment may best be served by placement of a jejunostomy tube (or similar device) prior to the initiation of treatment rather than waiting until there is further nutritional deterioration.

Candidiasis is best managed with antifungal agents, either systemic such as flucanozole 100 mg orally daily, or with topical antifungal solutions. Patients receiving antibiotics or steroids may be more likely to develop candidiasis and may develop it early in the course of their therapy.

The salivary glands are primarily affected by radiation in regard to saliva production. In some circumstances patients may develop swelling and discomfort in the glands after the first or second treatment due to a transient inflammatory response, but this usually subsides within a few days and can be treated with anti-inflammatory or pain medication. More importantly the salivary gland output is reduced, preferentially resulting in the reduction of the serous component. This results in thickened saliva that has a low pH and functions inadequately due to its viscosity and diminished amount compared to normal. There is inadequate lubrication and rinsing of the teeth following meals. The diminished pH also leads to the development of dental caries. Dental hygiene is extremely important in these patients and an adequate dental evaluation prior to, and after, treatment is essential. Radiation therapy will impact indefinitely on the oral health and dental care of the patient and therefore the dentist and oral hygienist need to become involved in the patient's care even before the inception of radiation.

There are a number of maneuvers that can be undertaken to try to ameliorate these radiation-associated problems (Fig. 15.1). Prior to treatment the patient can be placed on oral pilocarpine which appears to have some effect in reducing xerostomia. It appears to work more effectively if started before radiation and maintained throughout therapy. After the completion of radiation it may be prudent to continue pilocarpine for several weeks. Initiating treatment with pilocarpine after the completion of treatment is less effective, but a trial of three or four months after treatment can be given before it is deemed ineffective. If used after radiotherapy it appears to act primarily by stimulating minor salivary glands. It can be effective even in patients with severe xerostomia. Since all responders are usually identified by 12 weeks, prolonged administration is not warranted

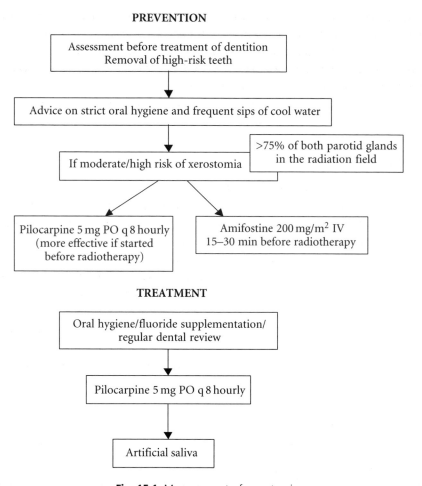

Fig. 15.1 Management of xerostomia.

in patients showing no improvement within that time period. Some patients experience sweating, nausea or vomiting and administration may need to be stopped if these side effects occur.

Another drug currently found to be effective in reducing the acute and chronic effects of head and neck irradiation is amifostine. It appears that the mucositis and xerostomia associated with radiation and chemoradiation can be diminished by using this agent, although administration is not done without some careful planning. Data suggest that patients receiving this agent experience improvement in their ability to carry out normal functions with reduced discomfort. Improvement seems to be most noted in regard to chronic xerostomia. Less oral toxicity should ultimately lead to better preservation of oral and dental health and ultimately in improved diet, nutrition, sleep, and overall quality of life.

Despite these interventions it is not unusual for patients to have some persistent chronic morbidity from the radiation. Xerostomia may persist for years and may never fully abate. Optimal dental care may require frequent and routine visits to the dentist for cleaning and fluoride treatments as well as timely intervention for dental caries. In fact, a fluoride gel can often be used as a topical application during the course of radiation and maintained for years afterwards. It helps to prevent the development of caries until normal salivary function returns.

15.4 **Thyroid**

Patients receiving therapeutic doses of radiation to the neck area are at risk for the development of hypothyroidism. The radiation causing this problem may be delivered as treatment for a primary head and neck cancer or for the treatment of Hodgkin's or non-Hodgkin's lymphoma. Cases of hypothyroidism have even developed after craniospinal irradiation and total-body irradiation for stem cell transplantation. Patients may develop subclinical or overt hypothyroidism and most will develop within 5 years of treatment. Since this may develop insidiously and years after radiation, the clinician must be alert to subtle signs or symptoms of this condition. Hyperthyroidism can also occur, though much less frequently, as a prelude to the eventual development of hypothyroidism.

Patients should have their TSH monitored yearly and overt or subclinical hypothyroidism should be treated with thyroxine.

15.5 **Mandible**

The effects of radiation on the mandible are of considerable importance as they can lead to the most troublesome complication of radiation to the head and neck region. It is known that radiation in high doses can interfere with the microvasculature supplying both oxygen and nutrients to metabolically active tissue. This is especially critical in bones with a limited vascular supply. Any interference with the vasculature to the bone can result in diminished healing and repair capacity following trauma of any sort. Infection in poorly vascularized tissue is also a major problem since the ability to eradicate infection is greatly compromised due to the hypovascularity. Following relatively high dose (>40 Gy) radiation to the mandible any trauma to the bone must be assiduously avoided. This of course includes injurious impact to the jaw as well as planned interventions such as dental extractions. General wisdom is to avoid all extractions after radiation to the mandible. However, if it is absolutely essential to do so, then a well-planned intervention must be coordinated. This usually involves the use of antibiotics both prior to, and after, extraction. It is felt that hyperbaric oxygen treatments may also be useful both prior to, and after, the procedure. The dental surgeon should ensure that no bone is left exposed following the extraction, thus the site is often oversewn to avoid leaving an exposed area that may be an avenue for infection. Even with cautious intervention there is still considerable risk for osteoradionecrosis, especially in patients with confounding risk factors, amongst which are alcoholism, poor nutrition and diabetes.

15.6 **Esophagus**

Like the mucosa in the oral cavity and pharynx the esophagus usually shows evidence of acute radiation effects within a few weeks of the initiation of therapy. Inflammation, mucosal denudation and the possibility of candidal infection are all likely to result in dysphagia that may worsen as the course of therapy continues. Interventions such as those described for oral mucositis are appropriate, keeping in mind that there may not be any evidence of candidiasis by routine examination. Often patients who have persistent dysphagia and/or odynophagia after they have been treated with sucralfate or viscous lignocaine are treated empirically for candidiasis. It is not necessary to subject the patient to endoscopy since, especially if the patient is also receiving chemotherapy or steroids, the likelihood for fungal infection is so high. In the rare circumstance when a patient has increasingly severe symptoms despite the usual interventions it may be necessary to resort to endoscopy to sort out the problem. Often this is inconclusive.

However, in some cases the diagnosis of viral infection can be made. Esophageal symptoms promptly resolve within a few weeks of completion of treatment.

High doses to a localized area are a risk of constriction due to fibrosis. Certainly increasing symptoms of dysphagia or obstruction after radiotherapy require endoscopic evaluation, especially in patients who have undergone treatment for an esophageal or mediastinal malignancy, both to rule out recurrence and also to perform bouginage for relief of symptoms, if appropriate.

15.7 **Lungs**

One of the greatest challenges to a radiation oncologist is to determine the volume and dose that can be tolerated by normal tissue in the treatment of the malignancy. Nowhere is this more crucial than in the treatment of the lungs where large volumes of treatment can have lethal consequences. The irradiated lung volume is a critical parameter to be considered in planning thoracic radiotherapy. The lung parenchyma has a relatively low tolerance of radiation and therefore planning must respect this sensitivity. The exact mechanisms of radiation pneumonitis have not been established. Nonetheless almost all plans for thoracic irradiation include a portion of normal functioning lung parenchyma. Therefore, it is expected that almost all patients receiving treatment to this area will show evidence of radiation damage that may produce symptoms.

Pulmonary injury secondary to radiation is a well-recognized syndrome. In almost all situations the radiographic consequences of radiation will be seen. The occurrence and extent of damage are related to the total dose of radiation, the volume of lung irradiated, the fractionation scheme and the use of chemotherapeutic agents. If doses of thoracic irradiation exceed lung tolerance (>15–$20\,Gy$) pulmonary reactions can be seen either radiographically, clinically, or both.

Clinically the patients may present one to three months after the completion of treatment with low-grade fever, a dry, non-productive cough, and dyspnea. The severity of the symptoms varies greatly depending upon the volume of functional lung affected and can range from barely perceptible to life-threatening. Radiographs at this time usually reveal areas of infiltrate that correspond to the borders of the treatment field. This area of pneumonitis may be generalized and not clearly defined in patients who have been treated by multi-field conformal approaches where it would be difficult to outline a sharp field border. Thus the classic description of a sharply defined border of pneumonitis may no longer be practical as a classic radiographic finding in radiation pneumonitis.

If acute radiation pneumonitis is complicated by a superimposed infection then the patient may have high fever, a productive cough and even hemoptysis. Intervention is standardized and includes supplemental oxygen, if required, as well as corticosteroids and antibiotics when super-imposed infection has been proven. The decision to give these patients corticosteroids may be difficult if the patient is a compromised host (prior chemotherapy and radiation) and if there is considerable concern of infection by an opportunistic infection. Prompt symptomatic improvement should be noted within 24 hours of initiation of treatment. Therefore, close follow-up is initially warranted and serial chest films should be taken over 4–7 days to document continued resolution of the infiltrates. Failure to see an improvement in the patient's symptoms or worsening pulmonary infiltrates should prompt further aggressive investigation that may include bronchoscopy and biopsy. This acute phase usually subsides over a few weeks and steroids can be slowly tapered over a period of 4–6 weeks. However in some patients the episode may be drawn out over several months and efforts to taper steroids may be fraught with difficulty. Occasionally, only a very slow taper meets with success. Rarely patients may need to remain on low doses of corticosteroids for long periods of time. This may be more likely in patients who have had antecedent chronic pulmonary disease.

Over the next few years continued changes occur in the field of radiation treatment. Gradual development of fibrosis is noted on radiographs where continued loss of lung volume and retraction may be noted. Pulmonary symptoms related to diminished volumes and diminished diffusion capacity may lead to the need for chronic pulmonary care and may include bronchodilators and supplemental oxygen. Unfortunately once pulmonary fibrosis has developed no intervention will improve matters. The best treatment is aimed at avoidance since the condition is irreversible.

15.8 Heart

Cardiac symptoms developing during radiation are unlikely. Yet heart disease occurring after irradiation of the mediastinum has been recognized for several decades. Pericardial disease, in its various forms, is the most common problem and there are reports of acute pericarditis, pericardial effusion and pericardial constriction. Acute pericarditis is occasionally seen when radiation has been delivered to a malignancy contiguous to the heart and tumor necrosis results in localized pericardial inflammation. Fever, pain and EKG abnormalities typical of pericarditis are seen and are non-specific. Pericardial effusion may develop in over a third of the patients who have received radiation to a significant cardiac volume (usually >60%), although most of these patients will be asymptomatic and only an echocardiogram may reveal this development. Pericardial disease that is functionally important should be detectable from history, physical examination and a chest radiograph revealing enlargement of the cardiac silhouette. Chronic effusion may lead to pericardial tamponade that would normally be treated by the surgical creation of a pericardial window. In rare circumstances the patient may present with pericardial constriction years after radiation without any antecedent history of acute pericardial disease.

Some instances of myocardial disease, coronary artery disease and valvular sclerosis have also been described in the medical literature. Acute cardiomyopathy is extremely rare unless tolerance doses are exceeded (>45 Gy to significant volume). This development would be more likely in patients receiving or having previously received moderate to maximal doses of potentially cardiotoxic agents, for example, anthracyclines.

15.9 **Brain**

The brain is usually spared any acute effects from radiation therapy. However, some early post-radiation reactions have been described. Primarily seen in children are a constellation of symptoms that have been designated as the *somnolence syndrome*. This syndrome is usually noted 6 weeks to 6 months following whole brain irradiation and is characterized by somnolence, lethargy, irritability and loss of appetite. No focal neurologic findings accompany these symptoms and the syndrome usually resolves within a few days to a few weeks. This syndrome is most commonly observed in children who have received cranial irradiation. No specific intervention is required.

Similar findings can be seen in patients, children and adults, who have undergone cranial irradiation for CNS tumors. However, following high dose radiation to localized areas of the brain for tumor, localized edema or tumor necrosis may develop and be responsible for the development of similar or more severe symptoms. Occasionally patients may have focal neurologic abnormalities on examination. There may be an exacerbation of focal signs that correspond to the edema or tumor changes. Often these signs will respond to steroid administration although relatively high doses may be required.

A number of late side effects of radiation have been described. Necrosis of brain tissue has been reported as soon as 6 months following brain irradiation but can be seen up to a few years after treatment. The physical findings correlate with the area of brain affected. Radiographic changes are generally limited to the areas of previous treatment and reflect diffuse edema. There may be some variable evidence of mass effect; that may confuse interpretation and may suggest tumor recurrence. Although MRI evaluation may show more extensive areas of white matter change, it may not be possible to attribute all the findings to radiation necrosis. Positron emission tomography using fluorine-18 deoxyglucose may be useful in separating disease recurrence from active tumor since it is expected that areas of necrosis are hypometabolic and therefore would not show increased activity in the areas of mass effect seen on conventional imaging. Nonetheless clinical differentiation may be difficult. Initial therapy is corticosteroid administration followed by surgical resection of focal areas of necrosis if there is evidence of unremitting edema. At times this intervention may document tumor recurrence as well.

Especially in elderly patients diffuse post-irradiation white matter changes can occur. Patients may demonstrate mild fatigue, barely discernible personality changes or, in some cases, debilitating dementia. Patients who have received chemotherapy may also develop leukoencephalopathy that may be variable in severity. Memory loss, gait disturbances, incontinence and dementia may be progressive and irreversible. These findings have been described primarily in elderly patients undergoing whole brain irradiation for brain metastases or as prophylactic irradiation following treatment of localized small cell lung cancer. Because of these observations the dose of whole brain irradiation as prophylactic therapy in small cell lung cancer has been lowered. Studies are also underway to determine if localized stereotactic irradiation using stereotactic linear accelerator-based radiosurgery or gamma knife radiosurgery for brain metastases is as effective as whole brain irradiation as initial intervention.

Careful psychologic testing has resulted in findings that document neurocognitive impairment in children receiving supratentorial radiation at an early age. Although this is most apparent in children receiving treatment before the age of 2 years, no doubt, changes can be well documented in children up to the age of 7 years or beyond. Memory deficits, learning disabilities and behavioral problems have been noted. Careful testing in cooperative patients may document actual IQ deterioration. No doubt these findings are a result of many factors impacting on the ill child; prolonged hospitalizations, removal from the family environment, hampered socialization and repeated exposure to frightening and painful procedures all have their impact. However, the role of radiation in contributing to these findings cannot be ignored and efforts are constantly underway to eliminate or at least diminish the dose of radiation administered to a child's CNS. In circumstances where it is clear that radiation is essential, an effort is made to delay treatment until after the age of 2 years, often by employing chemotherapy as a means of tumor control until radiation is administered.

15.10 **Spinal cord**

Radiation effects on the spinal cord are varied and are dependent on the dose and length of cord treated. Transient demyelination in the posterior columns and lateral spinothalamic tracts can result in a transient myelopathy seen within a few months to a few years following radiation therapy. Although neurologic examination is normal patients experience electric shock-like symmetric radiations down the spine to the extremities on neck flexion. Spontaneous resolution in 2–6 months is expected and no specific intervention is required. This syndrome does not presage further neurologic abnormalities. Patients undergoing radiation for Hodgkin's disease are most likely to be affected due to the long length of spinal cord in the field of treatment, although other patients who have received treatment to the upper thoracic area will occasionally report the same sensations.

More dire consequences result from higher doses (>45 Gy) to the spinal cord, especially if the dose is administered in few fractions to a long length of cord. Progressive neurologic signs and symptoms usually indicate a more significant amount of damage, probably to the microvasculature of the cord. Paresthesias, weakness, change in pain and temperature sensation and incontinence can all develop over time. Although there is white matter damage the vascular impairment may be the most important in the development of these findings. Diminishing blood supply and endothelial proliferation may result in cord infarction with sudden rapid development of paraplegia. In all cases of progressive findings suggestive of myelopathy it is essential to rule out epidural cord compression from tumor as a cause of the neurologic impairment since that is a problem potentially reversible with rapid surgical intervention and decompression. Late signs of radiation myelitis are occasionally manifested as high-intensity signals on T2-weighted images. Conversely, the MRI may be normal in the acute phase even if the patients have severe neurologic deficits.

15.11 **Eye**

Ocular changes from radiation are due to effects on the anterior chamber, the lacrimal glands, the cornea, the conjunctivae, the retina and the lens. Acute effects include conjunctivitis, chemosis, kerato-uveitis, and loss of eyelashes from epilation. Symptomatic treatment with saline solution eye drops is usually sufficient. In cases of intense inflammation a short course of steroid eye drops may be beneficial. Antibiotic drops are only employed if infection is present.

If lacrimal gland function has been disturbed by radiation then the dry eye syndrome may develop. Aggressive lubrication may need to be administered for long periods of time to prevent recurrent corneal ulceration. On the other hand patients may notice epiphora secondary to radiation fibrosis and closure of the nasolacrimal ducts. In this case probing and dilating the duct may be sufficient to relieve symptoms. In treatment plans that require high radiation doses to the nasolacrimal duct, it may be prudent to consider prophylactic stenting prior to radiation.

The lens may undergo subcapsular opacification as a result of radiation damage. Rarely will cataracts develop with doses less than 5 Gy, but are frequent with doses in excess of 12 Gy. Keeping the dose delivered to the eye, below the crucial level will avoid these problems. The incidence of cataracts is increased in patients who are also receiving treatment with steroids. If cataracts do develop they can be treated by ophthalmic surgery as employed for naturally occurring cataracts. The retina will tolerate doses in excess of

50 Gy and therefore visual impairment from radiation rarely occurs unless this level is exceeded. High doses may be required in treating tumors of the paranasal sinuses invading the orbit. Therefore, blindness may at times be considered an acceptable complication if it is an unavoidable side effect of a definitive, curative treatment attempt.

15.12 Stomach/intestines

Many of the acute side effects associated with treatment of the abdomen are related to the effect of radiation on the stomach and small and large intestine (Fig. 15.2). Nausea and vomiting are prominent symptoms of the treatment of the stomach and small intestine and may occur within 15 min to a few hours after treatment. Premedication with anti-emetics may prove helpful. As a general rule the larger the volume of upper abdomen in the field the higher the likelihood of nausea and vomiting. If the patient has persistent symptoms despite anti-emetics the daily dose of radiation may need to be lowered. Acute radiation enteritis or colitis develops when large portions of the bowel are in the field of treatment. Within a few weeks of the initiation of treatment patients may notice frequent stools, accompanied by cramping, bloating and tenesmus. As the treatment continues the stools may become loose and watery. Treatment is symptomatic and includes the introduction of a low-residue diet and antidiarrheal medications. If proctitis is significant then local soothing ointments can be used in the perianal area and rectal suppositories containing local anesthetics and steroid preparations may be of benefit.

The incidence of severe gastrointestinal toxicity is greater in patients with inflammatory bowel disease. Patients with Crohn's disease or ulcerative colitis may have more acute side effects requiring cessation of therapy before completion of the planned course of radiation. Late toxicity requiring hospitalization or surgical intervention is

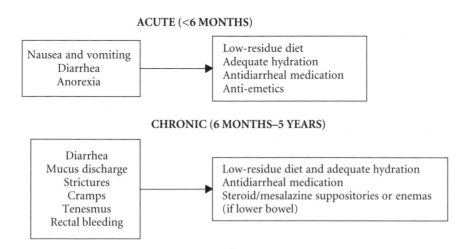

ACUTE (<6 MONTHS)

| Nausea and vomiting
Diarrhea
Anorexia | → | Low-residue diet
Adequate hydration
Antidiarrheal medication
Anti-emetics |

CHRONIC (6 MONTHS–5 YEARS)

| Diarrhea
Mucus discharge
Strictures
Cramps
Tenesmus
Rectal bleeding | → | Low-residue diet and adequate hydration
Antidiarrheal medication
Steroid/mesalazine suppositories or enemas
(if lower bowel) |

Fig. 15.2 Acute and chronic radiation enteritis.

also observed more frequently. Because of the enhanced toxicity in this group of patients undergoing radiation, careful use and planning of radiation is mandatory.

Late symptoms of stomach irradiation are somewhat vague and initially the patient may only have mild upper gastrointestinal symptoms, such as dyspepsia. Subsequently ongoing fibrosis may result in flattening of mucosal folds due to fibrosis, which may also result in antral narrowing. These changes are often preceded by mucosal ulceration. Occasionally perforation or significant bleeding occurs and surgical intervention is required. Progressive fibrosis results in continued contracture of the stomach and subsequently symptoms of early satiety may develop. In cases of persistent gastric symptoms patients can be treated with antacids or sucralfate and H_2-receptor antagonists.

Late injury to the bowel occurs from 6 months to 5 or more years following treatment, with late complications in the large bowel occurring earlier than small bowel problems. Chronic signs or symptoms associated with large bowel treatment include fibrosis and strictures, diarrhea, mucus discharge, rectal bleeding, tenesmus and cramps. If a patient has undergone both external beam and intracavitary radiation then there is a risk of fistula formation between the anterior rectal wall and the vagina and/or bladder. Bleeding can occur as a result of persistent non-healing mucosal ulceration or as a result of telangiectasia that form in the mucosa as a result of radiation injury.

Onset of small bowel injury is rarely noted before one year after the completion of radiation. The complications are similar to those encountered in the large bowel. Fibrosis may gradually develop resulting in symptoms due to intermittent partial small bowel obstruction. Patients experience bloating, cramps, nausea, vomiting and colicky pain. If significant ulceration develops there is a risk of bleeding or fistula formation. Entero-colic fistulae are more likely to develop in patients who have underlying bowel pathology, such as Crohn's disease.

Management in less severe cases includes the institution of a low-residue diet, stool softeners and anti-diarrheal agents. If bleeding sites can be identified by endoscopy then photocoagulation using endoscopic laser therapy is often effective. In some cases of extensive small bowel injury the presence of bile salts in the lumen may increase symptomatology; therefore the use of bile salt binding agents, such as cholestyramine may be effective. For lower bowel injury, treatments with topical steroid enemas or mesalamine suppositories are useful since they may reduce inflammation and promote healing.

Surgical intervention is rarely warranted, except to resect areas of persistent ulceration associated with uncontrolled bleeding or to resect areas of total or incapacitating obstruction. Controversy exists in regard to the proper surgical procedure on the small bowel since extensive resections may only result in increasing adhesions, bowel perforation with more fistulae formation and subsequently more morbidity. An alternative approach would involve bypassing the areas of obstruction.

15.13 **Kidney**

The renal tissue is particularly sensitive to the effects of radiation therefore it is important to clearly limit the volume and dose of radiation to the kidney ($<20\,Gy$). Symptoms of radiation damage are associated with the degree of renal dysfunction that has occurred and are indistinguishable from the signs and symptoms associated with acute or chronic renal failure.

Within 6 months of radiation, symptoms of acute renal failure may develop in patients who have developed radiation nephropathy. These include symptoms associated with fluid imbalance, anemia and hypertension. The hypertension may be mild or severe. Laboratory studies indicate an elevated creatinine and blood urea nitrogen and urinalysis may reveal proteinuria and hematuria. If renal dysfunction progresses some patients eventually require dialysis management of their renal insufficiency. Prevention of toxic doses to the kidneys is essential since there is no particular treatment that will reverse the problem and restore renal function.

15.14 **Bladder**

Damage to the bladder urothelium can occur in many of the same situations in which lower bowel injury occurs. Pelvic irradiation for rectal, prostate, gynecologic or bladder malignancies will result in variable exposure to the bladder. Acute symptoms are marked by urinary frequency, urgency, dysuria and diminished urinary volumes. At least acutely the smaller urine volumes are secondary to bladder urothelial inflammation and the increase in urinary frequency. Hematuria may be noted either microscopically or clinically and is due to the superficial inflammation. Higher doses may result in local areas of mucosal denudation and ulceration. Management is symptomatic. If there is evidence of a bacterial cystitis then appropriate antibiotics based upon culture and sensitivity studies should be initiated. Medications that may be effective include non-steroidal anti-inflammatory agents, as well as phenazopyridine HCL and anti-spasmodics.

After one to two years bladder fibrosis may result in a smaller bladder capacity. Also, as in the bowel mucosa, telangiectasia may form which can cause ongoing microscopic hematuria, or, at times, frank hematuria. In most cases of patients developing signs or symptoms following radiation, full urologic evaluation is warranted. This includes cystoscopy and cystometrics. Depending upon the information obtained drug therapy may be of benefit. Endoscopic cauterization may be employed to treat sites of active bleeding.

15.15 **Liver**

Hepatic damage from radiation is also relatively nonspecific in regard to physical and laboratory features. A hepatitis-like picture develops a month or so after the completion of radiation and the clinical picture is related to the volume of the organ treated. Patients complain of fatigue, vague upper abdominal pain and, at times, increasing abdominal girth. Jaundice is an uncommon finding but the liver enzymes are generally elevated. No specific therapy is warranted. If the dose of radiation is high enough to cause fibrosis (>25 Gy to the whole organ), this may develop as a late effect. In conformal field arrangements, treating only a part of the liver, this fibrosis is usually localized to the area of radiation and may not result in serious clinical problems if a crucial volume of the liver is not affected.

15.16 **Reproductive organs**

The male and female reproductive organs display varying degrees of sensitivity to radiation.

The male reproductive system effects are limited to effects on testicular function. Relatively low doses of radiation (doses in excess of 1 Gy) can result in azoospermia or oligospermia. It is wise to counsel patients to consider sperm banking prior to the initiation of treatment if this is appropriate and if the requisite delay in initiating treatment is acceptable. Even if adequate shielding of the testes is undertaken there may be enough internal scatter to result in sperm production defects. Recovery, if it occurs, may take years. Hormonal changes are usually not encountered unless fairly high doses are delivered to the testes.

Ovarian function can be affected by radiation and is reflected by both infertility and hormonal changes. In premenopausal women exposure to 15–20 Gy will result in infertility and premature menopause. Older premenopausal women may be more likely to develop symptoms at lower radiation doses.

The vaginal mucosa can reflect acute changes from treatment and, as at other mucosal sites, erythema and desquamation may occur within 2–3 weeks of beginning treatment. These local effects are dependent on dose and therefore patients receiving external beam and intracavitary treatments are more likely to develop severe changes. Confluent mucositis is a risk factor for the development of a candidal infection and antifungal therapy may be necessary. Fluconazole is helpful in dealing with this problem, which occurs frequently in patients in whom the whole length of the vagina is treated. Patients receiving chemotherapy are also especially vulnerable to developing fungal infections. The acute side effects of radiation subside within a month or so. Patients who have developed vaginal ulceration or necrosis will need longer healing times.

Atrophy and mucosal thinning with telangiectasia formation is seen months to years following treatment. If there has been significant tumor involving the rectovaginal septum or the anterior wall of the vagina, rectovaginal or cystovaginal fistula may develop. In these cases surgical debridement and diversion will be required.

In addition to the hormonal changes that influence vaginal lubrication, radiation may further affect sexual function by direct effects on the vagina. After high doses of radiation to the vagina by external beam and intracavitary radiation vaginal stenosis can develop. Not only can this make subsequent intercourse difficult; it also hinders adequate post-treatment examination. Regular use of a vaginal dilator after the acute effects of vaginitis have subsided is often successful in maintaining a vaginal lumen sufficient for intercourse as well as allowing routine vaginal examinations.

15.17 **Skin**

Often the first effects of radiation are noted by changes observed in the skin. Erythema develops within the first week or two and is followed by progressive changes of dry desquamation, moist desquamation and local hair loss. Treatment is symptomatic and is designed to soothe the pain, remove sloughed epithelium and promote healing. Patients should avoid bathing in hot water and sun exposure of treatment areas. Topical applications of moisturizers and/or hydrocortisone creams may ameliorate the sensitivity and pruritus. Any alcohol containing or irritating skin products and deodorants should be avoided.

Surfaces of the body where the beam of radiation is tangential to the skin seem to demonstrate the most pronounced acute changes. It is not unusual to observe more significant erythema and desquamation in regions such as the supraclavicular, axillary, vulval or perineal areas. Of course any region where there is a prominent tangential component of the radiation may demonstrate this effect, which accounts for the observation of more intense reaction in the infra-mammary area in breast cancer patients, for example.

Although most skin reactions subside within a few weeks of the completion of therapy, late effects can be seen in the skin, especially if high superficial doses of radiation have been administered. Almost all patients will demonstrate some degree of hyperpigmentation in the region irradiated. This more or less resolves after a few months, but some pigment changes may be observed for years in some patients. Thus, months after treatment one may observe subcutaneous fibrosis, thinning, atrophy and development of telangiectasias. The area may feel thickened and woody due to the fibrosis. Injury to these areas may result in ulceration or necrosis and healing may be slow and incomplete. Chronic ulceration may present a considerable challenge since even meticulous efforts at local care and infection control may not result in healing.

Although it is clear that concomitant chemotherapy may intensify the effects of radiation on the skin, even prior exposure to anthracyclines may result in a much more intense skin reaction. In addition, the administration of anthracyclines following radiation may also result in a "recall" of the previous skin reaction in prior sites of radiation.

Focal hair loss occurs within 7–10 days of starting radiation and hair growth will not be seen until several weeks after radiation has been discontinued. However, some patients receiving focal high doses (brain cancer patients) or receiving concurrent chemotherapy may develop irreversible alopecia.

Suggested reading

Alfonso, E.R., DeGregorio, M.A., Mateo, P., *et al.* (1997) Radiation myelopathy in over-irradiated patients: MR imaging findings. *Eur Radiol,* 7(3), 400–4.

Bentzen, S.M., Skoczylas, J.Z., and Bernier, J. (2000) Quantitative clinical radiobiology of early and late lung reactions. *Int J Radiat Biol,* 76(4), 453–62.

Etiz, D., Erkal, H.S., Serin, M., Kucuk, B., Hepari, A., Elhan, A.H., Tulunay, O., and Cakmak, A. (2000) Clinical and histopathologic evaluation of sucralfate in prevention of oral mucositis induced by radiation therapy in patients with head and neck malignancies. *Oral Oncol*, 36(1), 116–20.

Horiot, J.C., Lipinski, F., Schraub, S., Maulard-Durdux, C., *et al.* (2000) Post-radiation severe xerostomia relieved by pilocarpine: a prospective French cooperative study. *Radiother Oncol*, 55(3), 233–9.

Poulson, J.M., Vujaskovic, Z., Gillette, S.M., Chaney, E.L., and Gillette, E.L. (2000) Volume and dose-response effects for severe symptomatic pneumonitits after fractionated irradiation of canine lung. *Int J Radiol Biol*, 76(4), 463–8.

Rampling, R. and Symonds, P. (1998) Radiation myelopathy. *Curr Opin Neurol*, 11(6), 627–32.

Rubin, P., Constine, L.S., Fajardo, L.F., *et al.* (1995) Late effects of normal tissues (LENT) scoring system. *Int J Radiol Oncol Biol Phys*, 31(5), 1041–2.

Skwarchuk, M.W., Jackson, A., Zelefsky, M.J., Venkatraman, E.S., *et al.* (2000) Late rectal toxicity after conformal radiotherapy of prostate cancer (I): multivariate analysis and dose-response. *Int J Radiol Oncol Biol Phys*, 47(1), 103–13.

Tada, T., Minakuchi, K., Matsui, K., Kawase, I., Fukuda, H., and Nakajima, T. (2000) Radiation pneumonitis following multi-field radiation therapy. *Radiat Med*, 18(1), 59–61.

Trott, K.R. (1999) Chemoradiotherapy interactions and lung toxicity. *Ann Oncol*, 10(Suppl 5), S77–81.

Wasserman, T., Mackowiak, J.I., Brizel, D.M., Oster, W., Zhang, J., Peeples, P.J., and Sauer, R. (2000) Effect of amifostine on patient assessed clinical benefit in irradiated head and neck cancer. *Int J Radiat Oncol Biol Phys*, 48(4), 1035–9.

Willet, C.G., Ooi, C.J., Zietman, A.L., Menon, V., Goldberg, S., Sands, B.E., and Podolsky, D.K. (2000) Acute and late toxicity of patients with inflammatory bowel disease undergoing irradiation for abdominal and pelvic neoplasms. *Int J Radiat Oncol Biol Phys*, 46(4), 995–98.

Zierhut, D., Lohr, F., Schraube, P., Huber, P., *et al.* (2000) Cataract incidence after total-body irradiation. *Int J Radiat Oncol Biol Phys*, 46(1), 131–5.

Chapter 16

Drug-related Emergencies

Ultan McDermott, Bernard Pestalozzi, and
Markus Jörger

16.1 Introduction

Although cytotoxic agents that selectively target cancer cells are being developed, the majority of drugs in use tend to indiscriminately affect both cancer and normal cells. It is this that accounts for the different toxicities seen with the use of these agents. While many of the side effects are of short duration and cause no long-term morbidity, occasionally they can be so severe as to merit urgent action. It is these side effects that are the focus of this chapter. The chapter is divided into the different body systems affected and the management of drug-related toxicities specific to them.

16.2 Myelosuppression and neutropenic sepsis

Neutropenia as a result of myelosuppressive chemotherapy is common to most drug regimens. Any infections acquired while a patient is neutropenic are potentially life-threatening and this situation is the commonest drug-related emergency encountered by an oncologist. Its management is discussed in detail in Chapter 12.

16.3 Hypersensitivity reactions

Any cytotoxic agent can potentially cause a hypersensitivity reaction. Some drugs (e.g. taxanes) have a propensity to cause such reactions. Reactions may occur on first exposure (pseudo-allergic) and are mediated by massive histamine release from mast cells. More typically they occur on subsequent exposures following sensitization to the drug (type I hypersensitivity). The incidence of hypersensitivity reactions to the taxanes in particular is sufficiently high (5%) that routine premedication with antihistamines and corticosteroids is required. The onset of the reaction is often seen within minutes of starting the infusion.

Hypersensitivity reactions range from mild (urticaria only) to severe (anaphylactic reaction). Figure 16.1 lists the clinical features and management of hypersensitivity reactions.

Such reactions can be life-threatening and departmental protocols for their recognition and management should exist. Minor reactions can often be managed with antihistamines

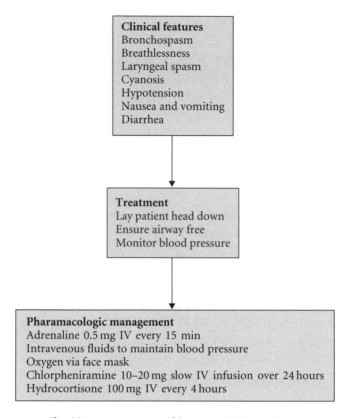

Fig. 16.1 Management of hypersensitivity reactions.

and additional corticosteroids alone but caution must be exercised if further exposure to the drug is planned (typically more prolonged infusions with increased prophylaxis against further reaction).

16.4 Cardiac toxicity

Cardiac toxicity may involve the myocardium/pericardium, the conduction system or the coronary blood vessels. Accordingly it tends to manifest as either myocardial dysfunction, angina or arrhythmias. Table 16.1 lists cytotoxic agents implicated in cardiac toxicity. When considering any of these agents for clinical use the patient's prior cardiac history is important.

16.4.1 Clinical presentation

Myocardial dysfunction—any damage to the myocardium impairs ventricular function, which in turn manifests as left ventricular failure. Symptoms of this include fatigue, exertional dyspnea, orthopnea and paroxysmal nocturnal dyspnea. Frank pulmonary edema will occur with the more advanced presentation. Investigations and treatment of any patient suspected of having significant myocardial dysfunction are shown in Fig. 16.2.

Table 16.1 Drugs associated with cardiotoxicity

Anthracyclines (doxorubicin, epirubicin, daunorubicin, idarubacin)

Cyclophosphamide, Ifosfamide

Taxanes (paclitaxel, docetaxel)

5-fluorouracil

Platinum agents (cisplatin)

Interferons

Vinca alkaloids (vincristine, vinblastine)

Retinoic acids

Mitomycin C

Mitoxantrone

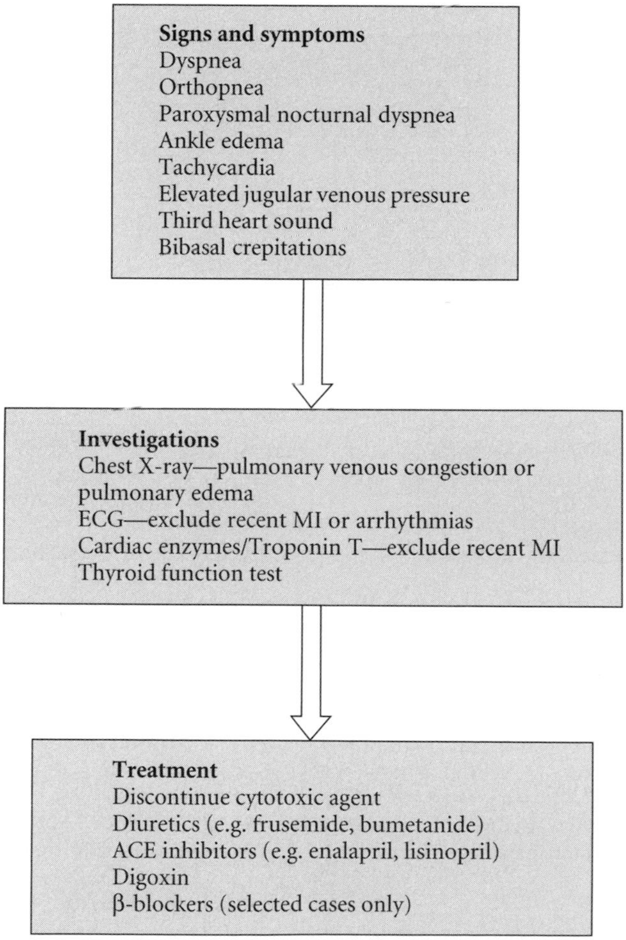

Signs and symptoms
Dyspnea
Orthopnea
Paroxysmal nocturnal dyspnea
Ankle edema
Tachycardia
Elevated jugular venous pressure
Third heart sound
Bibasal crepitations

↓

Investigations
Chest X-ray—pulmonary venous congestion or pulmonary edema
ECG—exclude recent MI or arrhythmias
Cardiac enzymes/Troponin T—exclude recent MI
Thyroid function test

↓

Treatment
Discontinue cytotoxic agent
Diuretics (e.g. frusemide, bumetanide)
ACE inhibitors (e.g. enalapril, lisinopril)
Digoxin
β-blockers (selected cases only)

Fig 16.2 Management of suspected myocardial dysfunction.

Chest pain—the onset of chest pain in any patient during or shortly after administration of any cardiotoxic agent must be investigated thoroughly. Typically angina is described as a 'crushing' sensation across the chest which may radiate into the arms. It is as a result of myocardial ischemia. It is more often seen in patients with a prior history of angina and tends to occur shortly after the chemotherapy administration. The most frequently cited example of exacerbation of underlying angina is with 5-fluorouracil (5-FU). The investigation and treatment of any patient suspected of having angina is shown in Fig. 16.3.

Arrhythmias—an abnormality of the cardiac rhythm is called a cardiac arrhythmia. Such a disturbance may cause sudden death, syncope, dizziness, palpitations or be entirely asymptomatic.

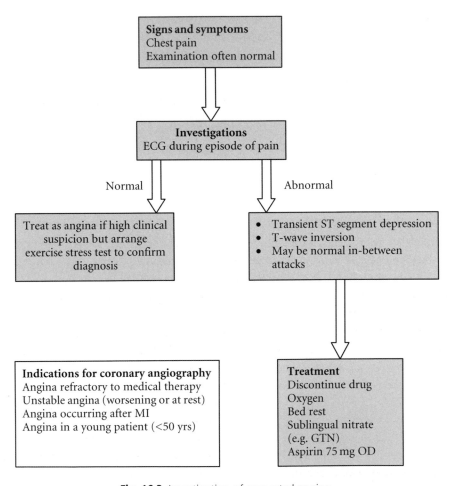

Fig. 16.3 Investigation of suspected angina.

There are two main types of arrhythmias:

1. Bradycardia, where the heart rate is slow (<60 beats per min).

2. Tachycardia, where the heart rate is fast (>100 beats per min). These tend to be symptomatic when the arrhythmia is fast and sustained. They can be further subdivided into supraventricular and ventricular arrhythmias. The latter are more likely to cause symptoms. Any tachycardia may exacerbate angina or precipitate heart failure in patients with prior ischemic heart disease or myocardial damage (e.g. previous myocardial infarction).

The primary investigation of any patient suspected of having an arrhythmia is an EKG but this can be normal if attacks are transient. A 24-hour Holter tape should be requested if there is still a high suspicion of arrhythmias based on the drug involved and the patient's history. The management of any arrhythmia should be discussed with a cardiologist.

Guidelines for safe use of cardiotoxic agents:

1. Ensure no significant cardiac history.

2. Limit cumulative dose to safe levels where known (e.g. cumulative doxorubicin dose <500 mg/m^2).

3. Baseline EKG and echocardiography prior to treatment—identifies patients with occult cardiac disease and allows comparison with any future investigations.

4. Radionuclide cardiac angiography (where available) allows modification of chemotherapy doses during treatment based on changes in the ejection fraction. In one study use of this technique reduced the incidence of cardiac failure from 21% to 3%.

16.4.2 **Anthracyclines**

The anthracyclines have been associated with cardiomyopathy since their earliest days. The incidence was as high as 30 percent in patients receiving more than 550 mg/m^2 of doxorubicin and considerably lower in those receiving less than this dose. This introduced the concept of a safe cumulative dose. There are recognized risk factors for cardiomyopathy with anthracycline use (Table 16.2).

Clinically the cardiac toxicity can be divided into acute and late presentations. The acute form occurs within days of treatment, occasionally heralded by transient arrhythmias. It takes the form of myocarditis and may lead to cardiac failure. For most patients, however, anthracycline-induced toxicity only comes to light months to years after completion of treatment. Diagnosis in this setting depends on the physician being aware of the late cardiotoxicity of the anthracyclines. Clinically the patient presents with fatigue, increasing dyspnea, and tachycardia. The investigation of choice in most centers is echocardiography, which may show a deterioration in systolic function. A previous echocardiogram prior to the anthracycline therapy is useful in this setting to determine the degree of loss of cardiac function. The primary mechanism by which doxorubicin

Table 16.2 Risk factors for cardiomyopathy with anthracyclines use

Age >70 yrs and female gender

Safe cumulative dose limit exceeded

Combination with other cardiotoxic agents

Prior heart disease, hypertension or liver disease

Mediastinal radiotherapy

causes cardiac damage is by binding to mitochondrial cardiolipin. This interrupts its binding to cytochrome c as well as facilitating the formation of free radicals.

Interest in the cardiotoxicity of anthracyclines has been renewed by the discovery of the monoclonal antibody trastuzumab (Herceptin), which has significant single-agent activity in metastatic breast cancer. When combined with anthracyclines 27 percent of patients developed heart failure. Prior treatment with anthracyclines also increased the incidence of heart failure (approx. 7%). Meticulous attention to both the patient's total anthracycline dose as well as cardiac history is essential.

16.4.3 Taxanes

Paclitaxel and docetaxel have both been reported as causing arrhythmias in phase I and II trials. The commonest arrhythmia is sinus bradycardia. Patients with a prior history of arrhythmias should be monitored closely with EKG while receiving treatment.

16.4.4 5-fluorouracil

The most frequent cardiotoxicity reported with use of this drug is precordial pain and ischemic EKG changes. Arrhythmias and myocardial dysfunction have also been reported, though less commonly. The risk of myocardial ischemia is highest (4–7%) in those patients with a prior cardiac history and typically occurs during, or shortly after, infusion of 5-FU.

Management of patients with chest pain entails discontinuation of 5-FU, administration of nitrates and EKG/cardiac enzymes/troponin-T levels to exclude a myocardial infarction. Symptoms often recur if the patient is rechallenged with the same agent.

16.5 Pulmonary toxicity

The number of chemotherapeutic agents implicated in pulmonary disease continues to grow (Table 16.3).

Chemotherapy-induced pulmonary toxicity affects not only the patient's health but also the physician's ability to deliver effective chemotherapy.

A number of mechanisms have been suggested in animal models of pulmonary damage, including:

(1) formation of reactive oxygen metabolites;

(2) oxygen free radicals arising from complex formation with Fe^{3+} ;

(3) excess collagen deposition and pulmonary fibrosis;

(4) inactivation of antiproteases in the lung leading to increased proteolytic enzyme activity;

(5) eosinophil accumulation in hypersensitivity reactions.

Histologic examination of lung biopsies from these studies shows many similar features, regardless of the drug involved. Vascular damage in the form of endothelial swelling and exudation of fluid into the intra-alveolar spaces is seen, as well as fibrosis secondary to fibroblast proliferation.

The predominant symptom is dyspnea, which typically develops over a number of weeks. The obvious exception to this is the rapid onset of the hypersensitivity reactions (usually over a short number of hours). Patients may also present with fever. Physical examination of the lungs may be entirely normal and prompt diagnosis in this situation relies on the physician having a knowledge of drugs implicated in pulmonary toxicity. Where signs are present they typically take the form of bibasal crepitations. Hemoptysis is unusual and should raise the suspicion of an alternate diagnosis.

In the setting of dyspnea, opportunistic infection and malignancy are prime candidates but can often rapidly be excluded by a chest X-ray. In drug-induced pulmonary toxicity

Table 16.3 Cytotoxic agents associated with pulmonary toxicity

Alkylating agents
Busulfan
Cyclophosphamide
Chlorambucil
Melphalan

Antimetabolites
Methotrexate
Mercaptopurine
Cytosine arabinoside
Gemcitabine

Nitrosoureas
Carmustine (BCNU)
Lomustine (CCNU)

Antibiotics
Bleomycin
Mitomycin

Miscellaneous
Procarbazine
Vinblastine
Vindesine
Retinoic acid
Etoposide
Paclitaxel

the classical finding is reticulo-nodular shadowing, but as with the clinical examination it may be entirely normal (Fig. 16.4)

A high-resolution CT scan of the chest remains the most sensitive technique to detect the early parenchymal changes due to drug toxicity. Pulmonary function tests frequently show a reduced diffusing capacity for carbon monoxide and should be carried out prior to commencing treatment with drugs which carry a significant risk of pulmonary toxicity (e.g. bleomycin). Such a baseline measurement is invaluable in determining the degree of toxicity which occurs.

Treatment primarily involves withdrawal of the implicated drug together with general supportive measures. With this approach some patients will improve both clinically and on their pulmonary function tests. A larger proportion will improve clinically but will be left with a permanent deficit in their diffusing capacity. Cases have been recorded of patients eventually requiring lung transplantation. For this reason, once the diagnosis is made vigilant follow-up is mandatory. Most centers will offer a trial of corticosteroids though no formal studies of their efficacy have been carried out.

16.6 Nephrotoxicity

By virtue of their role in the elimination and metabolism of many cytotoxic drugs, the kidneys are vulnerable to injury. This injury may range from an asymptomatic rise in the serum creatinine to acute renal failure requiring dialysis. Table 16.4 lists cytotoxic drugs and the risk of nephrotoxicity associated with their use.

When renal failure is detected (usually by a rise in the urea and creatinine) it is important to consider pre-renal, renal and post-renal causes (Fig. 16.5).

Although a number of cytotoxic agents may cause nephrotoxicity, the highest incidence and most severe cases are seen with the use of cisplatin. Hydration is important in reducing cisplatin-related nephrotoxicity. Normal saline is recommended as the chloride inhibits cisplatin hydrolysis in the kidneys. The concurrent use of diuretics or mannitol has not been shown to reduce the incidence of nephrotoxicity. Cisplatin should only be given to patients with a urinary output of at least 100 ml/hour during hydration.

The management of drug-induced nephrotoxicity consists primarily of discontinuing, or dose-reducing, the drug, correcting any significant electrolyte imbalances and in severe cases considering dialysis. Urgent indications for dialysis include hyperkalemia in conjunction with the renal failure, uremic pericarditis or symptomatic uremia.

Renal damage may be irreversible and therefore early detection is essential to prevent long-term morbidity. Any patient receiving a potentially nephrotoxic drug must have a glomerular filtration rate (GFR) calculated prior to each cycle of treatment. A decline in the GFR is often the earliest sign of nephrotoxicity.

16.7 Neurologic toxicity

Cytotoxic drugs have been implicated in both central and peripheral nervous system toxicity. There are, however, a number of causes for neurologic abnormalities and these

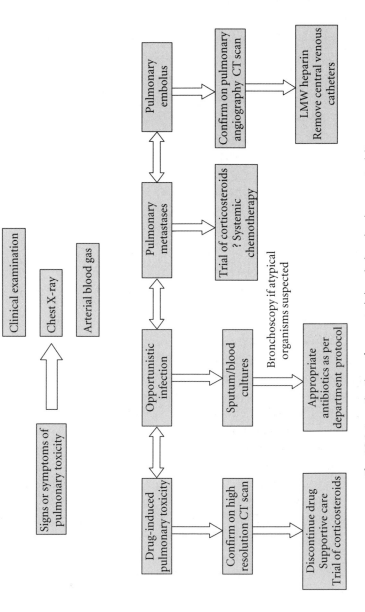

Fig. 16.4 Investigation of suspected drug induced pulmonary toxicity.

Table 16.4 Cytotoxic agents associated with nephrotoxicity

Drug	Likelihood of nephrotoxicity	Potentially irreversible
Cisplatin	High	Yes
Interleukin-2	High	No
Ifosfamide	High	Yes
Mitomycin	High	Yes
Streptozocin	High	Yes
Plicamycin	High	No
Dacarbazine	Low	No
Methotrexate (high doses)	High	No
Interferon	Low	Yes
Carboplatin	Low	No

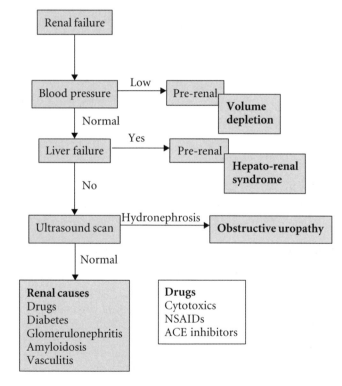

Fig. 16.5 Diagnosis of renal failure.

need to be considered alongside any cytotoxic drugs the patient may have received. The symptoms and signs vary depending on whether the agent affects the central or peripheral nervous system. The vinca alkaloids were the first class of cytotoxic drugs recognized as causing neurotoxicity. It is only recently that the actual mechanism for these toxicities is being discovered (Table 16.5).

Table 16.5 Incidence and mechanism of neurotoxicity

Cytotoxic drug	Incidence (%)	Proposed mechanism of neurotoxicity
Cisplatin	30	Accumulation of inorganic platinum
Paclitaxel	50–70	Microtubule effect
Vincristine	50	Disruption of microtubules in neurones
High dose Ara-C	15–37	Inhibition of neuronal deoxycytidine
Ifosfamide	10	? toxic metabolites
Methotrexate	8–12	Accumulation of homocysteine and adenosine
5-Fluorouracil	5	? related to DPD deficiency
Procarbazine	10–20	Unknown
Fludarabine	15	Unknown

The classical neurotoxic agent (and one of the first to be recognized as such) is vincristine. Its effects can be so disabling that a maximum dose of 2 mg per cycle of treatment is advocated in many regimens. As with other neurotoxic drugs, it commonly affects sensory elements of the peripheral nervous system, typically manifesting as symmetrical paresthesia of the hands and feet.

The combination of two neurotoxic drugs together can cause cumulative toxicity and should be avoided.

For many of these drugs, the neurotoxicity is self-limiting and tends to resolve gradually over time upon discontinuation of treatment. However, irreversible neurotoxicity has been reported with paclitaxel, docetaxel, ifosfamide, 5-FU, cytarabine and cisplatin.

Neurologic side effects of cytotoxics can be conveniently divided into those affecting the central and peripheral nervous systems. Some of the drugs discussed in this chapter have the propensity to affect both these systems.

16.7.1 Central nervous system (CNS) toxicity

This is usually related to the presence of high concentrations of the drug or toxic metabolite in the brain tissues. It is important to distinguish CNS toxicity secondary to cytotoxic agents to that arising from cerebral metastases, infections, electrolyte abnormalities or other drugs (Fig. 16.6).

The commonest manifestations of CNS toxicity are

1. Altered mental state—confusion, depression, drowsiness
2. Cerebellar dysfunction—ataxia, impaired co-ordination, dysarthria
3. Seizures
4. Myelopathy

16.7.2 Peripheral nervous system (PNS) toxicity

Peripheral nervous system toxicity commonly presents as a symmetrical paresthesia of the hands and feet. The toxicity is dependent on the total cumulative dose administered

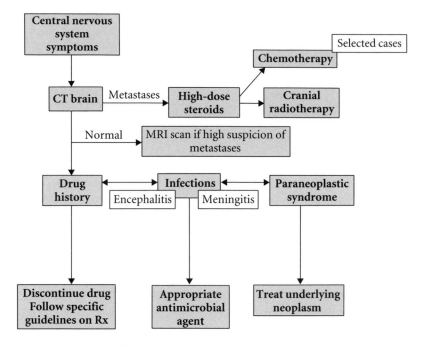

Fig. 16.6 Management of CNS toxicity.

to the patient and therefore tends to gradually worsen if treatment is continued. As noted above, even if drug-induced neurotoxicity is suspected, it is essential to exclude other causes of PNS abnormalities (Fig. 16.7). The mainstay of treatment of any peripheral drug-induced neurotoxicity is to discontinue or dose-reduce the suspected agent. Both pyridoxine (vitamin B6) and amitriptyline as well as narcotic analgesics have been used to alleviate some of the symptoms but no firm evidence as to their efficacy exists. Likewise the role of glutamate remains uncertain.

The commonest manifestations of PNS toxicity are:

1. Cranial
   (a) Ototoxicity—sensorineural hearing loss
   (b) Ophthalmoplegia
   (c) Facial palsy
2. Peripheral
   (a) Sensory—impaired sensation, paresthesia
   (b) Motor—weakness of specific muscle groups
   (c) Autonomic—postural hypotension

Cytotoxic drugs implicated in CNS and PNS neurotoxicity are detailed in Tables 16.6 and 16.7.

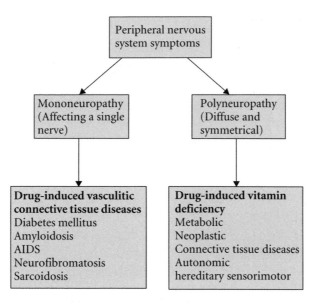

Fig. 16.7 Management of PNS toxicity.

Table 16.6 Drugs associated with central abnormalities

	Altered mental state	Cerebellar dysfunction	Seizures	Myelopathy
Cisplatin	−	−	+	−
Vincristine	−	−	+	−
Vindesine	−	−	+	−
Ara-C	+	+	−	−
Procarbazine	+	+	+	−
Ifosfamide	+	−	+	−
Methotrexate	+	−	−	+
5-Fluorouracil	−	+	−	−
Temozolamide	−	+	−	−
Fludarabine	+	−	−	−

A few of these agents deserve a particular mention either because of unusual presentations or treatments peculiar to that drug.

Ifosfamide

Toxicity is associated with visual and auditory hallucinations, confusion, agitation and personality change. Peripheral neuropathies may also occur. Significant abnormalities have been reported in up to 10 percent of patients, and especially those with recognized risk factors—renal dysfunction, low serum albumin, prior cisplatin therapy, CNS

Table 16.7 Drugs associated with peripheral abnormalities

	Sensory neuropathy	Motor neuropathy	Ototoxicity	Cranial neuropathy
Cisplatin	+	−	+	−
Paclitaxel	+	+	−	−
Vincristine	+	+	−	+
Vindesine	+	−	−	−
Etoposide	+	−	−	−
Ara-C	+	+	−	+
Methotrexate	−	−	−	+
Thalidomide	+	+	−	−
Procarbazine	+	−	−	−
Oxaliplatin	+	−	−	−

tumors and poor performance status. Management typically consists of discontinuing the drug and sedating with benzodiazepines. Concurrent administration with methylene blue reduces the risk of neurotoxicity.

Methotrexate

Meningeal irritation, paraparesis, or encephalopathy may all be manifestations of methotrexate toxicity. The neurologic dysfunction may be acute and transient or delayed in onset with personality changes. Treatment consists of active hydration to facilitate methotrexate clearance and leucovorin to circumvent the enzyme inhibition of methotrexate.

Vincristine

Vincristine is unique among cytotoxic agents in that neurotoxicity is the sole dose-limiting problem. Toxicity can affect the peripheral, central, or autonomic nervous systems. If a peripheral neuropathy occurs it tends to be mainly sensory and progress proximally as vincristine therapy is continued to involve the entire hands or feet. Even the subjective sensation of weakness in the arms or legs should raise the suspicion of neurotoxicity and prompt further investigation. Patients with hereditary neuropathies are especially prone to vincristine neuropathy. Acute, severe bone pain may occur shortly after drug administration but typically subsides after a few days.

Autonomic and cranial neuropathies may occur. Less common neurotoxicities include cortical blindness and laryngeal nerve (with vocal cord) paralysis, resulting in dysphonia.

The mainstay of treatment is to discontinue vincristine and wait for neurologic recovery. Symptoms may persist as long as 3 or 4 years after cessation of therapy, but they usually wane to a point where they are no longer troublesome to the patient. Empiric vitamin therapy is ineffective. Intestinal dysfunction from autonomic neuropathy may be improved by metoclopramide therapy.

Inadvertent intrathecal vincristine injection has been reported and produces a rapidly ascending, usually fatal, neuromyeloencephalopathy. Cerebrospinal fluid lavage dilutes and removes the drug and at present is the only treatment.

Cisplatin

Repeated administration may cause a sensory peripheral neuropathy in 30 percent of cases. Up to 30 percent of patients also develop ototoxicity though mostly in the frequency range above that of normal speech.

Paclitaxel

In a series of 812 patients receiving single agent paclitaxel 60 percent developed a peripheral neuropathy but only 3 percent were grades III or IV.

Oxaliplatin

Use of this cytotoxic agent has been associated with an unusual neurotoxicity—pharyngolaryngeal dysesthesia (dysphagia and dysphonia). A sensory neuropathy precipitated by cold temperature is also commonly seen.

16.8 **Hepatic toxicity**

The predominant hepatic injury secondary to cytotoxic agents is a form of chemical hepatitis, resulting from exposure to the parent drug or its active metabolites. Agents known to be involved are listed in Table 16.8.

Acute hepatic injury is often picked up on routine blood tests long before the patient becomes symptomatic. Typically the liver transaminases are elevated with or without a raised bilirubin.

It is important to recognize that these changes in liver biochemistry may also be the result of other drugs the patient may be receiving, liver metastases or viral and non-viral infections. Most viral infections are self-limiting and non-viral causes (Leptospirosis, Coxiella burnetii) are rare. Liver metastases may respond to high dose corticosteroids though ultimately only chemotherapy or hepatic resection in selected cases offer any durable response (Fig. 16.8).

Where drugs are the cause of acute hepatic toxicity, discontinuation usually results in the liver abnormalities returning to normal.

Rarely, fulminant hepatic failure may develop due to acute hepatic injury from any cause. Histologically there is massive hepatic necrosis. In this setting the patient is jaundiced with signs of hepatic encephalopathy (ranging from confusion and drowsiness to coma). Ascites and peripheral edema are common. Neurologic examination reveals spasticity and extensor plantar responses. The mortality rate from this condition can exceed 70 percent and prompt treatment is essential (Fig. 16.9). Patients should be transferred to a specialist liver unit once stable.

Dose modifications for liver dysfunction should be followed in patients receiving treatment with anthracyclines, vinca alkaloids, taxanes and irinotecan.

Table 16.8 Cytotoxic agents associated with hepatotoxicity

High potential for hepatotoxicity
Cytarabine
Interferons (in high doses)
Methotrexate (long-term therapy)
Streptozocin

High potential for hepatotoxicity with high doses
Busulfan
Cyclophosphamide
Cytarabine
Dactinomycin
Methotrexate
Mitomycin

Occasional irreversible hepatotoxicity
Busulfan (in high doses)
Cytarabine
Dacarbazine
Methotrexate
Mitomycin

Isolated instances of hepatotoxicity
Dacarbazine
Hydroxyurea
Interferons (in low doses)
Vincristine

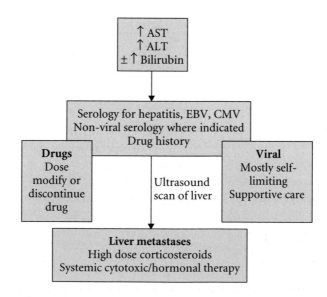

Fig. 16.8 Assessment of asymptomatic acute hepatic injury.

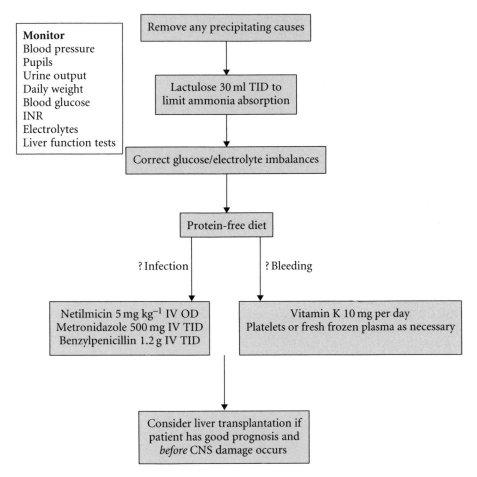

Fig 16.9 Management of hepatic failure.

16.9 **Extravasation**

The risks of cytotoxic drug extravasation (i.e. leak of a vesicant or irritant drug into tissues surrounding the venous blood system) have decreased considerably over the last decade, owing to improved drug administration and awareness. Leakage of these drugs can potentially cause significant tissue damage and must be managed rapidly if discovered. The management of extravasation is covered in Chapter 14.

Suggested reading

Cooper, J.A.D., White, D.A., and Matthay, R.A. (1986) Drug-induced pulmonary disease: I. Cytotoxic drugs. *Am Rev Respir Dis*, **133**, 321–40.

Ginsberg, S.J. and Comis, R.L. (1982) The pulmonary toxicity of antineoplastic agents. *Semin Oncol*, **9**, 34–51.

Kupfer, A., Aeschlimann, C., Wermuth, B., and Cerny, T. (1994) Prophylaxis and reversal of ifosfamide encephalopathy with methylene-blue. *Lancet*, **343**, 763–5.

Lefrak, E.A., Pitha, J., Rosenheim, S., *et al.* (1973) A clinicopathologic analysis of adriamycin cardiotoxicity. *Cancer*, **32**, 302–14.

Mal, H., Rullou, I., Mellot, F., Brugière, O., Sleiman, C., Menu, Y., and Fournier, M. (1999) Immediate and long-term results of bronchial artery embolization for life-threatening hemoptysis. *Chest*, **115**(4), 912–15.

Moertel, C.G., Fleming, T.R., Macdonald, J.S., Haller, D.G., and Laurie J.A. (1993) Hepatic toxicity associated with fluorouracil plus levamisole adjuvant therapy. *J Clin Oncol*, **11**, 2386–90.

Pinzani, V., Bressolle, F., Haug, I.J., *et al.* (1994) Cisplatin-induced renal toxicity and toxicity-modulating strategies: a review. *Cancer Chemother Pharmacol*, **35**, 1–9.

Schwartz, R.G., McKenzie, W.B., Alexander, S., *et al.* (1987) Congestive heart failure and left ventricular dysfunction complicating doxorubicin therapy: a seven year experience using serial radionuclide angiocardiography. *Am J Med*, **82**, 1109–18.

Singla, P.K. and Iliskovic, N. (1998) Doxorubicin-induced cardiomyopathy. *N Engl J Med*, **339**, 900–5.

Tyson, L.B., Kris, M.G., Corso, D.M., Choy, E., and Timoney, J.P. (1999) Incidence, course, and severity of taxoid-induced hypersensitivity reaction in 646 oncology patients. *Proc Am Soc Clin Oncol*, **18**, 585a (abstract).

Weiden, P.L. and Wright, S.E. (1972) Vincristine neurotoxicity. *N Engl J Med*, **286**, 1369–70.

Weiss, R.B., Donehower, R.H., Wiernik, P.H., *et al.* (1990) Hypersensitivity reactions from Taxol. *J Clin Oncol*, **8**, 1263–8.

Appendix

UK/US Drugs

Drug names are listed where they differ between the UK and the USA, and equivalents can be found. Other trade names may exist, but not all are tabulated. Certain drugs mentioned in the text are not licensed in both countries.

	UK generic name	UK trade name	US generic name	US trade name
A	Asparaginase	Crisantaspase	Asparaginase	Elspar
	Allopurinol	Zyloric	Allopurinol	Zyloprim
	Amitriptyline	Doxepin	Amitriptyline	Elavil
B				
C	Chlorpromazine	Largactil	Chlorpromazine	Thorazine
	Ciclosporin	Sandimmun	Cyclosporine	Sandimmune
	Cyclophosphamide	Endoxana	Cyclophosphamide	Cytoxan
	Cladribine	Leustat	Cladribine	Leustatin
	Ciprofloxacin	Ciproxin	Ciprofloxacin	Cipro
	Calcitonin	Miacalcic, Calsynar	Calcitonin	Miacalcin
	Ceftazidime	Fortum	Ceftazidime	Fortaz
	Clindamycin	Dalacin C	Clindamycin	Cleocin
	Chlorpheniramine	Piriton	Chlorpheniramine	Chlor-trimeton
D	Daunorubicin	Cerubidin	Daunorubicin	Cerubidine
	Docusate	Dioctyl	Docusate	Surfak, Colace
	Demeclocycline	Ledermycin	Demeclocycline	Declomycin
	Diclofenac Sodium	Voltarol	Diclofenac Sodium	Voltaren
E	Epirubicin	Pharmorubicin	Epirubicin	Ellence
F	Frusemide	Lasix	Furosemide	Lasix
	Flutamide	Drogenil	Flutamide	Eulexin
	Flumazenil	Anexate	Flumazenil	Romazicon
G				
H	Hydromorphone	Palladone	Hydromorphone	Dilaudid
I	Idarubicin	Zavedos	Idarubicin	Idamycin
	Irinotecan	Campto	Irinotecan	Camptosar
	Ifosfamide	Mitoxana	Ifosfamide	Ifex
	Insulin	Actrapid	Insulin	Velosulin
J				

	UK generic name	UK trade name	US generic name	US trade name
K				
L	Lomustine	CCNU	Lomustine	Ceenu
	Lebetalol	Trandate	labetalol	Normodyne
	Levofloxacin	Tavanic	Levofloxacin	Levaquin
	Lignocaine	—	Lidocaine	—
M	Mitomycin	Mitomycin C	Mitomycin	Mutamycin
	Metoclopramide	Maxolon	Metoclopramide	Reglan
	Mesna	Uromitexan	Mesna	Mesnex
	Metaraminol	Alprostadil	Metaraminol	Aramine
	Mirtazapine	Zispin	Mirtazapine	Remeron
	Chlormethine	—	Mustine	—
N				
O	Ofloxacin	Tarivid	Ofloxacin	Floxin
	Oestrogen	—	Estrogen	—
P	Phenoxybenzamine	Dibenyline	Phenoxybenzamine	Dibenzyline
	Phenytoin	Epanutin	Phenytoin	Dilantin
	Potassium Chloride	Slow K, Sando K	Potassium Chloride	K Dur
	Paracetamol	—	Acetaminophen	—
	Piperacillin/Tazobactam	Tazocin	Piperacillin/Tazobactam	Zosyn
	Paroxetine	Seroxat	Paroxetine	Paxil
Q				
R				
S	Sertraline	Lustral	Sertraline	Zoloft
	Sucralfate	Antepsin	Sucralfate	Carafate
T	Thioridazine	Melleril	Thioridazine	Mellaril
	Trazodone	Molipaxin	Trazodone	Desyrel
	Tramadol	Zydol	Tramadol	Ultram
	Levothyroxine	Eltroxin	Thyroxine	Synthroid
U	Ursodeoxycholic Acid	Ursofalk	Ursodeoxycholic Acid	Ursodiol
V	Valproic Acid	Epilim	Valproic Acid	Depakene
	Venlafaxine	Efexor	Venlafaxine	Effexor
W	Warfarin	Marevan	Warfarin	Coumadin
X				
Y				
Z				

Index

MSICU